J. Czernin, M. Dahlbom, O. Ratib, C. Schiepers

Atlas of PET/CT Imaging in Oncology

Springer-Verlag Berlin Heidelberg GmbH

J. Czernin, M. Dahlbom
O. Ratib, C. Schiepers

Atlas of PET/CT Imaging in Oncology

With a Foreword by Michael E. Phelps

With 647 Figures and 13 Tables

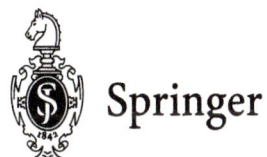

Springer

Authors

J. Czernin, MD
M. Dahlbom, MD
C. Schiepers, MD, PhD
Department of Molecular and Medical Pharmacology
David Geffen School of Medicine at UCLA
10833 Le Conte Avenue, AR-144 CHS
Los Angeles, CA 90095-6942
USA

O. Ratib, MD, PhD, FAHA
Department of Radiological Sciences
David Geffen School of Medicine at UCLA
100 Medical Plaza, Suite 100
Room 1-403
Los Angeles, CA 90095
USA

Contributors

T. Beyer
M. Seltzer
D. Townsend
C. Yap

ISBN 978-3-642-62141-3   ISBN 978-3-642-18517-5 (eBook)
DOI 10.1007/978-3-642-18517-5

Library of Congress Control Number: 2004102323

© Springer-Verlag Berlin Heidelberg 2004
Originally published by Springer-Verlag Berlin Heidelberg New York in 2004
Softcover reprint of the hardcover 1st edition 2004

Editor: Ute Heilmann, Heidelberg
Desk editor: Wilma McHugh, Heidelberg
Production editor: Bernd Wieland, Heidelberg
Cover design: F. Steinen, eStudio Calamar, Spain
Data conversion: AM-productions GmbH, Wiesloch

21/3111 – 5 4 3 2 1   SPIN 11414264
Printed on acid-free paper

Preface

Michael E. Phelps

The positron emission tomography (PET) scanner was developed to provide a molecular imaging technology for examining the biology of normal cellular function and its transformation to disease in the living subject. This is achieved by selecting targets of normal tissue and disease (proteins, RNA and DNA) of biochemical processes of interest and labeling a molecular probe selective for the target with a positron emitting radionuclide (e.g., F-18, C-11, N-13, O-15, I-124, Cu-64, Ga-68). Two examples relevant to cancer illustrate this. The first is 2-deoxy-2-[F-18] fluorodeoxy-D-glucose (FDG) that targets the glucose transporter protein and the enzyme hexokinase that phosphorylates glucose as the first step in the glycolytic pathway. FDG is a competitive substrate with glucose and provides the means to image the rate of glycolosis throughout the body. The second probe is 3'-[F-18] fluoro-3'-deoxythymidine (FLT) that targets the pyrimidine transporter and thymidine kinase that phosporylates thymidine. FLT is a competitive substrate with thymidine to provide the means to image DNA replication and thus cell proliferation. Both glycolosis and DNA replication are highly amplified in neoplastic degeneration.

Since PET is a quantitative imaging technique that can measure the tissue concentration of the imaging probe over time, it provides the means to translate biochemistry, biology and pharmacology laboratory assays into the examinations in living subjects. While x-ray computed tomography (CT) moved quickly to clinical applications after its invention, the first 15 years of PET were focused on research. This involved translating and validating a wide array of in vitro molecular assays into in vivo ones and using them to build a biological bridge between in vitro and in vivo biological sciences. In addition, PET was used to discover many aspects of normal biological functions and those of disease in living animals and the ultimate laboratory to study human disease, the patient. This built a scientific foundation for PET based on well-established principles of biochemistry and biology

and also established a scientific basis for the molecular imaging procedures employed in PET.

In about 2 million clinical PET studies there has not been one reported complication. This results primarily from the fact that PET employees a radiotracer technique in which the probe concentrations are typically in the range of femto moles per gram tissue so there are little to no significant mass effects exerted on biochemical or biological process.

While the scientific foundation of PET was being built there were also dramatic events taking place in biology in which disciplines were shifting to "molecular" – molecular biology, molecular genetics, molecular pharmacology, bio- and nanotechnologies, genomics, proteomics and systems biology that were all accompanied and enabled by revolutionary technology developments that made the new science possible. These efforts began to change the way people thought about and performed science and began building a new knowledge and technology base of molecular diagnostics and molecular therapeutics to establish the principles and practices of a new molecular medicine.

This new molecular world placed more emphasis on imaging proving an in vivo link in the discovery pathway to bring the new knowledge of the molecular basis of disease to the care of patients. From this came a growing discipline of molecular imaging, with PET in a leadership role in the in vivo applications. Many other imaging technologies have gathered around this theme to provide molecular and structure information, including optical imaging, magnetic resonance imaging (MRI), single photon computed tomography (SPECT), CT and ultrasound imaging. Molecular imaging is now becoming a robust field of its own.

As part of this change many in vivo imaging technologies and disciplines were also being merged at the instrument (e.g., PET/CT) or probe level (PET and optical reporter genes in the same gene construct) to gain the advantage of both. The goal is to combine molecular assays from different technologies, as well as combining biological and anatomical information. Further, molecular diagnostics and molecular therapeutics were merging together with common disease targets and building molecular probes (therapeutic and imaging) together to assist each other in the discovery process and in the care of patients.

PET/CT in cancer, the subject of this Atlas, illustrates many features of the evolutionary and revolutionary changes occurring. PET using FDG to image glycolosis reached a point in cancer where the literature showed that it was from 9 to 43% more accurate than anatomical imaging for diagnosing, staging, restaging and assessing therapeutic responses in a large number of different cancers and that the inclusion of PET in the clinical evaluation changed treatment in 15 to 50% of patients, depending on the clinical question. There are, however, specific cases where each technique is better than the other. In addition, PET/CT presents a picture of human anatomy upon which biological information within structures of the body is added. This combined information allows better delineation of disease within or between structures, as well as guiding surgical and radiation planning and biopsy by using both structure and biology identification and characterization. Therefore, it became clear that PET/CT is better than PET or CT alone.

PET/CT also provides advantages in the drug discovery process in evaluating pharmacokinetics and pharmacodynamics with PET with CT better defining the anatomical structures in which drugs actions take place, both at the disease target and throughout the organ systems of the body. These discovery-oriented studies will also define and evolve into new practice approaches in the way molecular diagnostics and therapeutics are employed together to improve patient selection through a more biologically informative picture of the patient, direct determination therapeutic doses and therapeutic outcomes.

This Atlas provides a thoughtful and well-illustrated educational approach for defining the principles and good practices of PET/CT. The addition of the CD-ROM allows teachers and students to manipulate and navigate through images as well as blending anatomical and biological information or concealing information to provide flexibility in individual teaching methods. The Atlas systematically provides clinical presentations of the cancers of the various organ systems from diagnosis to staging, recurrent disease and therapeutic response to help design the best patient management. It provides a comprehensive educational tool for radiologists and nuclear medicine specialists who want to learn about molecular PET/CTimaging.

Table of Contents

Introduction

J. Czernin, M. Dahlbom, O. Ratib, C. Schiepers, C. Yap

Positron Emission Tomography, introduced almost three decades ago by Phelps and Hoffman,[1] has only recently been accepted as the most important and innovative tool for cancer imaging. The diagnostic and prognostic accuracy of PET imaging with F-18 deoxyglucose (FDG) ranges from 80-90% for many cancers[2] and is superior to anatomical imaging. However, PET imaging is limited in its ability to assign molecular abnormalities to specific anatomical structures. This limitation has been recently overcome by the introduction of "in-line", "hybrid" PET/CT systems[3] that have dramatically increased the visibility of molecular imaging within the radiology and oncology community. PET/CT has introduced radiologists to the concept and importance of molecular imaging and helps to conceptualize the inherent limitations of size criteria for defining anatomical abnormalities as malignant or benign. The molecular information provided by PET enables radiologists for the first time to clearly characterize anatomical abnormalities as cancerous or not. On the other hand, molecular imaging benefits from the anatomical framework provided by CT. Hyper-metabolic lesions can now be assigned to specific anatomical structures.

Sales figures for PET/CT have surpassed those of "stand alone" PET systems and it is predicted that more than 90% of PET will be PET/CT in the near future.

The introduction of this technology results in new training requirements for radiologists and nuclear medicine specialists. Radiologists need to be familiar with the concept of molecular imaging while competence in cross-sectional anatomy is required from nuclear medicine.

The Atlas of PET/CT Imaging serves an educational purpose and is designed to teach radiologists and nuclear medicine specialists about important aspects of molecular imaging and nuclear medicine specialists about the benefits of anatomic imaging. It consists of a brief didactic portion and an extensive selection of interesting and challenging case examples.

The didactic portion of the book includes a review of the technical principles of PET and PET/CT imaging by M. Dahlbom and C. Schiepers who also discuss differences in PET and CT technology between different commercially available systems.

D. Townsend,[4] who introduced the PET/CT technology provides in chapter 3 the outlook for the future of dual modality imaging.

Different opinions have been voiced regarding the optimal imaging protocols. One school of thought believes that CT should only be used for attenuation correction and lesion localization while others demand that the most elaborate contrast and high-resolution studies should be performed. In any event, many of these debates have not resulted in a consensus and it appears likely that the specific expertise of the users will at least initially determine the implementation of specific imaging protocols. O. Ratib and T. Beyer will also discuss this and other issues related to image interpretation and navigation.

J. Czernin summarizes the clinical experience and research studies examining the impact and usefulness of PET/CT. A large number of abstracts thus far addressed the additional value of PET/CT over PET alone for staging and restaging of cancer. Recently a prospective study was published in the New England Journal of Medicine[5] that compared the diagnostic accuracy of integrated PET and CT to that of PET and CT alone in patients with non-small cell lung cancer. These and other studies are reviewed by in detail by J. Czernin.

A review of the normal FDG distribution in the human body, the pitfalls and normal variants by M. Seltzer and C. Schiepers is presented in chapter 7 and completes the didactic section.

The Atlas section illustrates the benefits but also pitfalls of combined PET/CT imaging. Examples of artifacts and physiological variants (brown fat, blood pool, thyroid uptake, muscle activity) are presented. The role of PET/CT for imaging cancers of the head and neck, solitary pulmonary nodules, lung cancer, cancers of the gastrointestinal tract, lymphoma, cancers of the skin, breast cancer, gynecological cancers, and cancers of the genito-urinary system is illustrated. Examples of benign diseases include inflammation, granuloma and benign tumors.

Each case includes a brief history, a specific teaching point that emphasizes image findings, and provides relevant clinical follow-up information and a brief list of relevant publications.

A special and unique feature of the Atlas, assembled and designed by O. Ratib, is an interactive CD-ROM that provides the original PET and CT images of each case in selected planes enabling the users to manually adjust the blending intensity of each modality in a fused image. In addition, users can display the clinical history, imaging techniques and diagnostic findings of each case as well as the corresponding specific teaching point. An "option" button allows turning on and off graphic annotations and legends for each image. The CD is designed to be an effective teaching tool through a user-friendly and intuitive graphic interface for navigating through 100 selected clinical cases covering many frequently encountered cancers.

The CD-ROM is also designed to become a convenient diagnostic companion for retrieving reference images of typical clinical cases that may be used as comparative studies for diagnostic interpretation of similar cases in clinical routine.

The convincing concept of merging molecular with anatomical imaging has driven the clinical acceptance of PET/CT. Initial data are emerging that strongly suggest that PET/CT imaging results in a higher diagnostic accuracy than PET imaging alone.[4,6-11]

The introduction of PET/CT demands a fresh look at the training requirements for specialists in the field of molecular-anatomical imaging. It is hoped that the Atlas of PET/CT imaging results in a better understanding of the capabilities of PET/CT, and in turn, to improved care and management of cancer patients.

References

1.   Phelps ME, Hoffman EJ, Mullani NA, Ter-Pogossian MM. Application of annihilation coincidence detection to transaxial reconstruction tomography. J Nucl Med. 1975;16(3):210-224.

2.   Czernin J, Phelps ME. Positron emission tomography scanning: current and future applications. Annu Rev Med. 2002;53:89-112.

3.   Beyer T, Townsend DW, Brun T, Kinahan PE, Charron M, Roddy R, Jerin J, Young J, Byars L, Nutt R. A combined PET/CT scanner for clinical oncology. J Nucl Med. 2000;41(8):1369-1379.

4.   Townsend DW, Cherry SR. Combining anatomy and function: the path to true image fusion. Eur Radiol. 2001;11(10):1968-1974.

5.   Lardinois D, Weder W, Hany TF, Kamel EM, Korom S, Seifert B, von Schulthess GK, Steinert HC. Staging of non-small-cell lung cancer with integrated positron-emission tomography and computed tomography. N Engl J Med. 2003;348(25):2500-2507.

6.   Israel O, Keidar Z, Bar-Shalom R, Gaitini D, Beck D, Amit A. Hybrid PET/CT imaging with FDG in management of patients with gynecologic malignancies. J Nucl Med. 2003;44(5 Suppl):129P.

7.   Antoch G, Stattaus J, Nemat AT, Marnitz S, Beyer T, Kuehl H, Bockisch A, Debatin JF, Freudenberg LS. Non-small cell lung cancer: dual-modality PET/CT in preoperative staging. Radiology. 2003;229(2):526-533.

8.   Cohade C, Osman M, Leal J, Wahl RL. Direct comparison of 18F-FDG PET and PET/CT in patients with colorectal carcinoma. J Nucl Med. 2003;44(11):1797-1803.

9.   Freudenberg LS, Antoch G, Schutt P, Beyer T, Jentzen W, Muller SP, Gorges R, Nowrousian MR, Bockisch A, Debatin JF. FDG-PET/CT in re-staging of patients with lymphoma. Eur J Nucl Med Mol Imaging. 2003;in press.

10.   Hany TF, Steinert HC, Goerres GW, Buck A, von Schulthess GK. PET diagnostic accuracy: improvement with in-line PET-CT system: initial results. Radiology. 2002;225(2):575-581.

11.   Fukui MB, Blodgett TM, Meltzer CC. PET/CT imaging in recurrent head and neck cancer. Semin Ultrasound CT MR. 2003;24(3):157-163.

Principles of PET/CT Imaging

M. Dahlbom and C. Schiepers

PET/CT imaging has rapidly gained clinical acceptance since Dr. David Townsend and his team[1] introduced the first hybrid PET/CT prototype consisting of a rotating PET component and a conventional single slice CT. The images obtained with this single gantry device were "mechanically" fused, providing anatomical information from CT that was near perfectly aligned with the functional information from PET. This prototype propelled dual modality imaging[2] and has proven clinically useful by improving both lesion localization and lesion characterization, thus increasing the accuracy for staging and diagnosing disease.[2-4]

Cancer patients undergo a number of different imaging studies throughout the course of their disease. Usually, the resulting images are reviewed on different display stations. The gathered information is synthesized and integrated by the interpreting physician(s). The multitude of images can also be coregistered or aligned retrospectively and fused using computer software. Post hoc image fusion, based on tomograms acquired at different institutions, on separate days, using varying equipment and protocols, is a tedious and time-consuming task.[5-10] Moreover, well-defined and reproducible landmarks are necessary to provide the coordinate system in which the images can be aligned, scaled and registered. Since patient positioning varies widely between PET and CT, e.g. arms up or down, different angles for head or neck relative to the patient axis, the post hoc fusion technique is prone to inconsistencies and errors. Also, there may be problems due to patient motion as well as involuntary motion of internal organs. Changes related to breathing and organ movement are inevitable, and cannot be controlled when a patient is imaged on different scanners and at different times, even when care is taken to ensure the same external body position of the patient (e.g. with external lasers).

PET/CT Instrumentation

In comparison to PET, CT utilizes radiation sources of significantly different energies and emis-

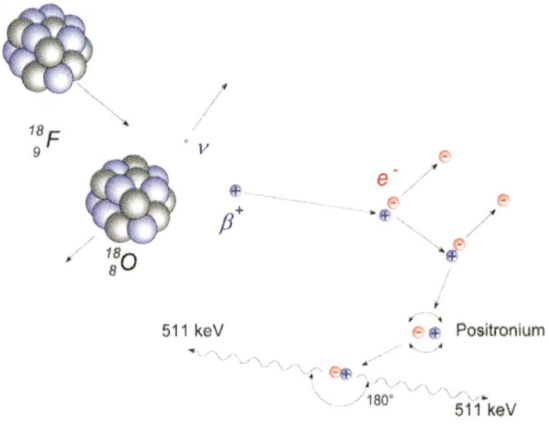

Figure 1. Illustration of positron decay and the creation of the two 511 keV annihilation photons. Following the decay of the instable 18F mother nucleus, a positron, a neutrino and a stable 18O daughter nucleus are created. The energy released in the decay is shared as kinetic energy between the three particles. The positron will travel some distance in the tissue and produce ionization and eventually lose most of its energy. It will then attract an electron and form positronium, which will annihilate within 10^{-12} s. In order to conserve energy and momentum, the annihilation photons both have an energy of 511 keV (total rest mass energy of the electron and the positron) and they are emitted 180 degrees apart (net momentum is zero).

sion rates. Each system also performs a different type of tomography: e.g., transmission by CT and emission by PET. Due to this, the detection and acquisition systems of the two modalities are different and highly specialized for the specific requirements of each modality.

PET uses coincidence detection for localization of the activity within the patient. During the decay of the injected isotope, positrons are emitted, which rapidly annihilate with electrons and the result is the creation of two annihilation photons, each having an energy of 511 keV. The high energy photons are emitted at an angle of 180 degrees (Figure 1). In a PET system, a large number of detectors, sensitive to these 511 keV photons, are placed around the imaged object (typical in a set of adjacent detector rings, of an axial FOV ranging from 15 to 40 cm). If a detection of a pair of 511 keV photons occurs simultaneously in a pair of detectors, then the system has recorded a coincidence (Figure 2). Knowing the location of the two detector elements in the system, one can determine that the radioactive decay occurred somewhere along the line connecting the two detector elements. By recording a large number of these coincidences, and using tomographic image reconstruction techniques, the activity distribution within the imaged object can be reconstructed.

In an ideal PET system only true coincidences should be detected. However, due to limitations in the detectors and its associated electronics, unwanted coincidence events are also recorded. The first type of events is the random or accidental event originating from two unrelated annihilation events. If not corrected for, the random coincidences generated form an undesirable contrast reducing background in the images and also compromising quantitation. Fortunately, there are accurate methods to measure and correct for random events, however, these result in increased image noise levels. Therefore, the random coincidence rate needs to be kept at a minimum. In contrast to the true coincidence rate which increases linearly with administered activity, the randoms rate increases with the square of the activity. Therefore, an increase in injected activity does not always translate into an improvement in image quality due to the increase in random events.

The second undesirable event type is the scattered event, where one or both of the two annihilation photons interact in the subject prior to being detected. This results in a mispositioning of the event since each interaction changes the direction of the photon. The presence of scatter in the reconstructed image reduces contrast and compromises the quantitative accuracy of the image. In contrast to the random events, scatter cannot be directly measured. Instead the scatter needs to be estimated from the acquired emission and attenuation data[11-14] and the accuracy of this correction has a direct impact on the image contrast, quantitation and quality.

Coincidence detection of annihilation photons requires a detection system that is sensitive to the relatively high photon energy (511 keV) and allows to accurately determine the energy of each photon that is detected at a fairly high count rate. In addition, these detectors need to have a fast response time, i.e., they need to be able to accurately determine a coincidence within 5-10 ns. This property is sometimes referred to as the coincidence time resolution and is specific to different detector materials. The time resolution has a direct impact on the randoms rate, i.e., a better or smaller time resolution will reduce the randoms rate, which in turn improves image quality. The time resolution for any given detector material is a function of both light decay time (how fast the scintillation light is generated in the detector) and the amount of light produced per absorbed photon. In general, the shorter the light decay time and the more light produced, the faster the detector. Some of the characteristics of the detector materials in current PET systems are listed in Table I.

In X-ray CT, scintillation detectors such as Cadmium Tungstate ($CdWO_4$) or Yttrium or Gadolinium ceramics are used.[15,16] However, due to

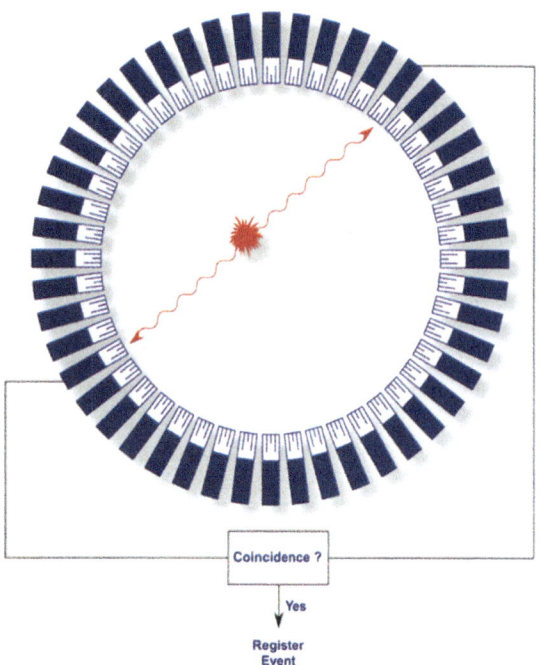

Figure 2. In a PET system a large number of detector elements are arranged around the subject. A coincidence is recorded if a pair of detectors simultaneously register the two annihilation photons. Knowing the location of the two detectors in the system, one can determine that the radioactive decay occurred somewhere along the line connecting the two detectors.

| TABLE 1. CHARACTERISTICS OF DETECTOR MATERIALS IN CURRENT PET SYSTEMS | | | | | |

Scintillator	Effective Atomic Number	Density [g/cm³]	μ_{511} keV [cm⁻¹]	Decay Time [ns]	Light Yield [per keV]
NaI	50	3.67	0.34	230	38
BGO	74	7.13	0.95	300	8
GSO	59	6.71	0.70	60	12-15
LSO	66	7.40	0.88	40	20-30

the high photon flux, not each individual photon can be analyzed. Instead, the signal produced from these detectors represents an average of several photon detections. In order to achieve a spatial resolution of 1 mm or less, very small detector elements have to be used (1 x 1 mm²). Due to the low energy of the X-rays, the entire photon energy can be absorbed in a small detector volume. Thus, high spatial resolution can be achieved without a significant loss in detection efficiency. However, these small detectors are not suitable for recording 511 keV photons, since only a small fraction of the emitted photons would be absorbed in the detector volume, therefore resulting in very poor detection efficiency. Conversely, due to their size, that would limit spatial resolution, detector systems designed for 511 keV would not be suitable for X-ray CT. Further, this detector system would have limited count rate capabilities.

Because of these quite different requirements for the detector systems, PET/CT scanners are composed of two distinct imaging systems, i.e., a PET and a CT scanner. Although these systems are integrated into a single gantry, the CT and PET images are typically acquired separately. The CT scan can be performed after the administration of a PET radiopharmaceutical because the CT detectors are insensitive to the annihilation radiation from the radiotracer and the detector signal is dominated by the X-ray detections due to the much greater photon flux.

Clinical CT and PET scanners are utilized to ensure diagnostic anatomical and molecular imaging capability.[2] Self-evidently, performing the studies during a single session enhances patient comfort and throughput.

Attenuation Correction

At 511 keV there is a high probability that at least one of the two 511 keV annihilation photons interacts in the tissue of the imaged patient. The result of these interactions is an attenuation of the photon flux. Since the probability for an interaction increases exponentially with the thickness of the subject, the greatest signal loss occurs in structures deep within the body. If the acquired data are not corrected for attenuation prior to reconstruction, deep structures will exhibit apparent lower uptake when compared to more superficial structures. There are, however, accurate methods to correct for attenuation, resulting in images that accurately represent the radioactivity distribution throughout the body. Most commonly the attenuation is measured directly using an external 511 keV source or a transmission source. A reference or blank scan is acquired prior to the positioning of the subject in the scanner. A transmission scan of the patient is then acquired for each bed position (Figure 3). The amount of attenuation through any section through the body is then calculated as the ratio of the blank and the transmission data. This method for measuring the attenuation employs the same principles that are used for generating CT images. The difference is that the photon source is a positron emitter, which generates 511 keV photons, rather than an X-ray tube. Furthermore, the photon flux from the transmission source is several orders of magnitudes less in comparison to an X-ray tube. Therefore the statistical quality of the PET transmission data is relatively poor, in comparison to X-ray CT. In order to acquire an attenuation correction of high enough statistical quality, a transmission scan can be fairly lengthy and typically increases the overall scan time by 50-100%.

On the other hand, a CT scan can be acquired of the whole body within 20 s using the later generation of multi-slice scanners. Furthermore, the quality of the CT images is typically not limited by photon statistics. It is therefore possible to use a set of CT images to derive an attenuation correction for PET, which would also be of very good statistical quality. However, since the CT images are derived from measurements of a polychromatic X-ray tube and an average energy of 60-70 keV, the image values (i.e., Hounsfield units) do not in general directly translate into attenuation values at 511 keV. Kinahan et al.[17] have shown that an accurate attenuation correction can be derived from a CT image by classifying the image into two main tissue types (i.e., soft and bone tissue), which is accomplished by simple thresholding (Figure 4). Different scaling factors are then applied to the two tissue images, which convert the Hounsfield units into attenuation values at 511 keV. The two scaling factors are necessary due to differences in mass attenuation coefficient between bone and soft tissue at low photon energies.

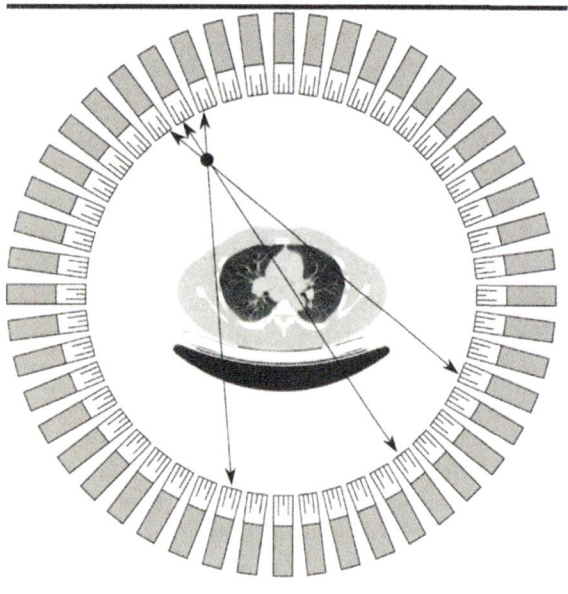

PET Transmission Scan

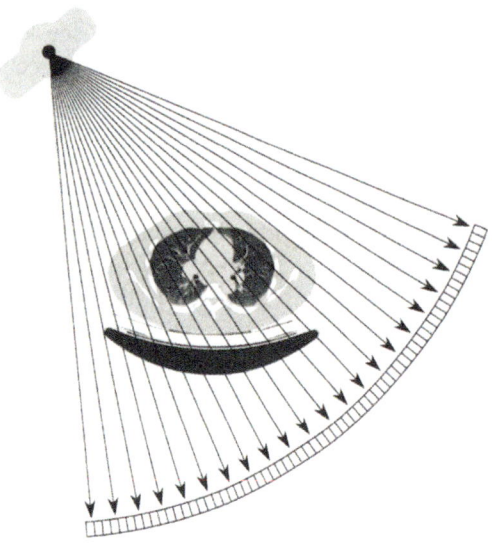

X-Ray CT Scan

Figure 3. Illustration of the similarities between a PET transmission scan (used for attenuation correction) and an X-ray CT scan. Both scans can produce a transaxial image, which represents the photon attenuation. In PET, a long-lived positron emitter is used as the source (e.g., [68]Ge/^{68}Ga rod source) and an X-ray tube is used in CT.

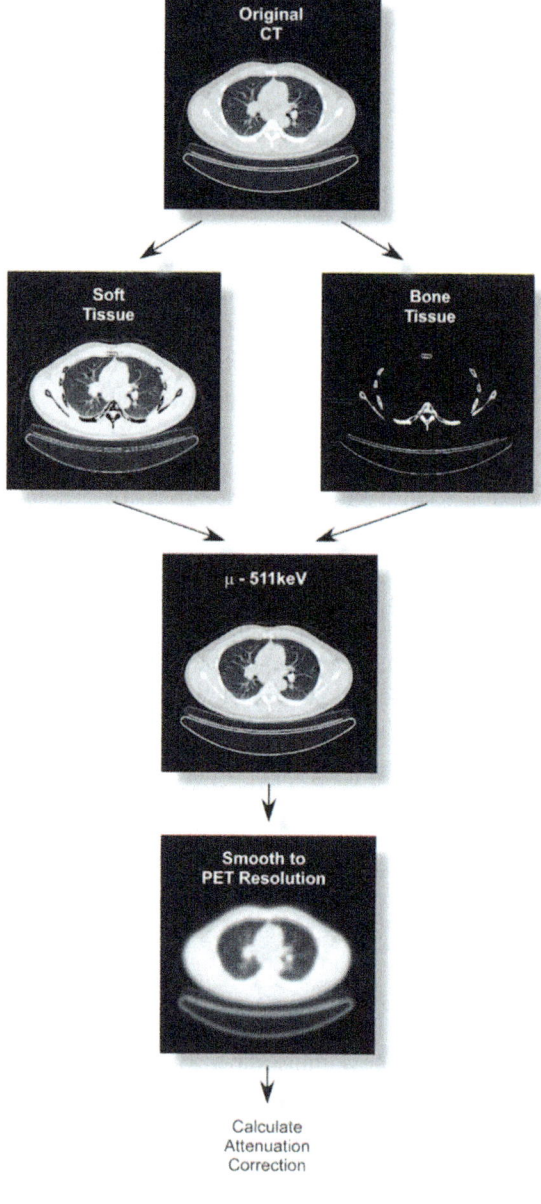

Figure 4. Since the X-ray CT image is derived from the attenuation of a polychromatic X-ray beam at a low energy (e.g., 80-140 kVp), it cannot directly be used to calculate the attenuation at 511 keV. In the method derived by Kinahan et al.[17] The bone tissue and soft tissues are separated using simple thresholding. Scale factors are applied to the two images that convert the Hounsfield units into linear attenuation coefficients at 511 keV. The scaled images are then combined and smoothed to the resolution of the PET scanner. From the smoothed image, the attenuation correction is then calculated for each line of response in the systems.

In routine PET/CT imaging, a low dose CT, i.e. 130 kVp, 10-40 mAs, usually provides images of adequate quality for the purpose of attenuation correction and anatomical localization.

Although the use of an X-ray CT has eliminated the problems of poor counting statistics of the measured attenuation correction, this method for attenuation correction is not without problems. In order to create an accurate attenuation correction, the PET and CT data have to be spatially registered. This is to a great extent solved by the integration of the PET and CT into a single unit. Furthermore, the patient should remain stationary between the two scans. Any misalignment of organs between the scans will result in inaccurate attenuation correction and may introduce artifacts. The most commonly seen artifacts are caused by respiratory motion on the CT that often creates a duplication of the dome of the liver that extends into the lungs. This artifact creates a similar artifacts and streaking on the PET volume (see chapter 5).

PET/CT Systems

All major vendors of PET scanners are marketing one or more PET/CT models, where the CT is typically a state of the art, multi-slice helical CT (2-16 slices). Apart from the number of slices of the CT, the greatest difference between these PET/CT systems is the PET detector material (e.g., Bismuth Germanate or BGO, Lutetium Oxyorthosilicate or LSO, Gadolinium Orthosilicate or GSO) and design (e.g., 2-D and/or 3-D acquisition mode, axial field of view or FOV) which are the primary factors that determines the system performance.[18]

Traditionally, PET systems acquire data in what is called the 2-D mode. This means that the coincidences that are recorded originate from a thin slice of the subject (Figure 5). To define this thin slice, and to eliminate scatter from the volume outside the slice, collimators or septa are placed on either side of the ring of detector elements. To acquire an image volume, the axial FOV has to be extended and several detector rings are placed next to each other. A drawback of this detection geometry is the relatively poor detection efficiency of the system. The detection efficiency of the system can be improved, by removing the inter-plane septa and allow each detector the record coincidences from the entire volume within the axial FOV, thus acquiring images in the 3-D mode. This improves the overall system sensitivity by a factor of 5-7. However, this sensitivity gain is partially offset by the increase in the number of detected scattered events and random events. In addition, the open geometry places a greater demand on the count rate capabilities of the scintillation detectors and the electronics.

BGO is the detector material that has been used in PET systems since the late 70's due to its high detection efficiency.[19] BGO is a relatively slow detector (determined by its light emission decay constant, see Table I) and it takes about 1 ms to process each detected event. Because of this relatively long processing time, this material is not suitable for use in PET system operating in 3-D mode at activity concentration in the FOV produced by typical clinical dosing regimen (e.g., 10-15 mCi). Because of the high dead time and excessive randoms rates induced

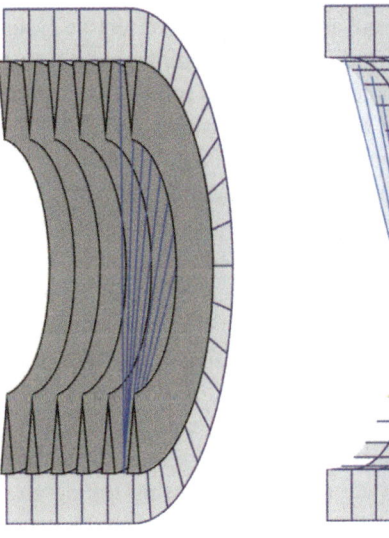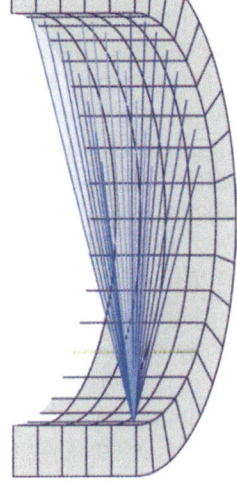

2-D Acquisition   **3-D Acquisition**

Figure 5. In the 2-D acquisition mode, coincidences are recorded from a thin slice of the subject. To define this slice, events are only recorded from detectors within the same detector ring (or a few neighboring detector rings). To eliminate scattered events originating from annihilations outside this slice, collimators or septa are placed between each detector ring. In the 3-D mode, the detectors record coincidences between all detector rings in the system (i.e., events are recorded from a 3-D volume). This improves the overall efficiency of the system, however, a substantial number of scattered events are recorded since the septa have to be removed in order to allow this detection mode. Furthermore, the open geometry requires detectors with shorter processing time due to the increase in photon flux.

by the high photon flux, a BGO system can only operate in 3-D mode efficiently at lower activity concentrations, thus offsetting the sensitivity gain of 3-D.

In the early 90's, the scintillator LSO was discovered,[20] which is a faster and brighter scintillator compared to BGO, with nearly the same detection efficiency. Because of these properties, this material is better suited for use in a system operating in 3-D acquisition mode, since it can handle the higher photon flux in 3-D mode without substantial great deadtime losses. Using LSO, the improved sensitivity of 3-D PET can be fully utilized at doses typically injected into patents scanned with 2-D BGO systems, primarily due to its better coincidence time resolution and shorter event processing time. Table I summarizes some of the key properties of the scintillators used in various PET systems.

The design of PET/CT systems is an area of rapid development and the most cost effective system configuration for different applications has yet to be determined. Table II summarizes some of the features of some current commercially available PET/CT systems. Common to current PET/CT systems is that PET and CT are two distinct systems that are axially offset relative each other. They share a common bed, and the two scans are performed sequentially (Figure 6). Knowing the relative offsets of the PET and CT systems, the same region of the subject can be scanned and later fused using specifically developed software.

Both the PET and CT scans produce image volumes that are registered in space. Both these image volumes are reconstructed using tomographic reconstruction techniques. CT is in general reconstructed using a method called filtered back projec-

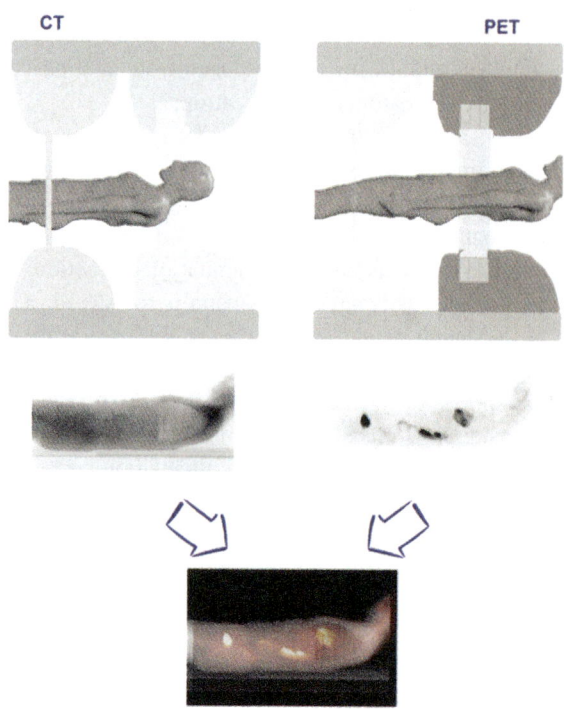

Figure 6. PET/CT typically consists of two distinct systems that are axially offset relative each other. Knowing the relative offset, the same region of the subject is imaged and later fused in software.

tion (FBP). This algorithm is well suited for reconstruction of data sets of very good statistical quality, such as X-ray CT. However, for PET data this algorithm is sub-optimal, especially for whole body scans, where the statistical quality of the data is frequently poor. PET data are in general reconstructed using iterative reconstruction techniques such as ML-EM,[21,22] OSEM[23,24] or MAP.[25,26] Common to these algebraic reconstruction methods is that they, through iterations, try to reconstruct an image that best fits the acquired data. These methods require considerable computational power, and the quality of the final image is highly dependent on the input parameters, such as number of iterations and smoothing factors.

The end result of the image reconstruction process is a large set of tomographic images that can be organized into a volume by stacking the slices on top of each other. A PET/CT scan from the pelvis up to the neck typically contains 200-300 transaxial slices and one of the main challenges is related to optimizing presentation and navigation through this data set. Frequently, a dual orthogonal volume view-

TABLE 2 FEATURES OF SELECT CURRENT COMMERCIALLY AVAILABLE PET/CT SYSTEMS					
	GE Discovery LS	GE Discovery ST	CPS BGO	CPS LSO	Philips Allegro
Detector Material	BGO	BGO	BGO	LSO	GSO
Patient Port [cm]	59	70	70	70	56.5
Detector Size [mm]	4x6x30	6.2x6.2x30	4.39x4.05x30	6.45x6.45x25	4x6x20
# of Detector Rings	18	18	32	24	
Detector Ring Diameter [cm]	92.7	92.7	82.4	82.4	90
# of Detector Elements	12,096	12,096	18,432	9,216	17,864
Transaxial FOV [cm]	55	60	58.5	58.5	57.6
Axial FOV [cm]	15.2	15.2	15.5	16.2	18
# of Slices	35	35	63	47	90

er is used, where the user can navigate through PET and CT volumes. Corresponding axial, coronal and sagittal images are displayed simultaneously as the user selects transaxial or axial cuts with a cursor (Figure 7). Since the cursors are linked, the same corresponding PET and CT slices are automatically displayed.

In addition, images can be fused together, so that, for instance, a coronal PET image displayed in pseudo color is overlaid on top of the CT image. By applying a varying the level of transparency, the uptake seen on the PET image can accurately be localized on the CT.

TABLE 3. COMMONLY USED β-EMITTING NUCLIDES	
Radionuclide	Half-Life
^{11}C	20.4 min
^{13}N	9.96 min
^{15}O	123 sec
^{18}F	110 min
^{68}Ga	68.3 min
^{82}Rb	78 sec

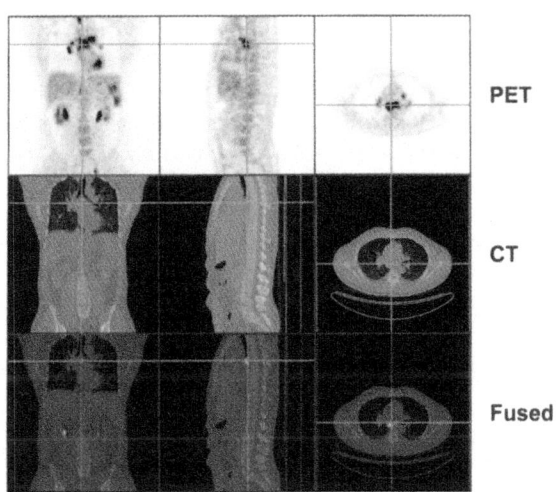

PET

CT

Fused

Figure 7. Example of a PET/CT navigation tool. The two top row shows coronal, sagittal, and transaxial PET and CT cross sections, respectively. The bottom row shows the fused images where the PET images are displayed in a hot metal pseudo color scale transparently overlaid on the CT images.

Patient Preparation and Protocol

For Oncology the most frequently used radiopharmaceutical is currently ^{18}F labeled fluorodeoxyglucose (FDG). Given the increased speed of image acquisition with the new PET/CT technology, radionuclides with a shorter half-life can be incorporated in the proteins, aminoacids, nucleic acids and enzymes, which biological pathways in the body can be followed and imaged. Table III provides an overview of the relevant β-emitting nuclides.

The standard patient preparation for a PET or a CT study is also applied to a routine PET/CT study. We currently recommend a 4-6 hour fasting period

prior to the scan and we inject 0.21 mCi/kg (7.7 MBq/kg) of ^{18}FDG intravenously. The PET imaging acquisition starts 60 minutes following the injection. For CT, the settings of the kVp, mAs, and pitch are also the same as for standard equipment. CT studies can be performed for lesion localization and attenuation correction (i.e., low current). However, if diagnostic CT studies are needed, i.v., contrast and high resolution scans are performed.

From the patient's point of view, the dual imaging study is beneficial. Preparation such as fasting has to be done only once, and all imaging is performed in a single session in the same imaging suite.

For an oncology study, typically, 0.21 mCi/kg (7.7 MBq/kg) of ^{18}FDG is administered to the patient, followed by a 60 min uptake interval. After voiding, the patient is positioned in the scanner. A scout scan or topogram is acquired to define the imaging filed. Subsequently, a helical CT scan is acquired without contrast. The complete CT scan duration is 30-90 s, depending on the axial field of view. The patient bed is moved axially into the PET field-of-view and a multi-bed PET scan is acquired over the same axial range as the CT. The duration of the PET scan is 6-28 min dependent on the number of bed positions, the type of detectors and mode of acquisition (2-D vs. 3-D). The CT data are used for attenuation correction, omitting the lengthy transmission scan with radioactive sources (2-5 min per bed position). If an i.v. contrast study is requested, the additional CT scan is performed after the standard PET-CT study is completed, to ensure correct attenuation correction.[17,27] The contrast CT is generally limited to a specific area of the body, e.g. chest or pelvis, in order to reduce the total radiation dose to the patient. The radiation dose from a whole body CT is significant. The total CT-PET-CT acquisition duration is generally less than 30 minutes.

At UCLA, a single gantry with a dual-slice CT and LSO-PET system is operational since August 2002 and more than 3,000 patient studies have been performed. The PET acquisition mode is 3-D only. We use a fixed CT protocol with 130 kVp, 130 mAs and pitch 1 with a total acquisition time of 80 seconds for a patient of average size. For PET, the [18]FDG dose is 0.21 mCi/kg (7.9 MBq/kg) and the acquisition time per bed related to patient weight, so-called weight-based acquisition (see Table IV).[28]

The contribution of breathing is less important for the abdomen than for the chest 29. Even the artifact caused by motion of the liver during CT acquisition (see for instance cases 1.5 on page 74), does not seem to pose a real clinical problem in staging of cancers with liver involvement. Non-attenuation corrected tomograms and projection images are always available to check for possible artifacts induced by mis-registered PET/CT slices. Metal implants or contrast may also induce artifacts.[30,31] Therefore, non-attenuation corrected images are routinely interpreted to check and eliminate possible imaging artifacts (see chapter 1). In order to reduce bowel uptake, some use pharmacological interventions to inhibit secretion and motility, but this does not seem necessary on a routine basis.

Our experience shows that the field of combined and correlative imaging is changing rapidly, and the nuclear medicine specialist should be prepared to participate in this evolving field of molecular imaging. For oncological applications, the importance of having a detailed anatomical framework that permits accurate interpretation of functional images cannot be over-emphasized. The requirements for such a reference framework will become increasingly important with the development of more specific tracers such as amino-acids, precursors, transporters, receptors and gene-imagers, where even the low-resolution anatomy seen on [18]FDG images will be absent.[32]

Summary

In this chapter the principles of PET/CT imaging were discussed. Development of new detector technology, systems design and processing algorithms have resulted in high-efficiency imaging systems such that the overall examination time can be drastically reduced when compared to conventional PET procedures. Importantly, this can be accomplished without compromising image quality.

Although patient preparation is similar for PET/CT and conventional routine CT or PET studies, the dual imaging session is beneficial for patients with regards to comfort and saved time. For the imaging specialist, this type of equipment increases patient throughput, and the technological innovations have led to superior image quality. The common scanning geometry results in near perfect registration of the PET and CT volumes, allowing accurate functional and anatomical image fusion. This in turn will improve lesion localization, and will increase the accuracy in diagnosing and staging of cancer.

References

1. Beyer T, Townsend DW, Brun T, Kinahan PE, Charron M, Roddy R, Jerin J, Young J, Byars L, Nutt R. A combined PET/CT scanner for clinical oncology. J Nucl Med. 2000;41(8):1369-1379.

2. Townsend DW, Cherry SR. Combining anatomy and function: the path to true image fusion. Eur Radiol. 2001;11(10):1968-1974.

3. Cohade C, Osman M, Leal J, Wahl RL. Direct comparison of 18F-FDG PET and PET/CT in patients with colorectal carcinoma. J Nucl Med. 2003;44(11):1797-1803.

4. Lardinois D, Weder W, Hany TF, Kamel EM, Korom S, Seifert B, von Schulthess GK, Steinert HC. Staging of non-small-cell lung cancer with integrated positron-emission tomography and computed tomography. N Engl J Med. 2003;348(25):2500-2507.

5. Bajcsy R, Lieberson R, Reivich M. A computerized system for the elastic matching of deformed radiographic images to idealized atlas images. J Comput Assist Tomogr. 1983;7(4):618-625.

6. Friston KJ, Frith CD, Liddle PF, Frackowiak RS. Plastic transformation of PET images. J Comput Assist Tomogr. 1991;15(4):634-639.

7. Gee JC, Reivich M, Bajcsy R. Elastically deforming 3D atlas to match anatomical brain images. J Comput Assist Tomogr. 1993;17(2):225-236.

8. Tai YC, Lin KP, Dahlbom M, Hoffman EJ. A hybrid attenuation correction technique to compensate for lung density in 3-D total body PET. IEEE Trans Nucl Sc. 1996;43(1):323-330.

9. Thompson P, Toga AW. A surface-based technique for warping three-dimensional images of the brain. IEEE Trans Med Imaging. 1996;15(4):402-417.

10. Bankman IN, ed. Handbook of medical imaging: processing and analysis. San Diego, CA: Academic Press, 2000.

11.   Levin CS, Dahlbom M, Hoffman EJ. A Monte Carlo correction for the effect of Compton scattering in 3-D PET brain imaging. IEEE Trans Nucl Sci. 1995;42(4):1181-1185.

12.   Ollinger JM. Model-based scatter correction for fully 3D PET. Phys Med Biol. 1996;41(1):153-176.

13.   Watson CC, Newport D, Casey ME, deKemp RA, Beanlands RS, Schmand M. Evaluation of simulation-based scatter correction for 3-D PET cardiac imaging. IEEE Trans Nucl Sci. 1997;44(1):90-97.

14.   Holdsworth C, Levin C, Dahlbom M, Farquhar T, Hoffman E. An investigation of Monte Carlo techniques to correct for scatter in PET thorax imaging. IEEE Nucl Sci Med Imaging. 1999.

15.   Kalender WA. Computed tomography: fundamentals, system technology, image quality, applications. Munich: MCD Verlag, 2000.

16.   Bushberg JT, Seibert JA, Leidholdt EM, Boone JM. The essential physics of medical imaging. 2nd ed. Philadelphia: Lippincott Williams & Wilkins, 2002.

17.   Kinahan PE, Townsend DW, Beyer T, Sashin D. Attenuation correction for a combined 3D PET/CT scanner. Med Phys. 1998;25(10):2046-2053.

18.   Melcher CL. Scintillation crystals for PET. J Nucl Med. 2000;41(6):1051-1055.

19.   Cho ZH, Farukhi MR. Bismuth germanate as a potential scintillation detector in positron cameras. J Nucl Med. 1977;18(8):840-844.

20.   Melcher CL, Schweitzer JS. Cerium-doped lutetium oxyorthosilicate: a fast, efficient new scintillator. IEEE Trans Nucl Sci. 1992;39(4):502-505.

21.   Shepp LA, Vardi Y. Maximum likelihood reconstruction for emission tomography. IEEE Trans Med Imaging. 1982;1(2):113-122.

22.   Lange K, Carson R. EM reconstruction algorithms for emission and transmission tomography. J Comput Assist Tomogr. 1984;8(2):306-316.

23.   Hudson HM, Larkin RS. Accelerated image reconstruction using ordered subsets of projection data. IEEE Trans Med Imaging. 1994;13(4):601-609.

24.   Meikle SR, Hutton BF, Bailey DL, Hooper PK, Fulham MJ. Accelerated EM reconstruction in total-body PET: potential for improving tumor detectability. Phys Med Biol. 1994;39:1689-1704.

25.   Mumcuoglu EU, Leahy RM, Cherry SR, Hoffman E. Accurate geometric and physical response modelling for statistical image reconstruction in high resolution PET. In: Del Guerra, A, ed.; 1996:1569-73 vol.3.

26.   Qi J, Leahy RM, Hsu C-H, Farquhar TH, Cherry SR. Fully 3D Bayesian image reconstruction for the ECAT EXACT HR+. IEEE Trans Nucl Sci. 1998;45:1096-1103.

27.   Dizendorf EV, Treyer V, von Schulthess GK, Hany TF. Application of oral contrast media in coregistered positron emission tomography-CT. Am J Roentgenol. 2002;179(2):477-481.

28.   Halpern BS, Dahlbom M, Quon A, Schiepers C, Waldherr C, Silverman DH, Ratib O, Czernin J. Impact of patient weight and emission scan duration on image quality and lesion detectability using PET/CT. J Nucl Med. 2004;In Press.

29.   Goerres GW, Burger C, Schwitter MR, Heidelberg TN, Seifert B, von Schulthess GK. PET/CT of the abdomen: optimizing the patient breathing pattern. Eur Radiol. 2003;13(4):734-739.

30.   Goerres GW, Hany TF, Kamel E, von Schulthess GK, Buck A. Head and neck imaging with PET and PET/CT: artefacts from dental metallic implants. Eur J Nucl Med Mol Imaging. 2002;29(3):367-370.

31.   Halpern BS, Dahlbom M, Waldherr C, Yap CS, Schiepers C, Silverman DH, Ratib O, Czernin J. Cardiac pacemakers and central venous lines can induce focal artifacts on CT corrected PET images. J Nucl Med. 2004;45.

32.   Phelps ME. PET: the merging of biology and imaging into molecular imaging. J Nucl Med. 2000;41(4):661-681.

A Future for PET/CT

D. Townsend

Introduction

Since the introduction of the first combined PET/CT scanner in 1998, diffusion of this technology into the clinical arena has been rapid, more reminiscent of the adoption of magnetic resonance (MR) imaging in the early eighties than the slower acceptance of positron emission tomography (PET). For almost two decades, PET was viewed primarily as a research tool until Medicare approval, in 1998, of PET imaging for the diagnosis and staging of a number of different cancers. With this approval, the role of PET in oncology increased significantly from 1999 onwards. Coinciding with the growth in PET, the first commercial PET/CT scanners appeared in the clinic in early 2001, further advancing the adoption of PET in oncology by bringing functional imaging with radioactive tracers directly to the radiological community. As the benefits of imaging anatomy and function in the same scanner has become more widely appreciated, the demand for the technology has increased to a point where, in less than three years, over 300 such units are now installed in medical institutions worldwide. The trend from PET to PET/CT is confirmed by vendors whose PET/CT sales now represent up to 80% of the PET market.

Imaging anatomy and function in a single scan is advantageous to both patient and physician. For the patient, it is a convenient, straightforward and complete procedure, while for the physician it provides accurately aligned images of function and anatomy from which functional abnormalities can be precisely localized and non-specific radiotracer uptake in normal structures can be distinguished from pathology. A number of recent studies have reported increased accuracy and physician confidence in reading PET/CT scans compared to PET only, beneficial aspects of PET/CT that directly impact patient management.

In less than four years, PET/CT scanners have evolved through a number of designs in which differ-ent performance levels of CT and PET are combined together. Currently, the overwhelming demand is for the highest level in both CT and PET, one that incorporates a sub second rotation, multi-slice CT and a high resolution, high count rate, dedicated PET scanner. These commercial designs place a CT scanner in front of the PET scanner with a common patient couch and involve little or no physical integration of the actual detector systems. Consequently, they allow the performance level of the CT and PET to be selected independently and even offer the possibility, in some cases, of field upgrades from CT or PET to PET/CT. Thus, combinations comprising 2, 4, 8 or even 16 row CT detectors with high-end dedicated PET scanners are currently the preferred PET/CT designs. The CT images are used not only for accurate anatomical localization of the PET tracer distribution but also to generate the attenuation correction factors that are applied to the PET emission data.

In view of the impact that combined PET/CT scanners have had on PET oncology within a relatively short time frame, it is of interest to review the evolution of recent designs and to explore possible future directions for this technology.

Advances in Current Designs

The first PET/CT prototype[1] was a mechanically integrated device with the CT and PET components mounted on the same rotating support; the device became operational in 1998. The first commercial scanners that followed successful clinical imaging with the prototype PET/CT[2-5] appeared in early 2001 and consisted of a CT scanner in tandem with a PET scanner, with little or no mechanical integration of the two systems beyond a common gantry cover.[6] This approach, with the CT and PET scanners kept separate, has been a characteristic feature of all commercial designs. The advantage of this design is flexibility in that different levels of CT and PET per-

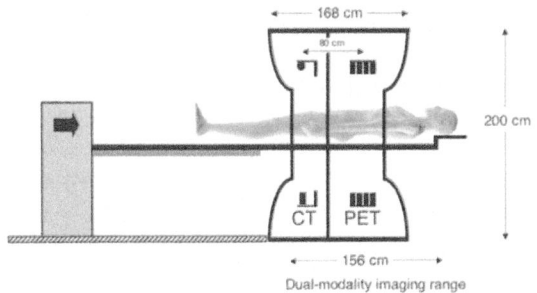

Figure 1. A schematic of a PET/CT scanner design currently marketed by Siemens as the biograph (Siemens Medical Solutions, Chicago, IL) and by CTI Molecular Imaging as the Reveal (CTI Molecular Imaging, Knoxville, TN). The design incorporates a multi-detector spiral CT scanner and an LSO PET scanner. The dimensions of the gantry are 228 cm wide, 200 cm high and 168 cm deep. The separation of the CT and PET imaging fields is about 80 cm. The co-scan range for acquiring both CT and PET is 156 cm (182 cm, feet first). The patient port diameter is 70 cm.

formance can be combined as required and upgraded independently. An upgrade path from CT or PET to PET/CT can, in some cases, also be envisaged. All designs incorporate a common patient couch that is designed to eliminate or minimize vertical deflection due to the weight of the patient and ensure accurate alignment of the CT and PET images. The major vendors have adopted different approaches to address this issue. One such design is illustrated schematically in Figure 1 (CPS Innovations, Knoxville, TN).

While the detector and data acquisition subsystems have been kept separate, attempts have been made to integrate the acquisition and to provide fused image display software. Combined scanners are operated from a single console with application-specific task cards selected for the CT and PET acquisition. While the early designs involved multiple computers for acquisition, image reconstruction, and image display, progress is being made in combining some of these functions into one computer, reducing complexity and increasing reliability. The most recent designs are simpler to operate, involve fewer computer systems, and are considerably more reliable. Indeed, poor reliability would be a major concern for the high patient throughput attainable with these scanners.

As mentioned, PET/CT designs have taken advantage of recent advances in both CT and PET

technology by maintaining separation of the imaging subsystems. While the CT scanners in the first PET/CT designs were single or dual slice, more recently [4, 8 and 16] slice systems have been incorporated into PET/CT scanners with rotation times reduced to 0.4 s. Such high performance, state-of-the-art CT can complete a whole-body scan in less than 30 s offering high throughput and flexibility for the respiration protocols. As multi-slice CT progresses to a greater number of slices and shorter rotation times, a critical review of the actual requirements of PET/CT for specific applications will be necessary. Many of the recent CT improvements are targeted at cardiology, whereas the role of PET/CT in cardiology has yet to be established. Indeed, oncology applications may be adequately addressed with a lower performance CT scanner, such as a 2 or 4 slice system.

The recent developments in PET scanner technology have been primarily oriented towards the introduction of new scintillators. For over two decades, PET detectors have been based on either thallium-activated sodium iodide (NaI(Tl)) or bismuth germanate (BGO). While NaI has high light output, it has low stopping power at PET photon energies (511 keV) and a long decay time. The low stopping power was overcome by BGO, first introduced for PET in 1977,[7] but at the expense of considerably reduced light output compared with NaI; the decay time for BGO is 30% longer than NaI. Some physical properties of these scintillators are compared in Table 1. The introduction of faster scintillators such as gadolinium oxyorthosilicate (GSO)[8] and lutetium oxyorthosilicate (LSO),[9] also compared in Table 1, offer enhanced PET scanner performance. LSO in particular outperforms BGO in almost every aspect, especially light output and decay time. The faster scintillators (Table 1) have lower dead time and give

Property	NaI	BGO	LSO	GSO
Density (g/mL)	3.67	7.13	7.4	6.7
Effective Z	51	74	66	61
Attenuation length (cm)	2.88	1.05	1.16	1.43
Decay time (ns)	230	300	35-45	30-60
Photons/MeV	38,000	8,200	28,000	10,000
Light yield (%NaI)	100	15	75	25
Hygroscopic	Yes	No	No	No

NaI: sodium iodide   BGO: bismuth germanate
LSO: lutetium oxyorthosilicate   GSO: gadolinium oxyorthosilicate

Table 1. Physical properties of different scintillators for PET.

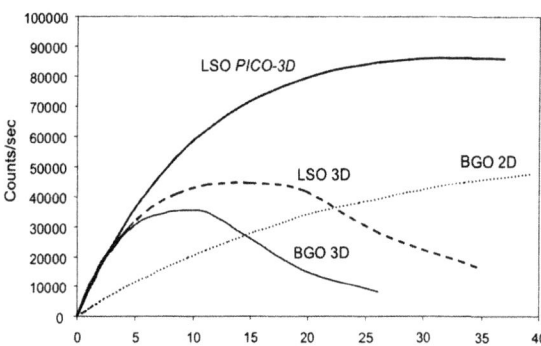

Figure 2. Noise Equivalent Count Rate (NEC) as a function of activity concentration in the NEMA NU-2001, 70 cm phantom. The curves are shown for the standard BGO ECAT EXACT with septa extended (BGO 2D), a BGO PET/CT scanner (BGO 3D), an LSO PET/CT scanner with standard electronics (LSO 3D), and an LSO PET/CT scanner with the new, high count rate PICO-3D electronics (LSO PICO-3D).

better count rate performance, particularly at high activity concentrations. This behaviour is confirmed in Figure 2 where the Noise Effective Count Rate (NEC)10 is shown as a function of activity concentration in the NEMA NU-2001 phantom for 2D and 3D BGO scanners compared with a 3D LSO scanner, without and with the new fast, PICO-3D electronics (CPS Innovations, Knoxville, TN). The curves show the expected behaviour with 3D superior to 2D and LSO out-performing BGO even at low activity concentrations. The new PICO-3D electronics, matched to the physical properties of LSO, show a significant improvement over the older design with peak NEC exceeding 80 kcps. All 3D measurements are for PET/CT scanners, whereas the 2D data are for the standard ECAT EXACT PET scanner (CPS Innovations, Knoxville, TN) with septa extended.

The current status of PET/CT scanners is perhaps best illustrated by a design in which a 16-slice CT scanner, the Sensation 16 (Siemens Medical Solutions, Forchheim, Germany) is combined with the recently-announced high resolution, LSO PET scanner (CPS Innovations, Knoxville, TN). The new PET scanner has unique 13 x 13 LSO block detectors each 4 mm x 4 mm in cross-section. The PICO-3D read-out electronics, adapted to the speed and light output of LSO, is operated with a coincidence time window of 4.5 ns and a lower energy threshold of 425 keV. The significance of these high resolution detectors is illustrated in Figure 3 for a patient with squamous cell carcinoma of the right tonsil. Following

treatment that included a right tonsillectomy, radical neck dissection and chemotherapy, the patient was restaged by scanning first on an ECAT EXACT (CPS Innovations, Knoxville, TN) with 6.4 mm x 6.4 mm BGO detectors, and then on the high resolution PET/CT scanner. A coronal section from the PET scan (Figure 3A) demonstrated a diffuse band of activity in the right neck (arrowed). The corresponding PET section from the PET/CT scan (Figure 3B) resolved this diffuse band into individual nodes in the neck of the patient (arrowed).

Currently there are more than six different designs of PET/CT scanner offered by the major vendors. All designs have in common a CT scanner in the front with a PET scanner behind and each combine varying levels of performance of the CT and PET components. The different performance ranges for some key operating parameters are summarized in Table 2.

CT-Based Attenuation Correction

A unique feature of combined PET/CT scanners is the use of the CT images to correct PET emission data for photon attenuation. The advantages of

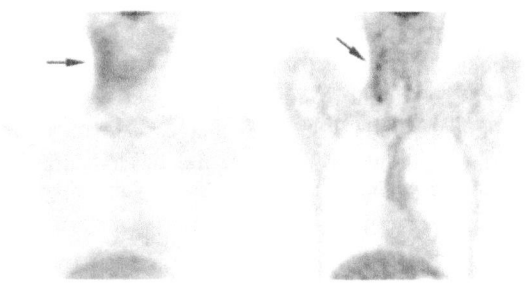

using the CT include low statistical noise and short scanning times compared with standard PET trans-

Table 3. A 52 year-old male patient, 135 lbs, diagnosed with squamous cell tonsillar cancer and a 4 cm positive node in the neck. The patient underwent pre-surgical chemotherapy, a right tonsillectomy and a right radical neck dissection for removal of the positive node and 45 additional nodes; all of the additional nodes had negative pathology. The patient suffered post-surgical infectious complications. A follow-up PET scan (A) acquired with arms down showed a diffuse band of activity in the right neck (arrowed) seen on a coronal section; a PET/CT scan (B) acquired with arms up and with the new high resolution detector blocks clearly resolved this diffuse band of activity into individual, sub clinical lymph nodes.

mission scans. Since the attenuation correction factors are energy-dependent, a scaling algorithm is required to transform the factors from the CT energy (~ 70 keV) up to the PET energy (511 keV). Scaling algorithms[11, 12] typically use a bilinear function to transform the attenuation values below and above a given threshold around 0 HU (Hounsfield Units), the CT value for water. While some PET/CT designs also offer optional standard PET transmission sources, the advantages of low noise and short CT scan times outweigh any of the perceived disadvantages of CT-based attenuation correction and few, if any, PET/CT installations still use standard PET transmission sources.

Two potential disadvantages of CT-based attenuation correction include CT and PET mismatch due patient respiration, and the use of intravenous or oral contrast when the CT scan is acquired with contrast for clinical purposes. Since clinical CT scans are acquired with breath hold at full inspiration while PET scans are acquired with the patient breathing quietly, there is a mismatch of the anatomical and functional images, particularly in the thorax and upper abdomen.[13] Such a mismatch can be reduced by allowing the patient to breath during the CT scan although this approach may introduce breathing artifacts into the CT scan, and can lead to interpretation errors in some cases.[14] Alternatively, a better match can be achieved by acquiring the CT scan at end or partial expiration when tolerated by the patient, thus eliminating CT breathing artifacts. The recent introduction of a 16-slice PET/CT scanner that can cover 100 cm axially in only 13 s facilitates the acquisition of end-expiration CT scans. To further improve the quality of the study, a respiration-gated PET scan can be acquired such that one of the gates corresponding to the end-expiration phase matches the CT scan. Preliminary PET/CT studies incorporating end-expiration breath-hold CT and gated PET show improved anatomical-functional image matching, particularly in the thorax, and more accurate lung tumor dimensions and uptake values from the PET scan. It is likely that gating will become a standard feature of future PET/CT scan protocols, particularly for lung cancer.

Iodinated contrast is used in CT to enhance attenuation values in the vessels (intravenous administration) and gastro-intestinal tract (oral administration). Contrast-enhanced pixels that are incorrectly scaled to 511 keV can potentially generate focal artifacts in the PET image through the CT-based attenua-

CT parameters		PET parameters	
detectors:	ceramic	scintillator:	BGO; GSO; LSO
slices:	1, 2, 4, 8, 16	detector size:	4 x 4 mm; 6 x 6 mm
rotation speed:	0.4 – 2.0 s	axial FOV:	15 – 18 cm
tube current:	80 – 280 mA	septa:	2D/3D; 3D only
heat capacity:	3.5 – 6.5 MHU	attenuation:	rod; point; CT-only
trans. FOV:	45 – 50 cm	trans. FOV:	55 – 60 cm
time /100 cm:	13 – 90 s	time/bed:	1 – 5 min
slice width:	0.6 – 10 mm	resolution:	4 – 6 mm
patient port:	70 cm	patient port:	60 – 70 cm

Table 2. A summary of some CT and PET parameters in current PET/CT designs

tion correction factors. This would be an undesirable outcome, particularly for tumor imaging. However, standard-of-care CT scanning generally dictates the use of either intravenous or oral contrast, or both as in the case of the abdominal and pelvic studies. An obvious way to avoid such problems is to perform two CT scans, a clinical CT with appropriate contrast administration, and a low-dose, non-contrast CT for attenuation correction and co-registration. The two scans could even be acquired with different breathing protocols, although this two-scan approach would further increase the radiation exposure to the patient. Recent results[15] have shown that the presence of intravenous contrast at normal concentrations actually has little effect on the CT-based attenuation correction factors. This is not generally the case for oral contrast where the larger intestinal volumes and wide range of concentrations can lead to over-correction of the PET data. However, Carney et al.[16] have shown that contrast-enhanced CT pixels can be separated from those of bone by a region-growing algorithm. Since the presence of iodinated contrast has a negligible effect (< 2%) on photon attenuation at 511 keV, the CT image pixels identified as oral contrast can be set to a tissue-equivalent value thus ensuring accurate attenuation correction factors for the PET data. This approach can, to a considerable extent, also reduce artifacts due to catheters and metallic objects in the patient.[17] As a consequence of this and other work, it is anticipated that PET/CT protocols will include CT and PET studies of clinical quality.

Towards Future PET/CT Designs

As mentioned, an advantage of limited integration of the CT and PET imaging components is that improvements and advances in either CT or PET can be more easily incorporated into new PET/CT designs. The evolution of PET/CT over the past three years has taken advantage of the independent developments occurring in the CT and PET fields. CT has emerged from an extended period of little innovation to one of rapid change with the development of spiral CT, multi-slice detector systems, short mechanical rotation times, and new X-ray tube technology. As multi-slice detectors increase from dual to 16-slice, to the recently-announced 32-slice, and even 64-slice with axial displacement of the X-ray focal spot, the prospect of 2D planar detectors and cone beam CT is becoming a reality. With rotation times of 0.4 s and below, rapid spiral scans can cover the entire thorax in 10 s, limiting artifacts due to cardiac motion.

The first PET/CT designs were single, dual or 4-slice CT scanners combined with PET technology from the early nineties. There was, therefore, a mismatch between the 60 s or less required for the CT scan and the 40 min or more for the PET scan. The CT scanner was idle for much of the time and patient throughput was limited to 4-5 patients per day maximum. However, PET scanner technology has been steadily improving over the past decade and the first clinical PET scanners based on fast scintillators such as GSO and LSO have rapidly found their way into the new PET/CT designs. Even a redesign of older BGO technology by one of the major vendors resulted in improved performance for their PET/CT scanner. As a consequence of these developments, the PET scan duration has been steadily decreasing to a point where a whole-body PET/CT scan can now be completed in less than 10 min,[18] thereby making more efficient use of the CT scanner and significantly improving patient throughput.

The 16-slice Sensation 16 LSO PET/CT scanner represents the current state-of-the-art with high sensitivity 3D acquisition mode, high count rate capability from the PICO-3D electronics, and now high spatial resolution with the 13 x 13, 4 mm x 4 mm LSO detectors. The device offers a flexible platform on which to refine specific protocols tailored to the patient and cancer type. Thus large patients may require higher levels of injected activity and longer imaging times to achieve diagnostic image quality, whereas for smaller patients, high resolution whole-body images can be acquired in 25 min or less. When required, the scanner is capable of short imaging times of less than 10 min.

The rapid diffusion of PET/CT technology into medical imaging departments is a reflection of

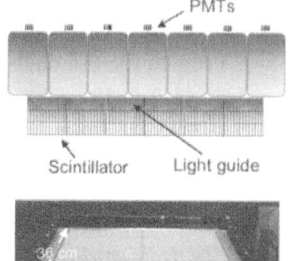
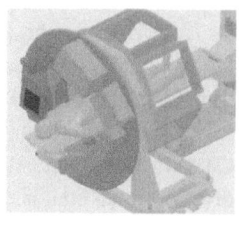

Figure 4. (A) A schematic of the LSO panel technology based on a quadrant-sharing approach using large phototubes (top) and a photo (bottom) of an actual panel, 36 cm x 52 cm in size; (B) a model of a possible integrated PET/CT design based on the LSO panels with the CT components mounted on the front of the assembly and up to six panel detectors mounted on the rear. The entire assembly can rotate at up to 30 rpm.

the acceptance of combined anatomical and functional imaging by radiologists, nuclear medicine physicians and other specialists. It is generally accepted that PET/CT scanners will become the imaging device of choice in oncology, and after observing the evolution of the early designs, the obvious questions are where is this technology going and what will be the designs of the future? The level of integration is a major issue with arguments for maintaining the current level of separate scanners in tandem as well as arguments for a completely integrated scanner that even go as far as a proposal to use the same detector material for both CT and PET.[19] The advantages of separate scanners in tandem, such as the current devices, include the ability to upgrade the CT and PET scanners individually as technology advances. It is also possible to envisage a family of PET/CT scanners where the CT and PET performance level is chosen to match the requirements and finances of the clinical department. Such an approach has many practical advantages.

The arguments for a more integrated system include the elimination of duplicate components such as mechanical supports and computers, a more compact system with a smaller footprint, and reduced cost and increased reliability by using common components for CT and PET. An integrated system would be an ambitious development requiring close interaction between the CT and PET manufacturers to combine common components. Recently, a large area

LSO panel detector has been proposed by Nahmias et al.[20] as an alternative to the conventional block detector, a standard in PET for two decades.[21] The panel design, shown schematically in Figure 4A, uses a quadrant-sharing approach with 5 cm photomultipliers bonded to the scintillator with the edges of the tubes positioned over the centers of the 5 cm x 5 cm blocks of LSO. The high light output from LSO allows the block to be cut into 12 x 12 small crystals and still maintain the ability to separate the detector elements. The concept is to mount three, four or five of these panel detectors in a hexagonal configuration and rotate the assembly at 30 rpm to acquire a full data set for 3D reconstruction. One of the completed panels with 10 x 7 blocks is shown in Figure 4A where the physical dimensions are 52 cm x 36 cm with the longer side mounted axially in the gantry. By mounting CT components on the front of the rotating support, as shown schematically in Figure 4B, an integrated system similar in design to that of the original prototype[1] could be developed, but with far superior performance. The peak NEC for the NEMA NU-2001 phantom has been measured to exceed 110 kcps for a five-panel PET system, at least 40% more than with current scanners.

The recent announcement of new X-ray tube technology, the Straton tube (Siemens Medical Solutions, Forchheim, Germany) could also impact an integrated PET/CT design. The new tube incorporates direct anode cooling and is a small, compact construction. The anode plate is only 12 cm in diameter and the need for heat storage capacity is eliminated. The tube has a substantially longer lifetime than a conventional tube and since it can withstand higher G-forces, rotation rates of 162 rpm are attainable. Such a compact design could play a significant role in future integrated PET/CT scanners.

Developing a PET/CT scanner that uses the same detector material for CT and PET is obviously a challenge. While this would result in the ideal integrated system, the technical demands on the detectors are very different for the two modalities. CT detectors operate in current integration mode, are very sensitive to photons around 70 keV, cover an axial range of 10-20 mm, and have pixel dimensions of 1 mm or less; PET detectors count individual incident photons, are especially sensitive to 511 keV photons, cover an axial range of 15-20 cm, and have pixel dimensions of 2-4 mm. Several other physical properties of the detector material, such as low afterglow for CT, are also important. While there are a few candidates for such a detector material – including LSO – designing a combined CT and PET detector array will be a challenge.

There is also work in progress to replace the phototubes used in current PET detectors with photodiodes, bonded to a scintillator such as LSO. When successful, the result will be a compact PET detector insensitive to magnetic fields and robust to fast rotation. From the PET/CT perspective, a more compact and robust PET detector will simplify integration and allow it to be rotated at rates up to 150 rpm that are attained by state-of-the-art CT scanners. Such a detector design could also open up the possibility for a PET/MR scanner, although that will be a major technical challenge, assuming there is a clinical demand for such a device.

To date, all commercial PET/CT designs combine a mid-to-high end CT scanner with a state-of-the-art, high end PET scanner. The price tag for such a scanner is close to the sum of the price tags for the individual devices. It is unlikely, even in the medium term, that the medical imaging market will accept such a pricing structure in the future and vendors will be under pressure to reduce costs. Cost reduction could be achieved through the development, as mentioned, of a more integrated system or by adopting lower performance, less expensive components. If, as predicted, the migration of PET to PET/CT continues at the present rate, there will be a significant demand for both mid-range and entry level PET/CT scanners for oncology.

Conclusions

As mentioned, an advantage of limited integration of the CT and PET imaging components is that improvements and advances in either CT or PET can be more easily incorporated into new PET/CT designs. The evolution of PET/CT over the past three years has taken advantage of the independent developments occurring in the CT and PET fields. CT has emerged from an extended period of little innovation to one of rapid change with the development of spiral CT, multi-slice detector systems, short mechanical rotation times, and new X-ray tube technology. As multi-slice detectors increase from dual to 16-slice, to the recently-announced 32-slice, and even 64-slice with axial displacement of the X-ray focal spot, the prospect of 2D planar detectors and cone beam CT is becoming a reality. With rotation times of 0.4 s and below, rapid spiral scans can cover the entire thorax in 10 s, limiting artifacts due to cardiac motion.

The first PET/CT designs were single, dual or 4-slice CT scanners combined with PET technology from the early nineties. There was, therefore, a mismatch between the 60 s or less required for the CT scan and the 40 min or more for the PET scan. The CT scanner was idle for much of the time and patient throughput was limited to 4-5 patients per day maximum. However, PET scanner technology has been steadily improving over the past decade and the first clinical PET scanners based on fast scintillators such as GSO and LSO have rapidly found their way into the new PET/CT designs. Even a redesign of older BGO technology by one of the major vendors resulted in improved performance for their PET/CT scanner. As a consequence of these developments, the PET scan duration has been steadily decreasing to a point where a whole-body PET/CT scan can now be completed in less than 10 min,[18] thereby making more efficient use of the CT scanner and significantly improving patient throughput.

The 16-slice Sensation 16 LSO PET/CT scanner represents the current state-of-the-art with high sensitivity 3D acquisition mode, high count rate capability from the PICO-3D electronics, and now high spatial resolution with the 13 x 13, 4 mm x 4 mm LSO detectors. The device offers a flexible platform on which to refine specific protocols tailored to the patient and cancer type. Thus large patients may require higher levels of injected activity and longer imaging times to achieve diagnostic image quality, whereas for smaller patients, high resolution whole-body images can be acquired in 25 min or less. When required, the scanner is capable of short imaging times of less than 10 min.

The rapid diffusion of PET/CT technology into medical imaging departments is a reflection of the acceptance of combined anatomical and functional imaging by radiologists, nuclear medicine physicians and other specialists. It is generally accepted that PET/CT scanners will become the imaging device of choice in oncology, and after observing the evolution of the early designs, the obvious questions are where is this technology going and what will be the designs of the future? The level of integration is a major issue with arguments for maintaining the current level of separate scanners in tandem as well as arguments for a completely integrated scanner that even go as far as a proposal to use the same detector

material for both CT and PET.[19] The advantages of separate scanners in tandem, such as the current devices, include the ability to upgrade the CT and PET scanners individually as technology advances. It is also possible to envisage a family of PET/CT scanners where the CT and PET performance level is chosen to match the requirements and finances of the clinical department. Such an approach has many practical advantages.

The arguments for a more integrated system include the elimination of duplicate components such as mechanical supports and computers, a more compact system with a smaller footprint, and reduced cost and increased reliability by using common components for CT and PET. An integrated system would be an ambitious development requiring close interaction between the CT and PET manufacturers to combine common components. Recently, a large area LSO panel detector has been proposed by Nahmias et al.[20] as an alternative to the conventional block detector, a standard in PET for two decades.[21] The panel design, shown schematically in Figure 4A, uses a quadrant-sharing approach with 5 cm photomultipliers bonded to the scintillator with the edges of the tubes positioned over the centers of the 5 cm x 5 cm blocks of LSO. The high light output from LSO allows the block to be cut into 12 x 12 small crystals and still maintain the ability to separate the detector elements. The concept is to mount three, four or five of these panel detectors in a hexagonal configuration and rotate the assembly at 30 rpm to acquire a full data set for 3D reconstruction. One of the completed panels with 10 x 7 blocks is shown in Figure 4A where the physical dimensions are 52 cm x 36 cm with the longer side mounted axially in the gantry. By mounting CT components on the front of the rotating support, as shown schematically in Figure 4B, an integrated system similar in design to that of the original prototype1 could be developed, but with far superior performance. The peak NEC for the NEMA NU-2001 phantom has been measured to exceed 110 kcps for a five-panel PET system, at least 40% more than with current scanners.

The recent announcement of new X-ray tube technology, the Straton tube (Siemens Medical Solutions, Forchheim, Germany) could also impact an integrated PET/CT design. The new tube incorporates direct anode cooling and is a small, compact construction. The anode plate is only 12 cm in diameter and the need for heat storage capacity is eliminated. The tube has a substantially longer lifetime than a conventional tube and since it can withstand higher G-forces, rotation rates of 162 rpm are attainable. Such a compact design could play a significant role in future integrated PET/CT scanners.

Developing a PET/CT scanner that uses the same detector material for CT and PET is obviously a challenge. While this would result in the ideal integrated system, the technical demands on the detectors are very different for the two modalities. CT detectors operate in current integration mode, are very sensitive to photons around 70 keV, cover an axial range of 10-20 mm, and have pixel dimensions of 1 mm or less; PET detectors count individual incident photons, are especially sensitive to 511 keV photons, cover an axial range of 15-20 cm, and have pixel dimensions of 2-4 mm. Several other physical properties of the detector material, such as low afterglow for CT, are also important. While there are a few candidates for such a detector material – including LSO – designing a combined CT and PET detector array will be a challenge.

There is also work in progress to replace the phototubes used in current PET detectors with photodiodes, bonded to a scintillator such as LSO. When successful, the result will be a compact PET detector insensitive to magnetic fields and robust to fast rotation. From the PET/CT perspective, a more compact and robust PET detector will simplify integration and allow it to be rotated at rates up to 150 rpm that are attained by state-of-the-art CT scanners. Such a detector design could also open up the possibility for a PET/MR scanner, although that will be a major technical challenge, assuming there is a clinical demand for such a device.

To date, all commercial PET/CT designs combine a mid-to-high end CT scanner with a state-of-the-art, high end PET scanner. The price tag for such a scanner is close to the sum of the price tags for the individual devices. It is unlikely, even in the medium term, that the medical imaging market will accept such a pricing structure in the future and vendors will be under pressure to reduce costs. Cost reduction could be achieved through the development, as mentioned, of a more integrated system or by adopting lower performance, less expensive components. If, as predicted, the migration of PET to PET/CT continues at the present rate, there will be a significant demand for both mid-range and entry level PET/CT scanners for oncology.

References

1. Beyer T, Townsend DW, Brun T, Kinahan PE, Charron M, Roddy R, Jerin J, Young J, Byars L, Nutt R. A combined PET/CT scanner for clinical oncology. J Nucl Med. 2000;41(8):1369-1379.
2. Charron M, Beyer T, Bohnen NN, Kinahan PE, Dachille MA, Jerin J, Nutt R, Meltzer CC, Villemagne V, Townsend DW. Image analysis in patients with cancer studied with a combined PET and CT scanner. Clin Nucl Med. 2000;25(11): 905-910.
3. Kluetz PG, Meltzer CC, Villemagne VL, Kinahan PE, Chander S, Martinelli MA, Townsend DW. Combined PET/CT imaging in oncology: impact on patient management. Clin Positron Imaging. 2001;3(6):223-230.
4. Meltzer CC, Martinelli MA, Beyer T, Kinahan PE, Charron M, McCook B, Townsend DW. Whole-body FDG PET imaging in the abdomen: value of combined PET/CT. J Nucl Med. 2001;42(5 Suppl):35P.
5. Meltzer CC, Snyderman CH, Fukui MB, Bascom DA, Chander S, Johnson JT, Myers EN, Martinelli MA, Kinahan PE, Townsend DW. Combined FDG PET/CT imaging in head and neck cancer: impact on patient management. J Nucl Med. 2001;42(5 Suppl):36P.
6. Townsend DW, Beyer T, Blodgett TM. PET/CT scanners: a hardware approach to image fusion. Semin Nucl Med. 2003;33(3):193-204.
7. Cho ZH, Farukhi MR. Bismuth germanate as a potential scintillation detector in positron cameras. J Nucl Med. 1977;18(8):840-844.
8. Takagi K, Fukazawa T. Cerium-activated Gd2SiO5 single crystal scintillator. App Phys Lett. 1983;42(1):43-45.
9. Melcher CL, Schweitzer JS. Cerium-doped lutetium oxyorthosilicate: a fast, efficient new scintillator. IEEE Trans Nucl Sci. 1992;39(4):502-505.
10. Strother SC, Casey ME, Hoffman EJ. Measuring PET scanner sensitivity: relating countrates to image signal-to-noise ratios using noise equivalent counts. IEEE Trans Nucl Sci. 1990;37(2):783-788.
11. Kinahan PE, Townsend DW, Beyer T, Sashin D. Attenuation correction for a combined 3D PET/CT scanner. Med Phys. 1998;25(10):2046-2053.
12. Burger C, Goerres G, Schoenes S, Buck A, Lonn AH, von Schultess GK. PET attenuation coefficients from CT images: experimental evaluation of the transformation of CT into PET 511-keV attenuation coefficients. Eur J Nucl Med Mol Imaging. 2002;29(7):922-927.
13. Beyer T, Antoch G, Blodgett T, Freudenberg L, Akhurst T, Mueller S. Dual-modality PET/CT imaging: the effect of respiratory motion on combined image quality in clinical oncology. Eur J Nucl Med Mol Imaging. 2003;30(4): 588-596.
14. Osman MM, Cohade C, Nakamoto Y, Marshall LT, Leal JP, Wahl RL. J. Clinically significant inaccurate localization of lesions with PET/CT: frequency in 300 patients. J Nucl Med. 2003;44(2):240-243.
15. Yau YY., Coel M, Chan WS, Tam YM, Wong S. Application of IV contrast in PET-CT: does it really produce attenuation correction error? J Nucl Med. 2003;44(5 Suppl):272P.

16.   Carney JP, Beyer T, Brasse D, Yap JT, Townsend DW. Clinical PET/CT scanning using oral CT contrast agents. J Nucl Med. 2002;43(5 Suppl):57P.

17.   Cohade C, Osman M, Marshall L, Wahl RL. Metallic object artifacts on PET-CT: clinical and phantom studies. J Nucl Med. 2002;43(5 Suppl):308P.

18.   Halpern B, Dahlbom M, Vranjesevic D, Ratib O, Schiepers C, Silverman DH, Waldherr C, Quon A, Czernin J. LSO-PET/CT whole body imaging in 7 minutes: is it feasible? J Nucl Med. 2003;44(5 Suppl):380P-381P.

19.   Nutt RE, Nutt R. Combined PET and CT detector and method for using same. US Patent No. 6,449,331. 2002.

20.   Nahmias C, Nutt R, Hichwa RD, Czernin J, Melcher C, Schmand M, Andreaco M, Eriksson L, Casey M, Moyers C, Michel C, Bruckbauer T, Conti M, Bendriem B, Hamill J. PET tomograph designed for five minute routine whole body studies. J Nucl Med. 2002;43(5 Suppl):11P.

21.   Casey ME, Nutt R. A multicrystal, two dimensional BGO detector system for positron emission tomography. IEEE Trans Nucl Sci. 1986;33(1):460-463.

PET/CT Image Acquisition Protocols and Imaging Data Workflow

O. Ratib and C. Yap

Integrated PET and CT imaging is changing the traditional PET imaging procedures and workflow and raises new technical challenges with regards to image acquisition and data management. The ability to combine morphological and molecular information in a single diagnostic procedure will progressively lead to changes in clinical pathways and patient management. It is therefore important to understand and adapt the underlying technical infrastructure and software tools to support those changes.

Visualization and interactive review of volumetric data from tomographic imaging techniques require adequate display and navigation tools for interpreting and referring physicians. Such display programs should facilitate rapid and convenient navigation through large, three-dimensional data sets. Traditionally, the interpretation of computer tomography (CT) studies was performed from two-dimensional sectional images printed side-by-side on large sheets of films. With the shift toward soft-copy reading it became rapidly evident that tiling sectional images side-by-side is not the most convenient solution for image display. Therefore, this approach was rapidly replaced by interactive tools allowing users to "browse" through stacks of cross-sectional images.[1]

With the improvement of spatial resolution of CT scanners, and the rapid improvement of processing power of diagnostic workstations it is now possible to interactively navigate through orthogonal planes in coronal, sagittal and oblique orientation. Radiologists have rapidly adopted these tools for diagnostic interpretation of tomographic studies in clinical routine. At a time of increasing economic restrictions on healthcare these software tools enhance physician's productivity by allowing faster navigation through very large data sets with limited user interaction.

Multimodality PET/CT scanners provide combined metabolic data from PET images near per-fectly mapped to anatomical data from CT. This adds an additional degree of complexity to the task of image interpretation using multidimensional visualization software tools. Integrated PET/CT images need to be analyzed in 5 or 6 dimensions: the three dimensional tomographic data are now extended to a fourth dimension representing the continuum between anatomy and function obtained by fusion of PET and CT images. The navigation along this dimension is performed by interactively adjusting the degree of "blending" or color overlay transparency of the functional PET data over the anatomical CT images. A fifth dimension consists of the large dynamic range of CT data allowing the user to visualize different tissue structures such as bones, soft tissue and lungs by adjusting the image contrast and intensity window. A sixth, or temporal dimension is added if PET or CT data are acquired dynamically, as is the case for quantitative PET studies of myocardial blood flow or glucose metabolism, or in the case of CT for cardiac cine sequences. The users need to navigate through these 5 or 6 d to explore spatial or temporal abnormalities. The workflow of such multidimensional large data sets needs to be managed appropriately and efficiently. Ironically, as the PET/CT imaging technology matured, the time required for image and data acquisition has decreased while at the time spent for reviewing and interpreting these large data sets has increased substantially.

PET/CT Imaging Protocols

Clinical utilization of PET/CT imaging requires the optimization of image acquisition and reconstruction techniques but also of the workflow of image distribution, image interpretation and image communication. PET/CT imaging is most frequently used for oncological applications such as diagnosing, staging, and restaging of cancer. With the rapid development of ultrafast multi-detector CT scanners combined with faster PET scanners, other applications such as cardiac PET/CT will soon emerge in clinical practice. For the purpose of this atlas we will however limit our attention to the methods and techniques applied to oncological indications.

Patient Preparation

To optimize imaging results patients need to be well prepared and informed about the diagnostic procedure. Patients who understand the imaging procedures will be more compliant with the sometimes demanding protocols. Planning should begin even before the patient arrives in the imaging suite. In addition to the clinical data obtained from the referring physician, information regarding patient height and weight (both factors can affect scanning time) and concomitant relevant diseases (e.g. diabetes mellitus) should be obtained.

Patients should refrain from solid food intake for about 6 hours. Patients may drink unsweetened beverages in the morning of the scan. Patients with afternoon appointments may have a light breakfast.

At the time of the study, important clinical data can generally be obtained from a short patient interview in particular regarding the recent medical history. Information regarding time and nature of previous treatments should be recorded. Patient history should also focus on indwelling catheters, metallic implants, and pacemakers.

Because the CT portion might include intravenous contrast a history of allergic reactions need to be obtained. In presence of or risk for renal dysfunction should be determined.

Serum glucose levels should be measured at the time of the study. Elevated serum glucose levels might explain poor image quality or might result in intravenous insulin application. The intravenous injection of [18]FDG should take place with the patient in the supine position. FDG is injected approximately 60 minutes prior to the study. Patients should remain in a relaxed position to minimize glucose metabolic activity in striated muscle. Patients should refrain from speaking to minimize pharyngeal muscle and vocal cord activity. We do not routinely induce muscle relaxation through the administration of benzodiazepines.

Voiding prior to the scan minimizes radioactivity accumulation in the urinary bladder. Patients are placed in the scanner in the "arms-up" position. If they are unable to keep their arms up for the 15-30

minutes of scanning patients can also be scanned with their arms down. In this case, special attention should be given to CT induced beam hardening effects on the reconstructed PET images.

To prevent misalignments between PET and CT images patients should be advised to minimize motion during the scan.

Breathing instructions are also important. For studies performed with free breathing patients should maintain a shallow breathing pattern and should avoid deep breathing and hyperventilation. Breath-holding might be important for some studies and should be practiced prior to imaging. The process of breath-holding in mid expiration or full inspiration needs to be demonstrated. Breathing training should always include several practice runs prior to the scan to ascertain patient compliance. When contrast CT is planned as part of the study, the patient must be informed of expected and unexpected side effects associated with intravenous contrast administration.

Image Acquisition

PET/CT whole body image acquisitions are shorter than PET image acquisitions. This is because PET/CT utilizes whole body CT data for attenuation correction thereby obviating the need for the time consuming conventional attenuation correction using germanium rod sources. A further breakthrough in PET/CT imaging resulted from the LSO-PET detector technology, which further shortens PET image acquisition times. These technological advances result in higher patient throughput and thus, in more economic utilization of the equipment.

Two distinct CT imaging protocols can be applied to PET/CT studies:

1) Low resolution and low dose CT images can be acquired for anatomical localization of metabolic abnormalities and for attenuation correction.

2) High resolution, breath-hold and contrast enhancement protocols are required for achieving the standard of care for oncology CT examinations.

There is however some controversy regarding the need for iodinated contrast material for the CT images since the most frequently used PET imaging probe, FDG, characterizes tissue with a much higher specificity than intravenous contrast. It is however of general consensus that iodinated contrast studies and breath-hold acquisition protocols for thoracic and

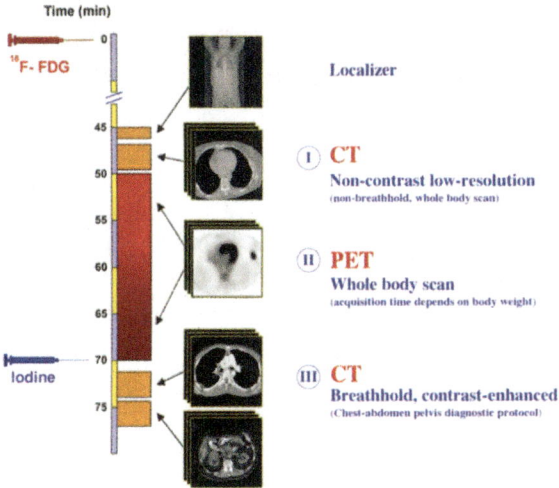

Figure 1. Timeline of a PET/CT procedure indicating the different image acquisition steps following an initial injection of FDG tracer, with an initial CT scan without contrast followed by the PET image acquisition that can vary depending on patient size, and followed by a complementary contrast CT study.

upper abdominal CT studies are necessary to maximize the diagnostic accuracy of CT. We have therefore elected to add a "diagnostic" CT acquisition after every standard PET/CT study when clinically indicated. Unlike the generic CT acquisition that is standard for all oncology PET/CT examinations, the diagnostic CT protocols vary depending upon the clinical indication and the anatomical region being investigated. Specific protocols are outlined below. The general timeline of CT and PET acquisition is shown in Figure 1.

Imaging Protocols

The standard PET/CT protocol includes a low-dose spiral CT acquisition from the base of the skull to mid thigh followed by a whole body PET study of the same region. The protocols presented here were developed for a commercially available "REVEAL" PET/CT scanner manufactured by CPS Innovations (Knoxville, TN). The device consists of a dual detector spiral CT scanner (Siemens Emotion Duo) and an LSO full ring PET scanner (ECAT ACCEL) combined into a single gantry.

The LSO-PET scanner provides higher count rate capability than conventional PET scanners and allows acquisitions as short as one minute per bed position without compromising image quality.[2]

A scout scan is performed first to determine the imaging field. This is followed by a whole body CT acquisition that can be accomplished in one minute with a dual slice CT system and within a few seconds using the new 16-slice CT devices.

Each subsequent PET acquisition covers 16.2 cm per bed position with an overlap of about 3.7 cm resulting in 6 to 7 bed positions for an average size patient to cover the whole body area from the base of the skull to mid thigh (Figure 2).

The PET images are acquired approximately 60 minutes after injection of 0.21mCi/Kg of FDG.

The acquisition time per bed position can be tailored to patient weight varying from 1 minute per bed position for patients under 130 Lbs (~60 kg) to 4 minutes per bed position for patient over 220 Lbs (~91 kg). Given the short acquisition time of both PET and CT data, patients are in general capable of maintaining the "arms up" position throughout the study.

The CT images are acquired with patients breathing in a gentle shallow fashion. This results in a good co-registration of CT and the non-breath-hold PET images. However respiratory motion frequently results in "mushroom" artifacts above the diaphragm due to different position of the diaphragm during the spiral CT acquisition. Because CT images are used for attenuation correction of PET images, the artifacts are also visible on the attenuation-corrected PET images.[3-5] These artifacts can be eliminated in cooperative patients that can be instructed to hold their breath at mid expiration position during acquisition of CT images.

Diagnostic contrast CT studies can be acquired immediately following the first combined PET/CT acquisition. Depending on the body region and underlying disease being investigated different protocols can be applied. The most common oncology protocol used in whole body CT evaluations of cancer patients is a combined thorax-abdomen-pelvis imaging sequence acquired after contrast injection (see Figure 2). The sequence starts with a high-resolution acquisition of chest images during full inspiration followed by breath-hold 20 seconds after the contrast injection. Subsequently, a first acquisition of the abdomen during the arterial phase and a second acquisition over the same region during the venous phase are acquired.

Finally, images over the pelvis are acquired 3 to 4 minutes after injection. With careful adjustment

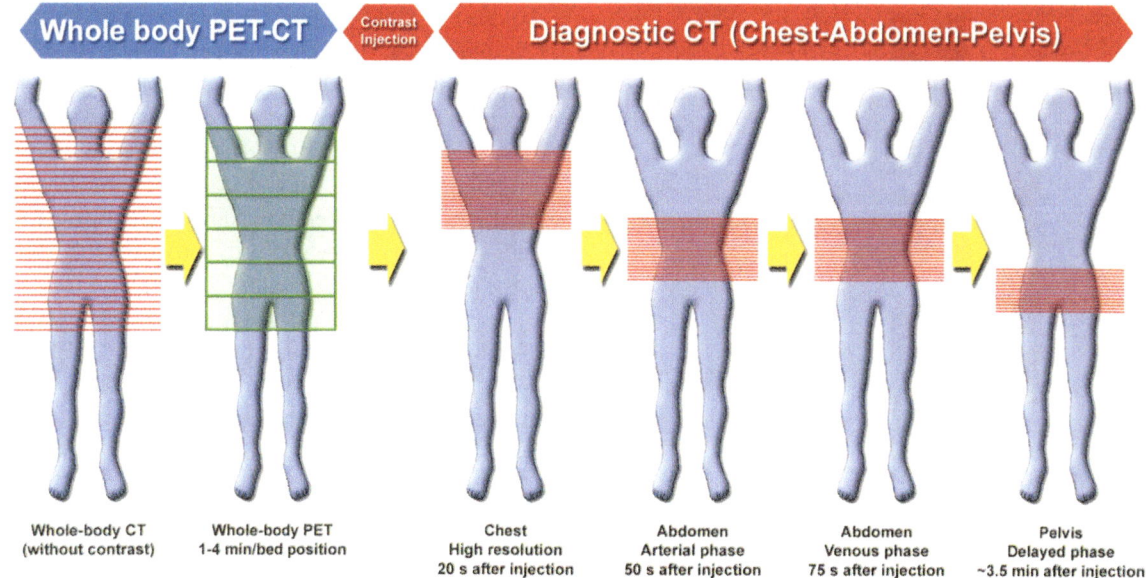

Figure 2. Diagram of coverage and position of image acquisition for the combined PET/CT study, followed by an optional chest-abdomen-pelvis diagnostic CT obtained after intravenous contrast injection.

of image acquisition parameters it is possible to acquire CT images of chest, abdomen and pelvis after a single injection of contrast material.

Another frequently requested protocol is a dedicated head-and-neck examination. For optimal evaluation of the neck area and to avoid beam-hardening artifacts, the images must be acquired with the patient in the "arms down" position. Therefore a second set of PET images must be acquired, since the whole body images are acquired in the "arms up" position. The details of the head and neck imaging protocol are described in Figure 3. The CT images are acquired 30 to 40 seconds after intravenous injection of 75 ml of contrast. When necessary, additional delayed phase CT images of the brain can be obtained after adequate time (usually around 5 minutes) is allowed for contrast material to cross the blood-brain barrier and reach the brain structures. A third set of matching PET images of the brain is then also acquired.

Image Reconstruction and Data Management

An important component of PET/CT imaging protocols is image reconstruction from the raw data acquired by the scanners. PET images can be reconstructed using different filters resulting in different image resolutions. Higher cut-off frequency filters result in sharper and crisper, yet more noisy images.

Lower frequency filters result in smoother images with less anatomical detail.

We have adopted different PET reconstruction parameters for images of the body and for images of the brain: whole body scans are reconstructed in 128 x 128 image matrix using iterative reconstruction methods (Ordered Subsets Estimation-Maximization, OSEM 2 Iterations 8 Subsets) with a 6-mm Gaussian post-reconstruction filter. The brain images are usual-

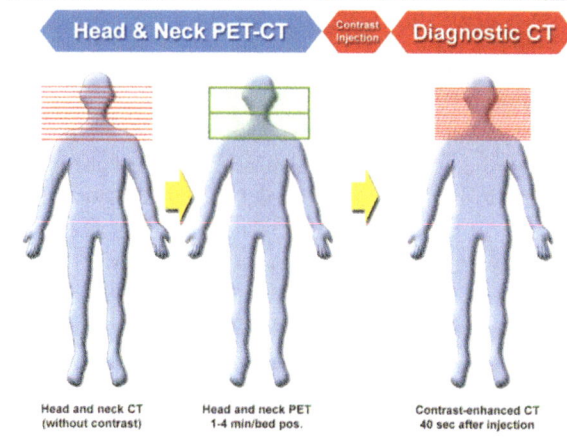

Figure 3. Diagram of complementary PET/CT and contrast-enhanced CT study of the head and neck that are acquired following the standard PET/CT acquisition when clinically indicated.

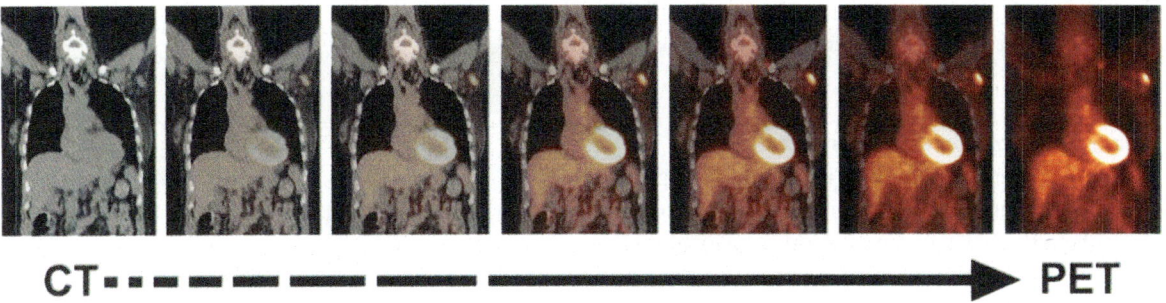

Figure 4. Example of fused PET/CT images showing different degree of image "blending" that allows the users to interactively navigate from the CT image to the PET image in continuous scale of what is being considered as a "fifth" dimension of the acquired data.

ly reconstructed using a higher resolution of 256 x 256 matrix using a filtered back projection technique and a 2-mm Gaussian post-reconstruction filter. The CT images can also be reconstructed with different parameters providing images of different resolution. The most important parameter is the reconstructed slice thickness. While thinner slices are particularly desirable for better quality of multi-planar reconstruction of coronal, sagittal and oblique planes, the thin slice reconstruction can result in an overwhelming number of images. Therefore a second set of images with thicker slices for easier and more convenient diagnostic interpretation is frequently generated. However, with the emergence of novel visualization tools that allow adjustment of slice thickness and image orientation on diagnostic workstations in real time, the need for different image reconstruction protocols with different slice thickness no longer exists.

PET images need to be reconstructed with and without attenuation correction. While attenuation correction is desirable to properly rescale regional tracer activity for differences in tissue attenuation, there are many situations in which CT images used for attenuation correction can introduce artifacts. This can result in "false" findings of increased or decreased tracer uptake. The most common sources of artifacts from CT-based attenuation correction are: image misregistration due to patient or respiratory motion, beam hardening effects and attenuation artifacts form high density objects such as metal implants and implanted devices. In those cases, the availability of non-attenuation corrected PET images is essential to properly differentiate between true pathological and "false" tracer uptake patterns.[6,7]

Image Storage and Communication

With the evolution towards multi-detector systems large data sets are generated. This represents a serious challenge for image storage and communication. Both PET and CT generate a set of "raw" data that can subsequently be reconstructed with different reconstruction parameters as described above. The reconstructed PET data are usually cross-sectional images of a given thickness and cover the whole segment being surveyed. Depending on the selected image resolution and slice thickness the resulting image set can vary in size. An average set of cross-sectional images of 5mm thickness for a whole body acquisition can vary from 7 Mbytes to 10 Mbytes depending on the patient size and the corresponding number of planes. These reconstructed images represent a much smaller volume of data than the corresponding raw data that can easily vary from 100 Mbytes to 160 Mbytes. Most institutions elect to store only the reconstructed images but not the raw data to avoid unnecessary overhead expenses.

The same principle applies to CT images particularly when derived from ultra-fast multi-detector CT scanners. These devices acquire very large sets of high resolution thin slice image data that can be reconstructed to different spatial resolutions. Sets of thin slices of approximately 1mm in thickness require over 300 images to cover the thorax and whole body images are composed of close to 1000 images of considerable size. For instance, whole body data sets that can vary in size from 150 to 500 Mbytes. High resolution scans using very thin slices are desirable to obtain isotropic three-dimensional data sets that can be re-sliced in any spatial direction with similar resolution. These large data sets represent a significant problem for image communication between different devices in a digital environment and incur significant costs associated with long-term data storage and archiving.

Image Visualization and Interpretation

Another challenging aspect of integrated PET/CT imaging is related to seamless navigation through and visualization of multi-dimensional imaging data. The inability to rapidly and efficiently navigate through these data sets remains a serious handicap for most interpreting physicians who need to adapt to time-consuming and awkward human-machine interactions.[8,9] None of the existing software package and image display program is ideally suited to complete this task. Most PET/CT workstations provide image fusion capability that allows color coded PET images to be mapped to CT images displayed in shades of gray.[8,10,11] Commercially available workstations provide tools for quantifying tissue density (Hounsfield units) and determining standardized uptake values of FDG (SUV). Size measurements can be performed routinely and CT images can be windowed to display different tissues (Figure 4).

Clinical Workflow

When PET/CT devices were deployed in clinical routine, two major technical challenges were identified: 1- the difficulty of optimizing new acquisition protocols and 2- the complex task of managing image data. These challenges are even more prominent for large multidisciplinary academic centers where the diagnostic procedures and interpretation tasks are often performed by highly specialized experts that often focus on specific imaging procedures applied to specific body regions. In such environment the PET/CT imaging procedures require major coordination efforts and consensus agreements between nuclear medicine specialists, oncology departments, thoracic, GI and GU, head and neck and neuro-radiologists. The logistics of maintaining an effective collaboration between all involved experts can be quite complex. Combined imaging protocols must be defined and implemented that are compliant with the requirements of each specialized area. Acquisition protocols that are applicable to PET/CT imaging can differ from the imaging protocols used on separate PET and CT scanners. Combining different CT acquisition procedures in a single patient examination often requires some compromise to arrive at feasible and mutually accepted protocols.

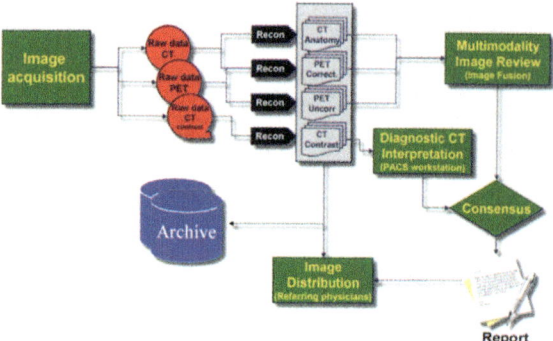

Figure 5. Workflow diagram showing the data flow from image acquisition, reconstruction in different modalities, interpretation by different interpreting physicians and generation of consensus report(s) that can be distributed to the referring physicians together with the images.

As another problem, nuclear medicine physicians interpret PET images while one or several sub-specialized radiologists might interpret the CT images. Thus, PET/CT studies need to be provided to different interpreting physicians who must review the different aspects of the study to generate a general consensus. Hence, the logistics of routing images to different interpreters and establishing an infrastructure allowing for timely image interpretation can be a very complex task.

At our institution PET/CT images are interpreted in the nuclear medicine department while radiologists read the diagnostic CT images. This can require multiple readers for interpreting a single whole body scan. Images are routed electronically to the different readers, but only a limited number of workstations is available for displaying integrated PET/CT images. Therefore, radiologists initially interpret the CT data, and the comprehensive study evaluation involving radiologists and nuclear medicine specialists takes place during a daily reading session around a specialized workstation. Thus, PET/CT image interpretation requires a significant amount of time and effort.

In smaller imaging centers and private practice settings the necessity of image interpretation by multiple interpreting physicians is more seldom and in most cases the CT study and the PET images are interpreted by the same individual, minimizing the need for complex image distribution and workflow.

Multi-Modality Image Navigation Tools

The navigation between the two modalities as well as the navigation through the volume of data is usually achieved through interactive manipulation of cursors and slide bars on a graphic user interface of the image display software. Using commercially available software, the time required for reviewing PET/CT studies can range from 10 minutes for a normal study to 30 minutes or more for a complex study with multiple lesions and abnormalities. This exceeds by far the average time that is required for a radiologist to review standard oncology CT studies. The best image display programs permit displaying multiple aspects of the study simultaneously. This includes the three orthogonal planes of the CT images, the reoriented PET images and the set of blended PET and CT images. In many instances an additional set of non-corrected and projection PET images also needs to be reviewed. The disadvantage of this approach is that individual images tend to become relatively small on the screen requiring the user to manually enlarge them for better visualization of details. Examples of multimodality image display programs are shown in Figures 6 and 7.

Another requirement for workstations is their ability to handle the large data sets in real time. For real time data navigation the data sets must be loaded in the computer memory. Some software programs achieve adequate real time performance by compromising the resolution of CT images either by reducing the spatial resolution from 512 x 512 to 256 x 256 pixels/slice). Alternatively, the dynamic range of the CT data can be reduced from 16 bits of gray shades per pixel to 8 bits (256 gray levels) per pixel. This however might render the quality of the CT images non-diagnostic. Display programs that can maintain the native high resolution of the CT data and scale the PET data to the CT resolution require computers with high processing power and large memory capacity. Even with high performance computers, the loading of a complete whole body PET/CT study can take up to several minutes.

Simple Techniques for Image Communication

Imaging findings need to be conveyed to referring physicians and other caregivers that rely on this information for patient management. Frequently, referring physicians receive a written report or, in some more sophisticated places, a written report including selected "snapshots" of pertinent findings. Some efforts are being deployed to find more convenient ways to provide more comprehensive image sets to caregivers. Such approaches would then allow the referring physicians to navigate through image data similar to the way interpreting physicians do. This is usually achievable by generating standard

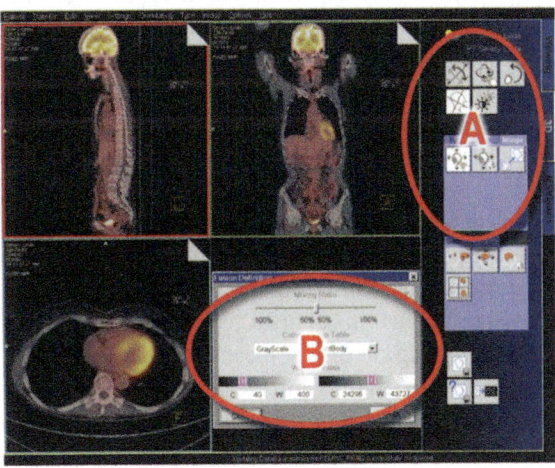

Figure 6. Example of a viewer-user interface that allows interactive navigation in three different orthogonal plane (using control panel located in A) while also adjusting the degree of color overlap of PET images over CT images (using adjustable slide bars in control panel B).

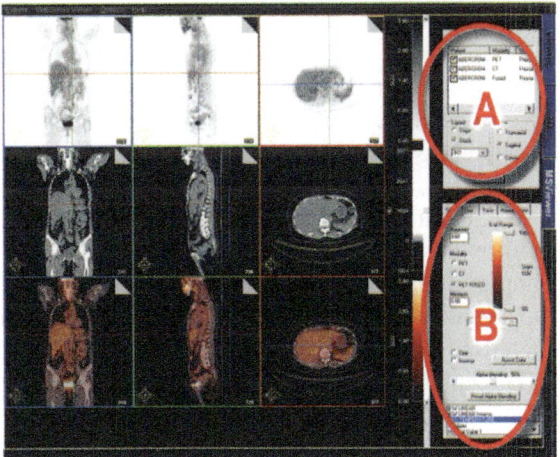

Figure 7. Example of a different layout of another multimodality viewing program that allows simultaneous display of the 3 orthogonal views of PET images (top), the corresponding CT images (middle) as well as the corresponding fused images (bottom). Images to be displayed are selected from a list located in (A) and the adjustment of image contrast window and level as well as PET/CT blending is obtained through adjustable scrollbars (B).

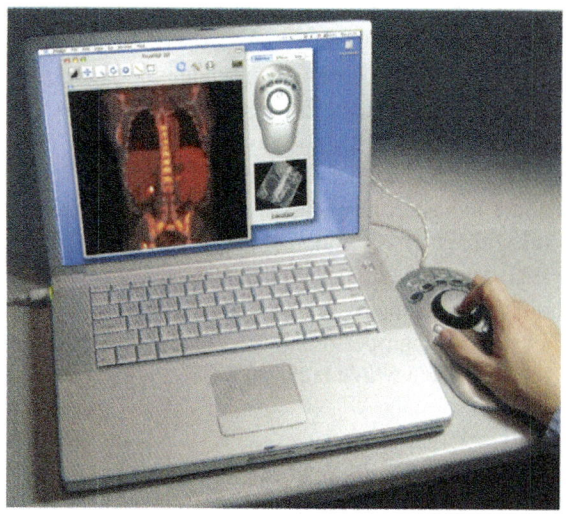

Figure 8. Prototype of a new multidimensional image navigation software (OsiriX) using a special multi-function jog-wheel allowing rapid interactive navigation through different dimensions of the image data.

video files such as AVI or QuickTime dynamic files that can be displayed on standard personal computers. However, these images are always selected by the interpreting provider and are thus an incomplete representation of the entire data set.

Future Perspectives

Combined PET/CT provide near perfectly co-registered functional and anatomical images in a single session. They represent the most important and comprehensive new imaging tool in oncology. On the other hand, continuing development of display software and image communication tools is required to utilize this technology to its highest potential for improved patient management.[12-20] These tools need to be tailored to the needs of patients, interpreting and referring physicians.

The computer infrastructure and software programs available for management and display of multimodality studies are still in their infancy. Currently available systems are simple evolutions from traditional multi-dimensional and nuclear medicine display programs and suffer from considerable limitations in performance and functional design. A new generation of diagnostic workstations might include specifically designed navigation devices similar to the ones used by the video-game industry to allow the user to navigate interactively through five or six dimension of

image data (Figure 8). Computer-assisted algorithms could guide users through the image data by automatically detecting areas of abnormal or suspicious metabolic activity or unusual morphological characteristics. There is a need for improving interfaces and navigation tools for users to efficiently navigate through image data. To become more widely adopted in clinical practice, the software programs will be more intuitive and simpler to use by physicians that are not necessarily computer experts.[21,22]

Imaging procedures have become a central component of clinical practice and clinical decision-making. The comprehensive imaging results of PET/CT studies would best be conveyed to referring physicians if images could be communicated in a seamless fashion. This approach would empower referring physician to interactively view the full set of registered data in a way similar to the image navigation used for diagnostic interpretation. This is particularly relevant in oncology where a community of physicians involved in patient management needs to visually assess subtle differences in localization, size, structure and topological distribution of pathological lesions in every region of the body. Thus, one message to the PET/CT manufacturers is to draw their attention to the fact that improving image communication and navigation tools will further enhance the adoption of PET/CT imaging in clinical routine.

Optimal utilization of PET/CT requires a multi-disciplinary approach that includes close interaction and collaboration between different disciplines and subspecialists. The current information management infrastructure and computer software lack the necessary tools to allow multiple users in different locations to jointly interpret the image data.

An important step for improvement of patient management is the collegial discussion between interpreting physicians and referring physicians, surgeons and oncologists. In a digital environment, such discussions occur in clinical conferences or tumor boards relying on digital means for presenting diagnostic images. Here again, the necessity for a convenient computer system that can be used to navigate through the multimodality images is critical.

The clinical success of PET/CT imaging will continue if technological advances include improvements in imaging equipment as well as tools for image display, communication and navigation.

The added value of providing better visualization of pathological processes through combined functional and anatomical information will result in better patient management.

References

1. Arenson RL, Chakraborty DP, Seshadri SB, Kundel HL. The digital imaging workstation. 1990. J Digit Imaging. 2003;16(1):142-162.
2. Halpern B, Dahlbom M, Vranjesevic D, Ratib O, Schiepers C, Silverman DH, Waldherr C, Quon A, Czernin J. LSO-PET/CT whole body imaging in 7 minutes: is it feasible? J Nucl Med. 2003;44(5 Suppl):380P-381P.
3. Goerres GW, Burger C, Kamel E, Seifert B, Kaim AH, Buck A, Buehler TC, von Schulthess GK. Respiration-induced attenuation artifact at PET/CT: technical considerations. Radiology. 2003;226(3):906-910.
4. Goerres GW, Burger C, Schwitter MR, Heidelberg TN, Seifert B, von Schulthess GK. PET/CT of the abdomen: optimizing the patient breathing pattern. Eur Radiol. 2003;13(4):734-739.
5. Beyer T, Antoch G, Blodgett T, Freudenberg LF, Akhurst T, Mueller S. Dual-modality PET/CT imaging: the effect of respiratory motion on combined image quality in clinical oncology. Eur J Nucl Med Mol Imaging. 2003;30(4):588-596.
6. Kamel EM, Burger C, Buck A, von Schulthess GK, Goerres GW. Impact of metallic dental implants on CT-based attenuation correction in a combined PET/CT scanner. Eur Radiol. 2003;13(4):724-728.
7. Goerres GW, Ziegler SI, Burger C, Berthold T, von Schulthess GK, Buck A. Artifacts at PET and PET/CT caused by metallic hip prosthetic material. Radiology. 2003;226(2):577-584.
8. Robb RA. 3-D visualization in biomedical applications. Annu Rev Biomed Eng. 1999;1:377-399.
9. Bidaut LM, Pascual-Marqui R, Delavelle J, Naimi A, Seeck M, Michel C, Slosman D, Ratib O, Ruefenacht D, Landis T, de Tribolet N, Scherrer JR, Terrier F. Three- to five-dimensional biomedical multisensor imaging for the assessment of neurological (dys) function. J Digit Imaging. 1996;9(4):185-198.
10. Cook GJ, Ott RJ. Dual-modality imaging. Eur Radiol. 2001;11(10):1857-1858.
11. Hanson DP, Robb RA, Aharon S, Augustine KE, Cameron BM, Camp JJ, Karwoski RA, Larson AG, Stacy MC, Workman EL. New software toolkits for comprehensive visualization and analysis of three-dimensional multimodal biomedical images. J Digit Imaging. 1997;10(3 Suppl 1):229-230.
12. Townsend DW, Beyer T, Blodgett TM. PET/CT scanners: a hardware approach to image fusion. Semin Nucl Med. 2003;33(3):193-204.
13. Bar-Shalom R, Yefremov N, Guralnik L, Gaitini D, Frenkel A, Kuten A, Altman H, Keidar Z, Israel O. Clinical performance of PET/CT in evaluation of cancer: additional value for diagnostic imaging and patient management. J Nucl Med. 2003;44(8):1200-1209.
14. Townsend DW, Beyer T. A combined PET/CT scanner: the path to true image fusion. Br J Radiol. 2002;75(Special Issue):S24-S30.
15. Hutton BF, Braun M, Thurfjell L, Lau DY. Image registration: an essential tool for nuclear medicine. Eur J Nucl Med Mol Imaging. 2002;29(4):559-577.
16. Hasegawa BH, Wong KH, Iwata K, Barber WC, Hwang AB, Sakdinawat AE, Ramaswamy M, Price DC, Hawkins RA. Dual-modality imaging of cancer with SPECT/CT. Technol Cancer Res Treat. 2002;1(6):449-458.
17. Ell PJ, von Schulthess GK. PET/CT: a new road map. Eur J Nucl Med Mol Imaging. 2002;29(6):719-720.
18. Beyer T, Townsend DW, Blodgett TM. Dual-modality PET/CT tomography for clinical oncology. Q J Nucl Med. 2002;46(1):24-34.
19. Kluetz PG, Meltzer CC, Villemagne VL, Kinahan PE, Chander S, Martinelli MA, Townsend DW. Combined PET/CT imaging in oncology. Impact on patient management. Clin Positron Imaging. 2000;3(6):223-230.
20. Wagner HN, Jr. Molecular medicine: from science to service. J Nucl Med. 1991;32(8):11N-23N.
21. Zhang J, Sun J, Stahl JN. PACS and web-based image distribution and display. Comput Med Imaging Graph. 2003;27(2-3):197-206.
22. Slomka PJ, Elliott E, Driedger AA. Java-based remote viewing and processing of nuclear medicine images: toward "the imaging department without walls". J Nucl Med. 2000;41(1):111-118.

Acquisition Schemes for Combined ^{18}F-FDG-PET/CT Imaging: An European Experience

Thomas Beyer, Gerald Antoch, Hilmar Kühl, and Stefan P Müller

Combined PET/CT imaging

For the past decade both, Computed Tomography (CT) and Positron Emission Tomography (PET) have been used widely, albeit frequently independently, in the management of cancer patients. To complement molecular and anatomical information such as obtained by PET and CT, respectively and thus facilitate a more accurate diagnosis[1] both, retrospective software-based approaches and, later, hardware-based approaches to combined dual-modality imaging have been introduced. Fully or semi-automated software algorithms allow registering almost any complementary images of the thorax, for example, in about a minute,[2] but often work only on axially limited image sets rather than whole-body studies. Hardware-based approaches to *anato-metabolic imaging*[1] in humans exist for combined PET/CT since 1998[3] but not yet for PET/MRT (Magnetic Resonance Tomography) imaging.[4]

Combined PET/CT tomographs allow acquiring molecular and anatomical information in a single examination without moving the patient in between,[3] thus minimizing any intrinsic spatial misalignment. The almost simultaneous acquisition of such complementary information has been shown to lead to additional diagnostic information.[5] Total examination times with PET/CT are much reduced in comparison to standard PET imaging times since the available CT transmission information is used for attenuation correction of the complementary PET emission data,[6] thus rendering lengthy standard transmission scans obsolete in PET/CT. This results in much reduced total examination times and in potentially reduced costs when 68Ge-based rod sources are not installed in the combined tomograph.[7] Taking together the benefits of intrinsically aligned PET and CT data, shorter scan times and logistical advantages in patient management with PET/CT, combined PET/CT imaging has become a state-of-the-art tool for patient management in clinical oncology.[8]

Standard PET/CT imaging protocol for oncology

FDG-PET/CT imaging

First clinical experience from applying PET/CT in oncology was based mainly on extending standard PET imaging using 2-[^{18}F]Fluoro-2-deoxy-D-glucose (FDG) by supplementing the limited anatomical background information of the PET with the intrinsically associated anatomy as imaged by the CT.[5,9,10] Initially combined imaging of the heart was not a primary concern of PET/CT imaging as illustrated by the incorporation of only mid-range CT components in the first generations of combined tomographs.[11] More recent PET/CT designs, however, also employ CT systems with up to 16 detector rows[12,13] and thus offer the potential of defining and evaluating acquisition protocol standards for imaging of the heart.

Protocol Step	PET/CT Advantage	Consequences
Patient Positioning	Patient is not moved between scans	Less stress on patients, and logistical benefit to the personnel
		Higher intrinsic accuracy of spatial registration of CT and PET
Topogram	Accurate definition of imaging range	Co-axial imaging range can be adapted to diagnostic needs, resulting in minimum time for sufficient diagnosis and for patient to remain still on bed
	CT and PET imaging range are matched	Ensure complementary information and avoid over-/underexposure of patient
Transmission Scan	CT replaces standard transmission scan	Reduced total scan time (by 30%)
		Reduced costs by avoiding the need for standard (decaying) TX sources and replacements thereof
	CT-based attenuation correction	Post-injection TX becomes standard, limited noise propagation into attenuation-corrected emission images

Table 1. Major advantages of combined PET/CT over PET protocols with or without an additional CT examination

FDG-PET/CT acquisition protocol design

For oncology purposes a standard PET/CT acquisition protocol, in essence, is a modern-day PET oncology imaging protocol, which consists of three steps: (1) Patient preparation and positioning, (2) Transmission scan, and (3) Emission scan. Additional CT scans, such as, e.g. a 3-phase liver CT or a high-resolution lung scan could be requested by the reviewing physician, but generally these CT scans are not used for attenuation correction. TABLE 1 summarizes the advantages of PET/CT imaging protocols in comparison to PET examinations with or without additional CT.

FDG-PET/CT acquisition procedure

An accurate localization scan is now available that precedes the transmission and emission acquisition (FIGURE 1). This localization scan is referred to as either a topogram or scout scan, and is similar to a conventional X-ray at a given projection angle. The topogram is acquired after the patient is positioned on the patient handling system of the combined PET/CT with the X-ray tube/detector-assembly locked typically in either frontal or lateral position (or any other position in between) and the patient pallet moving continuously into the gantry. In PET/CT imaging the topogram is used to define the axial examination range of the combined study. Thereby the axial extent of the complementary CT and PET acquisition are matched to ensure fully quantitative attenuation and scatter correction of the emission data, and to avoid any over- or under-scanning of the patient in case of limited or extensive disease. The patient is subsequently moved to the start position of the CT scan, which typically is acquired in spiral mode.[14] After the completion of the CT scan the patient is advanced to the field-of-view of the PET, to the rear of the combined gantry, where emission scanning commences in the caudo-cranial direction starting at the thighs to limit artefacts from the FDG excretion into the urinary system. Depending on the axial co-scan range and the emission time allotted for an individual bed position the combined scanning is completed in 30 min or less.[15] Since the CT images are reconstructed simultaneously and attenuation maps are calculated as soon as the CT images become available, the total post-acquisition data processing and image reconstruction is limited to the processing of the last bed position.

Classification of current PET/CT imaging protocols for clinical oncology

The acquisition parameters of the standard imaging protocol can be adjusted to account for specific imaging needs and, in particular, for clinical requirements on the CT image quality. Since the

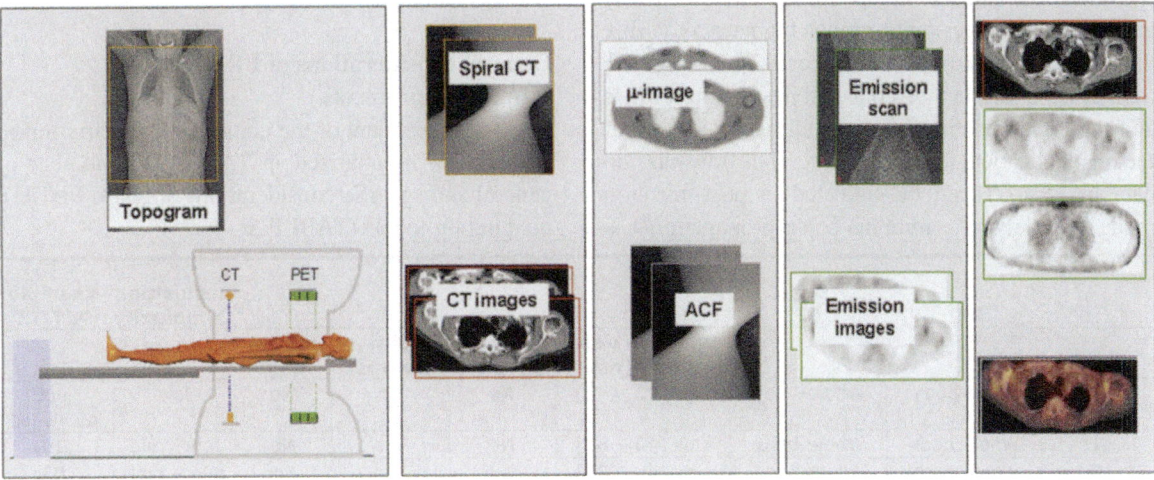

Figure 1. Standard FDG-PET/CT imaging protocol (from left to right). The patient is positioned on a common patient handling system in front of the combined gantry (A). First, a topogram is used to define the co-axial imaging range (A). The spiral CT scan (B) precedes the emission scan (D). The CT images are reconstructed on-line and used for the purpose of automatic attenuation correction of the acquired emission data (C). CT, PET with and without attenuation correction, and fused PET/CT images can be used for the clinical image review (E).

majority of imaging parameters in PET/CT relate to the set-up of the complementary CT acquisition protocol it appears reasonable to classify clinical PET/CT protocols and imaging scenarios with respect to the operation of the CT.

Today, with currently available 2nd and 3rd generation PET/CT systems five general imaging scenarios can be distinguished (TABLE 2). The least demanding facilitates the PET/CT as a fast PET using a low-dose CT scan for attenuation correction (I). In an alternative scenario the CT is operated at similar low-dose settings, but oral contrast agents are given to utilize the CT for additional anatomical labeling (II). In contrast, high-demand scenarios aim at high-quality scans in place of separate dedicated, and often region-specific, CT and PET exams (IV, V). Obviously, the complexity of these scenarios increases with the demands on the CT (e.g. V). From a brief survey of the available clinical PET/CT literature (e.g. references 10,16-21) it appears that class-II protocols are most frequently used, while class-IV and -V are the least frequently adopted protocols.

CT-based attenuation correction

Independent of the imaging scenario-of-choice all PET/CT protocols have in common that, based on the available CT transmission information, PET emission scans are corrected routinely for attenuation. X-ray transmission sources yield a much higher photon flux than standard transmission sources.[22] Therefore, CT transmission data can be collected in very short times and the contamination from the emission activity of the injected patient is insignificant. Thus transmission data in PET/CT can be collected in post-injection mode routinely.[3] In addition noise propagation[23] is limited due to the essentially noiseless CT transmission data.

However, X-ray photons are polychromatic, and therefore energy-scaling approaches are required to transform the CT transmission information into attenuation coefficients at emission energies different from those of the CT energy spectrum (e.g. 511 keV). The transformation of the CT transmission information to attenuation coefficients and, subsequently, to attenuation maps is based on work by LaCroix et al.[24] First the CT images are transformed into attenuation images at some estimated effective CT energy. Then, the attenuation image at the relevant emission energy is multiplied by the ratio of attenuation coefficients of water at that effective CT energy (40 – 70 keV) and the emission energy, respectively. While this simple scaling approach works well for soft tissues serious overestimation of the attenuation coefficients of cortical bone is observed.[24] To account for the larger energy differences between CT and PET the original scaling approach was modified.[6] Instead of a linear scaling with a single scale factor, a bi-linear scaling was developed[6, 25] to account for the non-linear energy dependencies of the Photoelectric and Compton effect, which dominate at lower (i.e. CT) and higher (i.e. PET) energies, respectively. Today all CT-based attenuation correction algorithms in commercial PET/CT systems are based exclusively on bi-linear scaling methods.[26, 27]

General considerations of FDG-PET/CT acquisition protocols

Independent of the choice of a specific image protocol as summarized in TABLE 2 a number of general and specific considerations apply to PET/CT imaging protocols (TABLE 3).[28]

	PET	CT	Effective dose per row [mAs]	IV contrast	Oral contrast	Breath hold	Acquisition Complexity	Example PET/CT
I	Whole-body[1]	Whole-body	Low [15 – 40]	No	No	No	low	not published
II	Whole-body	Whole-body	Low [40 – 80]	No	Yes	No	low - mid	(16)
III	Whole-body	Whole Body + Thorax	Low [40 – 80] Standard [~120]	No Yes	Yes	For Thorax CT	mid – high	(93)
IV	Whole-body	Whole-body	Standard [~130]	Yes	Yes	Limited	mid to high	(94)
V	Torso/Abdomen + Head/Neck	Torso/Abdomen + Head/Neck	Standard [~130] Standard [~200]	Yes Yes	Yes	Limited	high	(28)

[1] Whole-body refers to an imaging range of the upper neck to the upper thighs. It can be expanded to cover the entire body patient, bed travel permitting.

Table 2. Selected PET/CT imaging scenarios in clinical oncology.

Acquisition Step	General	Specific
Patient Preparation	Follow the guidelines for a standard PET exam with the same radioisotope, i.e. fasting patient, injected dose, quiet resting during uptake, uptake period, voiding before scan, etc. Educate patient on breath hold commands if required.	Question patient about previous allergic reactions towards contrast media and about oral anti-diabetic medications. Establish adequate renal function before using IV contrast. Patient must drink oral contrast agent during the uptake phase if the abdomen is to be included in the imaging field-of-view.
Patient Positioning	Use positioning aids for comfortable positioning. Remove jewelry and take off clothes with zippers. Raise and keep arms above the head.	
Topogram	Check for remaining high-density objects and remove (e.g. dental prostheses). Acquire CT in normal expiration if breath hold technique is desired.	
CT Scan	Follow breath hold protocol.	Follow contrast protocol.
PET Scan	Keep scan time reasonably short.	
Data Processing	Reconstruct PET without attenuation correction.	Additional CT reconstructions (e.g. lung, or bone window) may be required.
Image Review	Review uncorrected PET in case of artifacts.	Define strategies for joint report.

Table 3. General and specific imaging protocol considerations for each acquisition step of combined PET/CT. The general aspects should be followed irrespective of the clinical scenario (TABLE 2), while specific considerations apply to the more complex acquisition procedures only.

Patient preparation and positioning

For all oncology protocols patient preparation is similar to that for a standard PET exam as described in detail in.[29] In addition, patients are asked about allergies towards iodine-based CT contrast agents, should these be administered during the course of a PET/CT study. In patients with known mild reactions, the patient is pre-medicated while in case of known severe allergic reactions no IV contrast is given. Typically the serum creatinine value is obtained to assess adequate renal function of the patient who is anticipated to receive IV contrast. Oral contrast agents do not require testing or special pre-medication but patients must drink up to 1.5 L of the contrast solution during the FDG uptake phase depending on which oral contrast is given.

Prior to the PET/CT exam patients should remove all metal (e.g. bracelets, dental braces, pants with zippers, etc), which may lead to scatter artefacts on the CT transmission scan (FIGURE 2). Patients must be positioned comfortably on the patient examination pallet with their arms raised above their head, if possible, which is standard practice in CT to avoid well-known truncation and banding artefacts (FIGURE 3).

CT and PET acquisition

In most cases the CT is performed as a single spiral acquisition and the patient is given breath hold commands in selected scenarios to better match the position of the organs of maximum mobility between the CT and the PET scan.[30-32] The subsequent PET acquisition follows closely that of a standard emission scan. Emission data can be acquired in 2D (with septa extended into the field-of-view) or in 3D (septa retracted), but most commercial PET/CT systems today[12] employ fully-3D PET[33] only and provide a 2D-PET option only upon request. The introduction of fast PET scintillation detectors based on LSO or GSO[34, 35] combined with more powerful detector and acquisition electronics[36] offer dramatic reductions in total scan time for a whole-body acquisition to 10 – 15 min.[29]

Alternative PET tracer

Although clinical routine PET/CT is used synonymously with FDG imaging, there are a number of promising new radiopharmaceuticals. For example, C-11 acetate, C-11 choline,[37] and F-18 Fluorocholine have been suggested for prostate cancer imaging. Ga-67 DOTATOC or F-18 Fluoro-DOPA have been proposed to image neuroendocrine tumors. I-124 is a specific tracer for imaging thyroid tissue and thyroid carcinoma.[38, 39] Considering the potential of PET/CT in the context of biologically oriented radiotherapy treatment planning,[40] there may be great promise in radiopharmaceuticals for assessing hypoxia (F-18 MISO or Cu-64 ATSM) to achieve biological con-

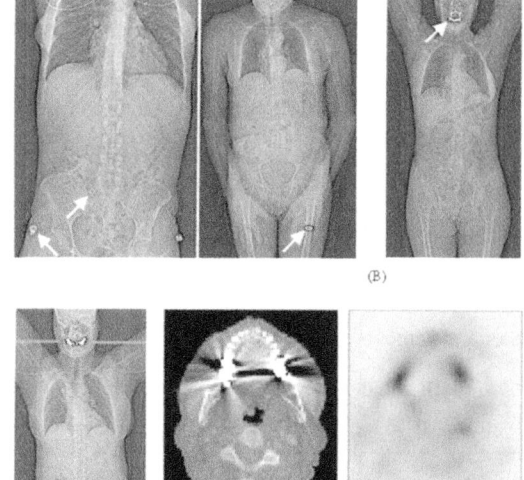

Figure 2. Topograms should be used to detect residual and removable high-density objects that may cause artefacts on subsequent CT, such as buttons, zippers, or jewelry. When high-density objects such as dental implants (B) cannot be removed, the resulting CT and corrected PET images should be reviewed with caution (C).

formity. Depending on the choice of the PET tracer emission acquisition protocols must be adjusted with respect to the scan time, injected activity, uptake time, etc. In addition, the time of the examination with respect to the start, or end of therapy must be adequately defined according to the existing guidelines for using PET imaging during the course of therapy.

Image reconstruction and review

Based on the standard acquisition scheme that involves a transmission and an emission scan, all PET images are reconstructed after (CT-based) attenuation correction. The reconstruction method of choice is based on iterative reconstruction techniques that involve an attenuation-weighted ordered subset approach[41, 42] or a RAMLA approach.[43]

In either case artefacts on CT images may propagate into the corrected PET images. These artefacts may arise from the spatial mismatches between the CT and the PET information due to respiratory or other involuntary patient motion. In addition high-density artefacts on CT from high-density objects, or focal CT contrast accumulations may lead to corresponding artificial tracer uptake patterns in the corrected PET images. It is thus important to understand the pitfalls of CT-based attenuation correction and the

resulting uptake patterns in PET/CT images.[44-46] In case of CT-induced artefacts it is recommended to review also the PET images without attenuation correction, and to dynamically adjust the blending of the reconstructed CT and the PET image sets during the review.

CT protocol considerations in the context of combined PET/CT imaging
Respiratory motion

In the majority of patients respiratory motion results from abdominal respiration, when breathing with the diaphragm dominates over thoracic respiration together with large excursions of the ventral thoracic wall.[47] With the lower thorax and the liver being the areas most affected by respiration,[48] CT examinations of the chest, abdomen and pelvis are performed routinely with instructing the patient on either a breath hold or co-ordinated breathing. With multi-row CT it is possible to scan the entire chest within a single full-inspiration breath hold, which is the more preferred respiratory state. The reason for using full-inspiration breath hold is the prolonged period that patients can tolerate to sustain without breathing. In addition pulmonary pathologies are much better identified in the completely inflated lung. Alternatively, thoracic CT examinations can be performed in expiration or end-expiration breath hold, which is followed during CT-guided intervention.

Limiting respiration-induced motion artefacts

Several PET/CT groups have described respiratory motion and the resulting discrepancy of the spatial information from CT and PET as a source of potential artefacts in corrected emission images after CT-based attenuation correction.[30, 49, 50] These artefacts become dominant when standard full-inspiration breath hold techniques are transferred directly from clinical CT to combined PET/CT examination protocols scanning without further adaptations (FIGURE 4A). In the absence of routinely available respiratory gating options[51] the anatomy of the patient captured during the CT scan must be matched best to the PET images that are acquired over the course of multiple breathing cycles. Reasonable registration accuracy can be obtained, for example, with the spiral CT scan being acquired during shallow breathing.[30, 31] In a recent retrospective study we found a significant reduction in respiration artefacts on CT and PET images patients breathing quietly during the CT and the PET exam on a 4- and 16-row PET/CT system in comparison to a 2-row PET/CT (submitted to the SNM 2004). Alternatively, a limited breath hold protocol can be adopted with either a 1- or a 2-row system, or when dealing with uncooperative patients. Patients are then required to hold their breath in expiration only for the time that the CT takes to cover the lower lung and liver, which is typically less than 15 s.[32]

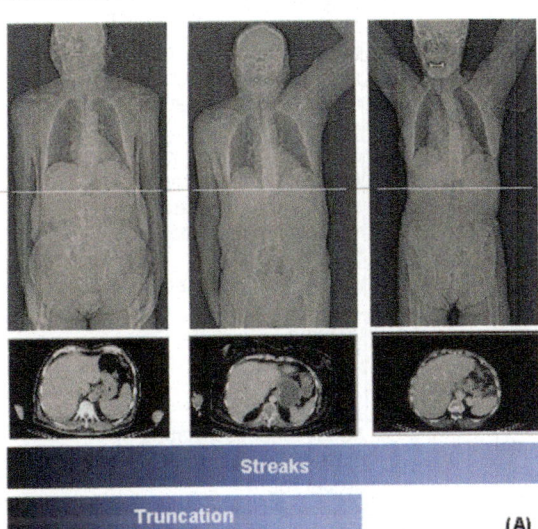

Streaks

Truncation

(A)

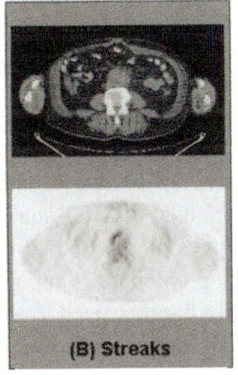
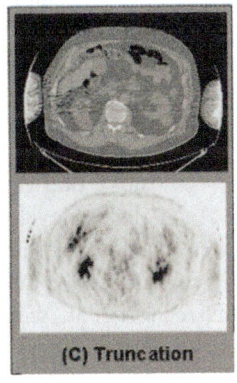

(B) Streaks

(C) Truncation

Figure 3. (A) Topogram scans of three patients with different positions of the arms. Transverse CT images (50 ± 150 HU) at the level of the mid-liver illustrate the magnitude of streak and truncation artefacts. Leaving the arms close to the body yields streak artefacts (B), and in case of larger patients serious truncation effects (C), which both propagate into the corrected PET image. (B and C courtesy Heiko Schöder, MD, Memorial-Sloan Kettering Cancer Center).

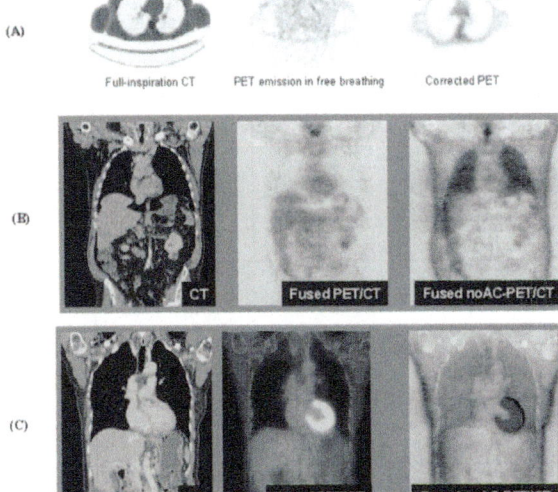

(A) Full-inspiration CT · PET emission in free breathing · Corrected PET

(B) CT · Fused PET/CT · Fused noAC-PET/CT

(C) CT · Fused PET/CT · Fused noAC-PET/CT

Figure 4. Mismatches in respiration between CT and PET can lead to serious artefacts such as a "disappearing chest wall" in (A) where the CT and the PET were acquired in full inspiration and during shallow breathing, respectively. Serious artefacts may also be observed in the region of the diaphragm when uncoordinated breathing is accepted during the CT (B). These artefacts are not seen on the whole-body emission images generated over many respiratory cycles (noAC). Special breathing protocols have been proposed to minimize respiration-induced artefacts (C).

Breath hold commands (in normal expiration, for example) can be combined with very fast CT scanning, and therefore may help reduce respiration mismatches over the entire whole-body examination range (FIGURE 4C). Nevertheless, when respiration commands are not tolerated well and significant respiration-induced artefacts are suspected,[52] it is advisable to reconstruct the emission data without attenuation correction and to review the two sets of fused PET/CT images very carefully.

Standard use of CT contrast agents

Clinical CT examinations are almost routinely performed with contrast enhancement to selectively increase the visibility of tissues and organs for an easier and more accurate assessment of disease and existing alterations of the anatomy of the patient. According to their administration CT contrast agents[53] fall into oral and intravenous agents (TABLE 4). Oral contrast agents can be separated further into positive, negative, and water-equivalent contrast

Contrast	Category	Constituents	Enhancement [HU] vs non-enhanced CT	References for CT	Implications for PET/CT	References for PET/CT
Oral Positive		Barium	200 - 700	(95)	May lead to overestimation of m-map resulting in possibly false uptake patterns but little effect on SUV in corrected PET (outside the immediate location of artifact).	(65)
		Iodine	200 - 500	(96)	May lead to overestimation of m-map resulting in possibly false uptake patterns but little effect on SUV in corrected PET (outside the immediate location of artifact).	(64)
	Water-equivalent	Water	0		No artifacts associated. Application preferred for upper abdomen studies since only poor small bowel distension.	
		Water, osmotic (mannitol), thickening agent (locust bean gum, pending patent)	30-Oct		No artifacts associated. Suitable for whole-body imaging.	(67)
	Negative	Air		(97)	No artifacts associated. Extensive patient preparation.	
IV Positive		Iodine up to 400 mg/mL	parenchyma: 40-90, vessels: 100–300	(98)	Bolus passage in thoracic vein may induce focally increased concentrations of contrast that may translate into false positives on corrected PET.	(63)

Table 4. Classification of CT contrast agents and implications for their application in PET/CT (based on [Speck, 1999 #1]).

agents depending on the resulting changes in the CT attenuation values of the enhanced structures and organs in reference to the attenuation of water (i.e. soft tissue). Negative oral contrast (e.g. air) is used only rarely. Instead most oral contrast media used in radiology today are positive or water-equivalent materials. Positive water-soluble oral contrast agents for CT imaging are based on iodine, which has a high density and expresses only low toxicity.[53] However, iodine-based dispensions (e.g. Gastrografin) are expensive and thus insoluble barium-based suspensions are often preferred. In conventional CT barium sulfate is used in concentrations of 1.5 %. Depending on the choice of iodine- or barium-based contrast patients are asked to drink up to 1.5 L of the contrast dis-/suspension prior to the CT exam (FIGURE 5).

Positive oral contrast is not known to affect the blood glucose level. In combined PET/CT studies, however, slight increases in physiologic uptake patterns of FDG in the descending colon were reported by Dizendorf et al., which were hypothesized to arise from an increased peristalsis in the presence of large quantities of dense contrast.[54] More importantly, serious artefacts were reported in PET/CT studies of patients who underwent a colonoscopy only days before the combined examination.[55] These artefacts are due to the excessively high attenuation values on CT that arise from accumulations of barium sulfate (concentration of up to 50%), and frequently render the CT and PET/CT images diagnostically useless in the areas affected by the coral contrast.

The other group of CT contrast agents are IV contrast agents, which are mostly non-ionic iodine-based substances that yield a positive enhancement of vascular structures (e.g. angiography,[56] and highly vascularized tissues (e.g. liver[57]). Several studies have demonstrated a substantial diagnostic benefit of IV contrast enhancement over native protocols.[58-61] The anatomical structures can be delineated well on enhanced studies, and the sensitivity for the detection of pathological lesions as well as the characterisation of these lesions can be increased (FIGURE 6A).

Nevertheless, to achieve a diagnostic benefit in contrast-enhanced CT a number of - frequently competing - parameters during the IV application of the contrast agent must be considered. With different CT tomographs at hand and with different levels of expertise the best choice of contrast volume, or the duration of the contrast infusion, and the time elapsed following the infusion, to name a few, is discussed extensively, and often controversially, in the literature.[62] The application of IV contrast agents thus mandates the careful optimization and adjustment of a variety of injection parameters (TABLE 5).[56] Today only the advantages and pitfalls of CT contrast applications have been discussed in the context of PET/CT with CT-based attenuation correction. Little or no data is available, however, on the affect of specific contrast application parameters, such as the flow rate, the total contrast volume applied and the usefulness and feasibility of an additional saline flush.

Alternative CT contrast protocols

The unmodified transfer of standard CT contrast protocols into the context of PET/CT has been shown to yield CT and PET images with contrast-related artefacts if attenuation correction is performed based on the acquired CT data.[63]

Several authors have described their observations of biased CT-based attenuation map in case the CT images were acquired in the presence of positive oral contrast. Depending on its concentration attenuation coefficients were overestimated by 26 %[64] up to 66 %.[65] However, the resulting overestimation of the standardized uptake values (SUV) in the corresponding regions on the corrected PET was only 5 % and thus was clinically insignificant assuming the contrast materials were distributed evenly.[54] Nevertheless, the concentration of the oral contrast agent in the colon can vary significantly as reported by Carney et al.66 and may lead to a degradation of the diagnostic accu-

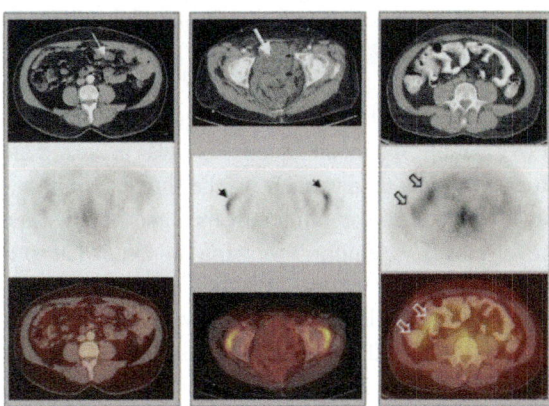

Figure 5. PET/CT without (A) and with (B, C) oral contrast agents. CT, corrected PET, and fused PET/CT images are shown from top to bottom. Water-based oral contrast yields good small bowel distention (B, white arrow) without introducing high-density artefacts. Small arrows indicate muscle uptake. Positive oral contrast may result in areas of increased FDG uptake on corrected PET images (C).

racy of the corrected PET data. Therefore, threshold-based segmentation algorithms to segment and replace contiguous areas of high-density contrast enhancement on CT images prior to the attenuation correction procedure have been developed.[64-66] These algorithms have been shown to correct, or at least reduce any overestimation in the transformed attenuation maps and, in turn, in the corrected PET images, but also require a significant amount of user interaction and processing time, which render theses algorithms sub-optimal for routine applications.

Unlike segmentation techniques that aim at retrospective modifications and corrections of the measured CT-based attenuation map alternative contrast application schemes represent a straightforward approach to avoiding artefacts from high concentrations of positive oral (and IV) contrast agents prospectively. Antoch et al. have presented a water-based oral contrast agent, resulting from previous developments for improved MRT contrast enhancement, for PET/CT imaging.[67] This contrast agent (TABLE 4) is based on a combination of water, 2.5% mannitol, and 0.2% of locust bean gum[67] and allows for good differentiation of bowel loops from surrounding structures (FIG 7A). Unlike iodine or barium, water-equivalent oral contrast agents do not increase the CT attenuation and thus do not lead to an overestimation of the PET activity in the corrected images.

While alternative contrast materials are inadequate for vascular enhancement, high-density artefacts from the bolus injection of IV contrast agents63 can be avoided by alternative acquisition protocols. For example, diagnostic quality CT was achieved and focal contrast enhancement in the thoracic vein was avoided under the condition of the caudo-cranial, i.e. reverse, CT scanning following a somewhat prolonged scan delay after the administration of the IV contrast (FIGURE 7B).[68] Alternatively, a more general solution would be to acquire only a non-enhanced CT for attenuation correction and anatomical labeling (TABLE 2, I-II). However, then additional CT scans with contrast enhancement might be required for accurate delineation of lesions, thus leading to additional patient exposure and more logistical efforts.

Metal artefacts

High-density implants, such as dental fillings, pacemakers, prostheses, or chemotherapy infusion ports may lead to serious artefacts in CT images.[69, 70] These CT artefacts (FIGURE 2) have been shown to propagate through CT-based attenuation correction into the corrected PET emission images where artificially increased tracer uptake patterns may then be generated.[46, 71, 72] It is therefore recommended that PET images from PET/CT are routinely correlated with the complementary CT, and that these PET data are interpreted with care when lesions are observed in close proximity to artefactual structures on CT. Until robust metal artefact correction algorithms[70.73] become available routinely in PET/CT the additional evaluation of the emission data without CT-based attenuation correction is also recommended.[72]

Truncation artefacts

Spiral CT technology today offers a transverse field-of-view of 50 cm, and thus falls short 10 cm from the transverse PET imaging field.[12] This difference may lead to truncation artefacts in the CT images[74] and to a systematic bias of the recovered tracer distribution when scanning obese patients, or when positioning patients with their arms down (FIGURE 3). If not corrected for truncation, CT images appear to mask the reconstructed emission data with the tracer distribution being only partially recovered outside the measured CT field-of-view.

To reduce the amount of truncation on CT and to minimize the frequency of these artefacts, whole-body or chest patients should be positioned according to CT practice with their arms raised above their head. By keeping the arms outside the field-of-view the amount of scatter[75] and patient exposure are also much reduced. Given the short acquisition times of a PET/CT36 most patients tolerate to be scanned with their arms raised for the duration of the combined exam.

A number of algorithms have been suggested to artificially extend the truncated CT projections and to recover the truncated parts of the measured attenuation map in cases where truncation is observed. If applied to the CT images prior to CT-based attenuation correction these correction algorithms will help to recover completely the tracer distributions measured with the complementary emission data.[76] Further work is needed, however, to make such algorithms routinely available for clinical diagnostics.

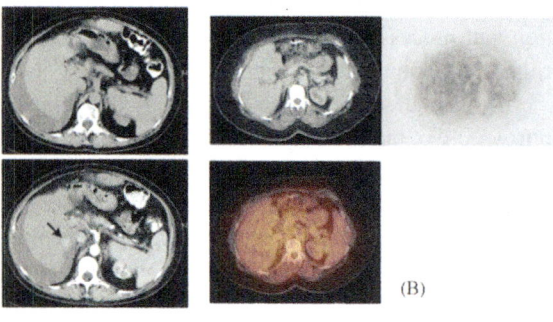

(A)

(B)

Figure 6. (A) Hepatocellular carcinoma metastasis on non-enhanced CT (top) and after application of 100 mL of iodinated (300 mg iodine per mL, flow 3 mL/s) IV contrast (bottom). The lesion is seen only after IV contrast administration (arterial phase). (B) 58 y/o female with hepatic metastasis from uveal melanoma. The contrast-enhanced CT clearly showed a lesion in the right liver lobe, while PET was negative for disease. Diagnosis of metastatic disease was based on the CT data when evaluating fused images and proven by histopathology.

CT exposure settings

With CT being used clinically for 25 years now a number of standardized scanning protocols exist that include the definition of CT acquisition parameters. The choice of parameters includes the tube voltage (kVp), tube current (mA), time for a full rotation of the X-ray tube detector assembly (s), slice collimator setting (mm), and table feed per rotation (mm). Each parameter contributes to the final CT image quality (FIGURE 8) and to the exposure of the

Consideration	Decision	Trend	Discussion	Reference	Implications for PET/CT	References
Contrast enhancement	yes/no	Yes: in most cases	Better vessel delineation, higher T/B contrast	(60)	IV contrast may cause artefacts in corrected PET.	(84)
Repeated scanning	mono-, bi-, or triple-phase	bi-/triple-phase for liver, mono-phase for extended imaging ranges	Helpful in differentiation of lesions	(61) (57)	Multi-phase scanning requires higher-end CT and advanced protocol flexibility.	(12)
Contrast volume	0 – 150 mL	Adapt to patient weight	Less volume reduces toxicity and saves costs	(99)	Higher volume may increase likelihood/significance of artefacts	Not investigated.
Contrast flow rate	1 – 3 mL/s	Lower rates (1.5 mL/s), or different rates when breaking up the total volume	Affects time to, and duration of peak enhancement	(100,101,102)	CT must be fast to follow the contrast agent. Optimize rate for whole-body CT.	Not yet investigated.
Concentration of iodine	280 – 350 mg/mL	Lower concentrations (300 mg/mL) preferred	Lower concentration reduces toxicity and saves costs	(98)	Higher concentration may increase likelihood/significance of artefacts	Not yet investigated.
Saline flush	yes / no	yes	Substitute last ~30%IV contrast volume with saline; reduces toxicity and saves cost	(103,104)	Requires dual-injector system. CT must be fast enough.	Not yet investigated.
Scan delay	20 – 50 s	Yes, delay time adapted to organ/range	Improves optimum enhancement	(105)	Match CT speed to scan delay and organ/range of interest.	(68)
Bolus tracking	yes / no	Used frequently	Optimizes enhancement, semi-/automatic	(106)	Requires higher-end CT and advanced protocol flexibility.	Not yet investigated.
Injection needle	21 – 23 G	Use larger needles	Tradeoff flow with costs	(107)	Careful patient preparation	n.a.

Table 5. Variables of IV contrast agent protocols in clinical CT imaging, and implications for PET/CT

patient.[77] A recent survey among German radiologists, for example, showed an average effective dose to the patient of about 5 – 8 mSv when comparing 14 standard examinations using multi-row CT.[78] This dose will increase to about 18 mSv[79] [our data submitted to SNM 2004] when larger axial imaging ranges are being covered in high-quality imaging scenarios (TABLE 2, V).

Various approaches to CT scanning have been suggested to reduce patient exposure while keeping CT image quality at diagnostic levels. These efforts aim at (a) reducing the absolute tube current, (b) modulating the tube current, such that the photon flux is increased in the lateral views and decreased significantly in the anterior and posterior direction, and (c) additional radiation protection. In detail, Kalra et al. reported on a 50 % reduction in X-ray tube current without degrading clinical image quality in abdominal CT of normal-weight patients up to 90 kg.[80] Tube current modulations have been shown to reduce effective patient exposure by as much as 20 % in adults[81] and 23 % in children.[82] And a 40 % reduction in skin dose can be achieved by the use of eye lens protectors during head and neck imaging.[83]

With patient exposure from CT being at least 100 times higher than from an equivalent PET transmission scan[22, 79] the question arises on the best use of the CT in a PET/CT scenario. To avoid overexposing patients some users have therefore chosen to adopt low-dose CT protocols as part of their PET/CT scenario (TABLE 2, I-III). While patient exposure from CT can be reduced to a little over 1 mSv and thus to a fraction of the exposure from the FDG administration the overall diagnostic quality of the CT (and PET/CT) will be limited (FIGUFRE 8). An alternative solution would be to start a PET/CT examination with an emission scan and selectively perform additional CT scans over limited axial imaging ranges where a lesion was seen on the PET. Such protocols, however, await further modifications to the commercially available acquisition software packages.

Towards efficient and high-quality PET/CT protocols

Imaging scenarios and reasoning

Almost five years after the introduction of the first PET/CT tomograph dual-modality molecular-anatomical imaging has become a very popular imaging modality for cancer patient work-up. However, with PET/CT still being a novel imaging technique and with only a small number of standardized studies having been performed on its true diagnostic accuracy[16,17,21] no standards for combined imaging protocols exist as of today. The lack of carefully conducted prospective trials with sufficiently large patient populations to assess the diagnostic advantage of PET/CT over either PET or CT alone has contributed much to a very subjective use of the new imaging modality. The availability of standalone CT and PET, which have been part of the patient work-up procedures for a long time further invigorate this.

Nevertheless, many cancer patients today are referred for a PET/CT examination only after already having undergone a separate CT, thus obviating the need for a potentially useful high-quality CT exam portion as part of the PET/CT in the majority of cases. Furthermore, site-specific regulations and, sometimes, traditions frequently prohibit an active communication and routine collaboration of the nuclear medicine and radiology professionals, thus limiting the understanding of both the CT and the PET capabilities of a combined PET/CT system in the hand of a single professional user. These observations have lead to a rather diverse variety of PET/CT usage scenarios in clinical practice as seen from TABLE 2.

The benefits and challenges of CT-based attenuation correction

This diversity is further enhanced by the lack of a common understanding of the sources of potential image artefacts, which may degrade the diagnostic quality of the PET/CT examination. These artefacts are mostly related to image distortions, which are introduced during the CT portion of the combined PET/CT exam, and which then may propagate through CT-based attenuation correction into the corrected PET emission images. In many cases these artefacts are generated from the unmodified use of standard CT acquisition parameters and CT contrast application schemes. The sources of these artefacts are, however, well understood and alternative imaging protocols, particularly in the presence of CT oral and IV contrast agents have been proposed to yield radiological-equivalent images. Although choosing an adequate CT contrast protocol often is a trade-off between radiological requirements and technical practicalities the successful modification of standard contrast application schemes[68,84] has contributed to a readiness of radiologists to substitute a clinical CT scan by a combined PET/CT examination. To facilitate this particular adoption of PET/CT in radiology practice in the future the flexibility of the acquisition software must be enhanced to integrate specific CT contrast protocols, such as multi-phase scanning (TABLE 5).

Nevertheless, the optimization of PET/CT acquisition protocols has lead to widespread acceptance of CT-based attenuation correction as part of a combined PET/CT or PET examination (TABLE 2). All but one commercial PET/CT vendor today offer combined systems with the exclusive use of the CT as the method-of-choice to perform attenuation correction. By using the CT scan instead of a lengthy PET transmission measurement the time for the acquisition of the attenuation data for a whole-body study is reduced to a minor fraction of the total examination time (1 min, or less). With the CT acquisition not being biased in post-injection mode transmission data are acquired routinely after injecting the patient, and corrective data processing as in post-injection PET transmission scenarios[85,86] is no longer required.

It is a well-known paradigm in nuclear medicine that attenuation correction is essential to remove distortions of the reconstructed tracer distribution and to recover the true appearance (and extent) of lesions, as discussed by Zasadny et al. for the case of lung cancer PET imaging.[87] Accurate, i.e. quantitative recovery of tracer distributions can only be achieved if an attenuation map is generated - either from independent transmission measurements or from calculations, which is used to correct for the self-absorption of the emitted photons.[88] Therefore attenuation correction is also of essence for efficient therapy moni-

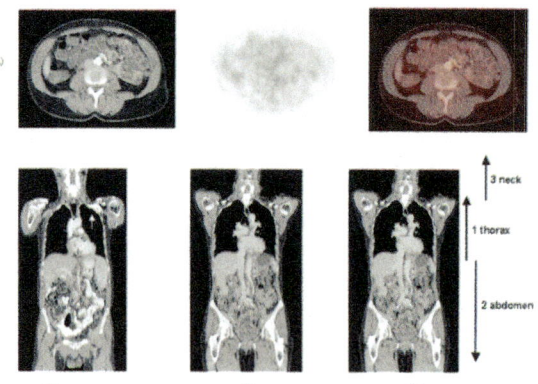

Figure 7. (A) CT protocols with water-equivalent oral contrast allow for good small bowel distension and artefact-free PET images.[67] (B) A standard bolus injection of IV contrast and scanning from the head towards the feet in a single spiral may lead to CT artefacts in the thoracic veins due to bolus passage of the IV contrast agent. Alternative IV contrast injection and scanning direction schemes (C) have been demonstrated to result in better diagnostic quality CT. Ideally one would split the whole-body CT in three shorter but contiguous scan ranges, for which the CT scan parameters (e.g. direction, slice width, table feed, delay) are adjusted individually (D).

toring.[89,90] However, only with the introduction of PET/CT tomography attenuation correction has become an integral part of routine PET imaging and with its routine availability will help making PET/CT a very suitable tool for efficient therapy monitoring. In the future standards will need to be defined to make reasonable use of the X-ray transmission scan, which – even at low tube current settings – represents an order of magnitude increase in patient exposure compared to a standard PET transmission scan.

Image review

It is well known that complex imaging technology often leads to a more efficient examination of the patient but results in more data and diagnostic information to review. This observation has been described by Roos et al. who analyzed the changes in clinical workflow resulting from the replacement of a single-row CT with a multi-row CT.[91] They conclude that with the introduction of the multi-row CT patient handling and acquisition times were reduced but that the new technology resulted in a data explosion, which in turn led to increased image processing and handling times. This issue can be extended to PET/CT, where a single examination yields more data (and more information) than either modality alone, in particular in case of high-quality imaging scenarios when separate CT and PET scans are replaced by an equivalent high-quality combined examination (TABLE 2). The easiest way to utilize both, the CT and the PET image sets is to fuse them, however, at the cost of a somewhat reduced image contrast. A better way to review PET/CT images is a correlated representation side-by-side or separately with a linked cursor. Such viewing option mandates a high-performance computer platform and reviewers with excellent capabilities for orientation in three-dimensional coordinate systems. It was repeatedly pointed out that nuclear medicine physicians must broaden their knowledge of cross-sectional anatomy, while radiologists need to gain a deeper understanding of the physiology behind the human anatomy. Obviously cross-fertilizing imaging expertise would benefit the review of PET/CT images, independent on whether a single reviewer is a radiology or nuclear medicine professional.

In the near future significant enhancements of the PET/CT data handling and viewing software are expected to facilitate a broader clinical acceptance of this imaging modality with the diagnostic and refer-

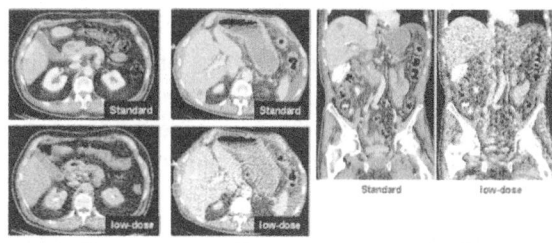

Figure 8. CT image quality from standard and low-dose spiral CT acquisitions. (A) CT was acquired on dual-row CT with 130 kVp and 120 mAs (standard) and 15 mAs (low dose). (B) CT was acquired on 16-row CT with 80 kVp and 120 mAs (standard) and 30 mAs (low dose). (C) Coronal view of (B); very little anatomical detail is seen.

ring physician and therapist. Already today PET/CT is used for longitudinal monitoring of therapy response, and therefore efficient and accurate image alignment and visualization tools are required to view and process PET/CT image volumes of the same patient over time. Similarly with the expected increase in images and image information from the use of the latest and future generations of PET/CT tomographs intelligent software tools[92] are needed to direct the physicians to potentially malignant sites.

Conclusion

Still being at its infancy and with only a few prospective studies being conducted yet on the efficacy of PET/CT in oncology imaging, PET/CT already has revolutionized medical imaging. Based on the success of PET, PET/CT imaging has quickly generated a high interest by diagnosticians and therapists. Through collaborative efforts to optimize dual-modality acquisition protocols, high-quality PET/CT examinations have become feasible. Contrast-enhanced CT data as part of the combined PET/CT examination provide additional information when compared to non-enhanced PET/CT. The benefit of shorter total scan times, increased patient comfort and promising gains in the clinical utility of PET/CT will lead to a dramatically increasing spread of this technique. At the same time the sources for image artefacts and pitfalls are identified and understood, and they will be addressed by ongoing technical and methodological developments. Acquisition protocols need to evolve steadily and to be adjusted to the technical capabilities of the most recent dual-modality systems. Thereby the judicious choice on an appropriate optimized protocol - matched to the clinical diagnostic task – will help avoid or minimize artefacts. Only when all clinical professionals and technical personnel is involved in this process, and when industry responds to the recent demands of the PET/CT community this new technology will yield a positive return on investment.

Acknowledgement

The clinical success and the generation of optimized clinical protocols at the University Hospital Essen is based largely on our technologists Mrs Bärbel Terschüren, Sandra Pabst, Janina Marchese, Lydia Schostock, Dorothea Porsch-Plottek, Sandra Heistrüvers, and Mr. Slavko Maric, and by the involved physicians Drs Jörg Stattaus, Thomas Egelhof, and Lutz Freudenberg.

References

1. Wahl RL, Quint LE, Cieslak RD, Aisen AM, Koeppe RA, Meyer CR. "Anatometabolic" tumor imaging: Fusion of FDG PET with CT or MRI to localize foci of increased activity. J Nucl Med. 1993;34(7):1190-1197.

2. Slomka PJ, Dey D, Przetak C, Aladl UE, Baum RP. Automated 3-dimensional registration of stand-alone 18F-FDG whole-body PET with CT. J Nucl Med. 2003;44(7):1156-1167.

3. Beyer T, Townsend DW, Brun T, Kinahan PE, Charron M, Roddy R, Jerin J, Young J, Byars L, Nutt R. A combined PET/CT tomograph for clinical oncology. J Nucl Med. 2000;41(8): 1369-1379.

4. Townsend DW, Cherry SR. Combining anatomy and function: the path to true image fusion. Eur Radiol. 2001;11(10):1968-1974.

5. Kluetz PG, Meltzer CC, Villemagne VL, Kinahan PE, Chander S, Martinelly MA, Townsend DW. Combined PET/CT imaging in oncology: Impact on patient management. Clin Positron Imaging. 2000;3(6):223-230.

6. Kinahan PE, Townsend DW, Beyer T, Sashin D. Attenuation correction for a combined 3D PET/CT scanner. Med Phys. 1998;25(10):2046-2053.

7. von Schulthess GK. Cost considerations regarding an integrated CT-PET system. Eur Radiol. 2000;10(Suppl 3):S377-S380.

8. Czernin J, Schelbert H. eds. PET/CT: Imaging function and structure. J Nucl Med. 2004;45(Suppl 1):1S-103S.

9. Charron M, Beyer T, Bohnen NN, Kinahan PE, Dachille M, Jerin J, Nutt R, Meltzer CC, Villemagne V, Townsend DW. Image analysis in patients with cancer studied with a combined PET and CT scanner. Clin Nucl Med. 2000;25(11):905-910.

10. Bar-Shalom R, Yefremov N, Guralnik L, Gaitini D, Frenkel A, Kuten A, Altman H, Keidar Z, Israel O. Clinical performance of PET/CT in evaluation of cancer: Additional value for diagnostic imaging and patient management. J Nucl Med. 2003;44(8):1200-1209.

11. Beyer T, Townsend DW, Blodgett TM. Dual-modality PET/CT tomography for clinical oncology. Q J Nucl Med. 2002;46(1):24-34.

12. Beyer T, Townsend DW. Dual-modality PET/CT acquisition systems for clinical oncology. In: Oehr P, Biersack HJ, Coleman RE, eds. PET and PET/CT in Clinical Oncology. Heidelberg: Springer; 2003:9-28.

13. Townsend DW, Beyer T, Blodgett TM. PET/CT scanners: a hardware approach to image fusion. Semin Nucl Med. 2003;33(3):193-204.

14. Kalender WA. Computed Tomography: fundamentals, system technology, image quality, applications. Munich: MCD Verlag; 2000.

15. Halpern B, Dahlbom M, Waldherr C, Quon A, Schiepers C, Silverman DH, Ratib O, Czernin J. A new time-saving whole-body protocol for PET/CT imaging. Mol Imaging Biol. 2003;5(3):182.

16. Hany TF, Steinert HC, Goerres GW, Buck A, von Schulthess GK. PET diagnostic accuracy: improvement with in-line PET-CT system: initial results. Radiology. 2002;225(2):575-581.

17. Lardinois D, Weder W, Hany TF, Kamel EM, Korom S, Seifert B, von Schulthess GK, Steinert HC. Staging of non-small-cell lung cancer with integrated positron-emission tomography and computed tomography. N Engl J Med. 2003;348(25):2500-2507.

18. Bristow RE, del Carmen MG, Pannu HK, Cohade C, Zahurak ML, Fishman EK, Wahl RL, Montz FJ. Clinically occult recurrent ovarian cancer: patient selection for secondary cytoreductive surgery using combined PET/CT. Gynecol Oncol. 2003;90(3):519-528.

19. Cohade C, Osman M, Leal J, Wahl RL. Direct comparison of 18F-FDG PET and PET/CT in patients with colorectal carcinoma. J Nucl Med. 2003;44(11):1797-1803.

20. Antoch G, Stattaus J, Nemat AT, Marnitz S, Beyer T, Kuehl H, Bockisch A, Debatin JF, Freudenberg LS. Non-small cell lung cancer: dual-modality PET/CT in preoperative staging. Radiology. 2003;229(2):526-533.

21. Antoch G, Vogt FM, Freudenberg LS, Nazaradeh F, Goehde SC, Barkhausen J, Dahmen G, Bockisch A, Debatin JF, Ruehm SG. Whole-body dual-modality PET/CT and whole-body MRI for tumor staging in oncology. JAMA. 2003;290(24): 3199-3206.

22. Zaidi H, Hasegawa B. Determination of the attenuation map in emission tomography. J Nucl Med. 2003;44(2):291-315.

23. Holm S, Toft P, Jensen M. Estimation of the noise-contributions from blank, transmission and emission scans in PET. IEEE Trans Nucl Sci. 1996;43(4):2285-2291.

24. LaCroix KJ, Tsui BMW, Hasegawa BH, Brown JK. Investigation of the use of X-ray CT images for attenuation correction in SPECT. IEEE Trans Nucl Sci. 1994;41(6):2793-2799.

25. Fleming JS. A technique for using CT images in attenuation correction and quantification in SPECT. Nucl Med Commun. 1989;10(2):83-97.

26. Burger C, Goerres G, Schoenes S, Buck A, Lonn AH, von Schulthess GK. PET attenuation coefficients from CT images: experimental evaluation of the transformation of CT into PET 511-keV attenuation coefficients. Eur J Nucl Med Mol Imaging. 2002;29(7):922-927.

27. Kinahan PE, Hasegawa BH, Beyer T. X-ray-based attenuation correction for positron emission tomography/computed tomography scanners. Semin Nucl Med. 2003;33(3):166-179.

28. Beyer T, Antoch G, Müller S, Egelhof T, Freudenberg LS, Debatin J, Bockisch A. Acquisition protocol considerations for combined PET/CT imaging. J Nucl Med. 2004;45(Suppl 1):25S-35S.

29. Hamblen SM, Lowe VJ. Clinical 18F-FDG oncology patient preparation techniques. J Nucl Med Technol. 2003;31(1):3-7.

30. Goerres GW, Kamel E, Heidelberg TN, Schwitter MR, Burger C, von Schulthess GK. PET-CT image co-registration in the thorax: influence of respiration. Eur J Nucl Med Mol Imaging. 2002;29(3):351-360.

31. Goerres GW, Burger C, Schwitter MR, Heidelberg TN, Seifert B, von Schulthess GK. PET/CT of the abdomen: optimizing the patient breathing pattern. Eur Radiol. 2003;13(4):734-739.

32. Beyer T, Antoch G, Blodgett T, Freudenberg LF, Akhurst T, Mueller S. Dual-modality PET/CT imaging: the effect of respiratory motion on combined image quality in clinical oncology. Eur J Nucl Med. 2003;30(4):588-596.

33. Bendriem B, Townsend D. The theory and practice of 3D PET. In: Cox PH, ed. Developments in Nuclear Medicine (Vol 32). Dordrecht: Kluwer Academic Publishers; 1998.

34. Karp JS. Against: Is LSO the future of PET? Eur J Nucl Med Mol Imaging. 2002;29(11):1525-1528.

35. Nutt R. For: Is LSO the future of PET? Eur J Nucl Med Mol Imaging. 2002;29(11):1523-1525.

36. Townsend DW, Carney JP, Yap JT, Hall NC. PET/CT today and tomorrow. J Nucl Med. 2004;45(Suppl 1):4S-14S.

37. Blumstein NM, Feigl F, Glatting G, Hautmann H, Gottfried HW, Wahl A, Reske SN. How effective is [11C]choline PET/CT in detecting primary prostate cancer in biopted patients? J Nucl Med. 2003;44(5 Suppl):133P.

38. Bockisch A, Brandt-Mainz K, Gorges R, Muller S, Stattaus J, Antoch G. Diagnosis in medullary thyroid cancer with [18F]FDG-PET and improvement using a combined PET/CT scanner. Acta Med Austriaca. 2003;30(1):22-25.

39. Freudenberg LS, Antoch G, Gorges R, Knust J, Pink R, Jentzen W, Debatin JF, Brandau W, Bockisch A, Stattaus J. Combined PET/CT with iodine-124 in diagnosis of spread metastatic thyroid carcinoma: a case report. Eur Radiol. 2003;13:L19-L23.

40. Bradley JD, Perez CA, Dehdashti F, Siegel BA. Implementing biologic target volumes in radiation treatment planning for non-small cell lung cancer. J Nucl Med. 2004;45(Suppl 1):96S-101S.

41. Hudson HM, Larkin RS. Accelerated image reconstruction using ordered subsets of projection data. IEEE Trans Med Imaging. 1994;13(4)601-609.

42. Voltini F, Zito F, Bruno A, Castellani M, Canzi C, Matheoud R, Schiavini M, and gerundini P. Image quality changes of whole-body PET studies due to different OS-EM parameter choices. Eur J Nucl Med. 2000;27:1187.

43. Daube-Witherspoon ME, Matej S, Karp JS, Lewitt RM. Application of the row action maximum likelihood algorithm with spherical basis functions to clinical PET imaging. IEEE Trans Nucl Sci. 2001;48(1):24-30.

44. Goerres GW, von Schulthess GK, Hany TF. Positron emission tomography and PET CT of the head and neck: FDG uptake in normal anatomy, in benign lesions, and in changes resulting from treatment. Am J Roentgenol. 2002;179(5):1337-1343.

45. Yeung HW, Grewal RK, Gonen M, Schoder H, Larson SM. Patterns of 18F-FDG uptake in adipose tissue and muscle: a potential source of false-positives for PET. J Nucl Med. 2003;44(11):1789-1796.

46. Bujenovic S, Mannting F, Chakrabarti R, Ladnier D. Artifactual 2-deoxy-2-[18F]fluoro-D-glucose localization surrounding metallic objects in a PET/CT scanner using CT-based attenuation correction. Mol Imaging Biol. 2003;5(1):20-22.

47. Onishi H, Kuriyama K, Komiyama T, Tanaka S, Ueki J, Sano N, Araki T, Ikenaga S, Tateda Y, Aikawa Y. CT evaluation of patient deep inspiration self-breath-holding: how precisely can patients reproduce the tumor position in the absence of respiratory monitoring devices? Med Phys. 2003;30(6):1183-1187.

48. Suramo I, Paivansalo M, Myllyla V. Cranio-caudal movements of the liver, pancreas and kidneys in respiration. Acta Radiol Diagn (Stockh). 1984;25(2):129-131.

49. Beyer T, Townsend DW, Nutt R, Charron M, Kinahan PE, Meltzer CC. Combined PET/CT imaging using a single, dual-modality tomograph: a promising approach to clinical oncology of the future. In: Wieler HJ, Coleman RE, eds. PET in Clinical oncology. Steinkopff Darmstadt: Springer; 2000:101-124.

50. Osman MM, Cohade C, Nakamoto Y, Wahl RL. Respiratory motion artifacts on PET emission images obtained using CT attenuation correction on PET-CT. Eur J Nucl Med Mol Imaging. 2003;30(4):603-606.

51. Nehmeh SA, Erdi YE, Rosenzweig KE, Schoder H, Larson SM, Squire OD, Humm JL. Reduction of respiratory motion artifacts in PET imaging of lung cancer by respiratory correlated dynamic PET: methodology and comparison with respiratory gated PET. J Nucl Med. 2003;44(10):1644-1648.

52. Osman MM, Cohade C, Nakamoto Y, Marshall LT, Leal JP, and Wahl RL. Clinically significant inaccurate localization of lesions with PET/CT: frequency in 300 patients. J Nucl Med. 2003;44(2):240-243.

53. Speck U. Contrast Media. Overview, Use and Pharmaceutical Aspects. 4th revised ed. Berlin: Springer; 1999.

54. Dizendorf EV, Treyer V, von Schulthess GK, Hany TF. Application of oral contrast media in coregistered positron emission tomography-CT. Am J Roentgenol. 2002;179(2):477-481.

55. Beyer T. Design, construction, and validation of a combined PET/CT tomograph for clinical oncology. In: Department of Physics. University of Surrey: Surrey; 2000:303.

56. Fleischmann D. High-concentration contrast media in MDCT angiography: principles and rationale. Eur Radiol. 2003;13:N39-N43.

57. Kopp AF, Heuschmid M, Claussen CD. Multidetector helical CT of the liver for tumor detection and characterization. Eur Radiol. 2002;12(4):745-752.

58. Albertyn LE. Rationales for the use of intravenous contrast medium in computed tomography. Australas Radiol. 1989;33(1):29-33.

59.   Cho JS, Kim JK, Rho SM, Lee HY, Jeong HY, Lee CS. Preoperative assessment of gastric carcinoma: value of two-phase dynamic CT with mechanical iv. injection of contrast material. Am J Roentgenol. 1994;163(1):69-75.

60.   Delorme S, Knopp MV, Kauczor HU, Raue F, Buhr H, van Kaick G. An optimized examination protocol for contrast-enhanced cervical and mediastinal CT. Clin Imaging. 1996;20(1):31-36.

61.   Conrad R, Pauleit D, Layer G, Kandyba J, Kohlbecher R, Hortling N, Baselides P, Schild H. Spiral CT of the head-neck area: the advantages of the early arterial phase in the detection of squamous-cell carcinomas. Rofo Fortschr Geb Röntgenstr Neuen Bildgeb Verfahr. 1999;171(1):15-19.

62.   Feuerbach S, Lorenz W, Klose KJ, Gmeinwieser J, Lackner KJ, Landwehr P, Grabbe E, Kloppel R. Contrast medium administration in spiral computed tomography: the results of a consensus conference. Institute for Radiodiagnosis, Regensburg. Rofo Fortschr Geb Rontgenstr Neuen Bildgeb Verfahr. 1996;164(2):158-165.

63.   Antoch G, Freudenberg LS, Egelhof T, Stattaus J, Jentzen W, Debatin JF, Bockisch A. Focal tracer uptake: a potential artifact in contrast-enhanced dual-modality PET/CT scans. J Nucl Med. 2002;43(10):1339-1342.

64.   Dizendorf E, Hany TF, Buck A, von Schulthess GK, Burger C. Cause and magnitude of the error induced by oral CT contrast agent in CT-based attenuation correction of PET emission studies. J Nucl Med. 2003;44(5):732-738.

65.   Nehmeh SA, Erdi YE, Kalaigian H, Kolbert KS, Pan T, Yeung H, Squire O, Sinha A, Larson SM, Humm JL. Correction for oral contrast artifacts in CT attenuation-corrected PET images obtained by combined PET/CT. J Nucl Med. 2003;44(12):1940-1944.

66.   Carney J, Beyer T, Brasse D, Yap JT, Townsend DW. Clinical PET/CT scanning using oral CT contrast agents. J Nucl Med. 2002;43(5 Suppl):57P.

67.   Antoch G, Kuehl H, Kanja J, Lauenstein T, Schneemann H, Hauth E, Jentzen W, Beyer T, Goehde S, Debatin J. Introduction and evaluation of a negative oral contrast agent to avoid contrast-induced artefacts in dual-modality PET/CT imaging. Radiology. 2004:In Press.

68.   Beyer T, Antoch G, Rosenbaum S, Freudenberg L, Fehlings T, Stattaus J. Optimized IV contrast administration protocols for diagnostic PET/CT imaging. Eur Radiol. 2004:Abstract.

69.   Duerinckx AJ, Macovski A. Polychromatic streak artifacts in computed tomography images. J Comput Assist Tomogr. 1978;2(4):481-487.

70.   deMan B, Nuyts J, Dupont P, Marchal G, Suetens P. Metal streak artifacts in X-ray computed tomography: a simulation study. IEEE Trans Nucl Sci. 1999;46(3):691-696.

71.   Kamel EM, Burger C, Buck A, von Schluthess GK, Goerres GW. Impact of metallic dental implants on CT-based attenuation correction in a combined PET/CT scanner. Eur Radiol. 2003;13(4):724-728.

72.   Goerres GW, Ziegler SI, Burger C, Berthold T, von Schulthess GK, Buck A. Artifacts at PET and PET/CT caused by metallic hip prosthetic material. Radiology. 2003;226(2):577-584.

73.   Glover GH, Pelc NJ. An algorithm for the reduction of metal clip artifacts in CT reconstructions. Med Phys. 1981;8(6):799-807.

74.   Carney J and Townsend D. CT-based attenuation correction for PET/CT scanners. In: von Schultess G, ed. Clinical PET, PET/CT and SPECT/CT: Combined Anatomic-Molecular Imaging. Lippincott, Williams and Wilkins; 2002.

75.   Carney JP, Townsend DW, Kinahan PE, Beyer T, Kalender WA, Kachelriess M, DeMan B, Nuyts J. CT-based attenuation correction: the effects of imaging with the arms in the field of view. J Nucl Med. 2001;42(5 Suppl):56-57P.

76.   Schaller S, Semrbitzki O, Beyer T, Fuchs T, Kachelriess M, Flohr T. An algorithm for virtual extension of the CT field of measurement for application in combined PET/CT scanners. Radiology. 2002;225(P):497.

77.   Kalender WA, Schmidt B, Zankl M, and Schmidt M. A PC program for estimating organ dose and effective dose values in computed tomography. Eur Radiol. 1999;9(3):555-562.

78.   Brix G, Nagel HD, Stamm G, Veit R, Lechel U, Griebel J, Galanski M. Radiation exposure in multi-slice versus single-slice spiral CT: results of a nationwide survey. Eur Radiol. 2003;13(8):1979-1991.

79.   Wu TH, Huang YH, Lee JJ, Wang SY, Wang SC, Su CT, Chen LK, Chu TC. Radiation exposure during transmission measurements: comparison between CT- and germanium-based techniques with a current PET scanner. Eur J Nucl Med Mol Imaging. 2004;31(1):38-43.

80.   Kalra MK, Prasad S, Saini S, Blake MA, Varghese J, Halpern EF, Thrall JH, Rhea JT. Clinical comparison of standard-dose and 50% reduced-dose abdominal CT: effect on image quality. Am J Roentgenol. 2002;179(5):1101-1106.

81.   Tack D, De Maertelaer V, Gevenois PA. Dose reduction in multidetector CT using attenuation-based online tube current modulation. Am J Roentgenol. 2003;181(2):331-334.

82.   Greess H, Nomayr A, Wolf H, Baum U, Lell M, Bowing B, Kalender W, Bautz WA. Dose reduction in CT examination of children by an attenuation-based on-line modulation of tube current (CARE Dose). Eur Radiol. 2002;12(6):1571-1576.

83.   Hein E, Rogalla P, Klingebiel R, Hamm B. Low-dose CT of the paranasal sinuses with eye lens protection: effect on image quality and radiation dose. Eur Radiol. 2002;12(7):1693-1696.

84.   Antoch G, Freudenberg LS, Beyer T, Bockisch A, Debatin JF. To enhance or not to enhance? 18F-FDG and CT contrast agents in dual-modality 18F-FDG PET/CT. J Nucl Med. 2004;45(Suppl 1):56S-65S.

85.   Smith RJ, Karp JS, Muehllehner G, Gualtieri E, Benard F. Singles transmission scans performed post-injection for quantitative whole body PET imaging. IEEE Trans Nucl Sci. 1997;44(3):1329-1335.

86.   Watson CC, Schäfer A, Luk WK, Kirsch CM. Clinical evaluation of single-photon attenuation correction for 3D whole-body PET. Trans Nucl Sci. 1999;46(4):1024-1031.

87.   Zasadny KR, Kison PV, Quint LE, Wahl RL. Untreated lung cancer: quantification of systematic distortion of tumor size and shape on non-attenuation-corrected 2-[Fluorine-18]fluoro-2-deoxy-D-glucose PET scans. Radiology. 1996;201(3):873-876.

88.   Bailey DL. Transmission scanning in emission tomography. Eur J Nucl Med. 1998;25(7):774-787.

89. Coleman RE. For: Is quantitation necessary for oncological PET studies? Eur J Nucl Med. 2001;29(1):133-135.

90.   Eary JF, Krohn KA. Positron emission tomography: imaging tumor response. Eur J Nucl Med. 2000;27(12):1737-1739.

91.   Roos JE, Desbiolles LM, Willmann JK, Weishaupt D, Marincek B, Hilfiker PR. Multidetector-row helical CT: analysis of time management and workflow. Eur Radiol. 2002;12(3):680-685.

92.   Ratib O. PET/CT image navigation and communication. J Nucl Med. 2004;45(Suppl 1):46S-55S.

93.   Ratib O. PET/CT Image Navigation and Communication. J Nucl Med. 2004; 45: 46S-55.

94.   Antoch G, Freudenberg LS, Stattaus J, Jentzen W, Mueller SP, Debatin JF, Bockisch A. Whole-body positron emission tomography-CT: optimized CT using oral and IV contrast materials. Am J Roentgenol. 2002;179(6):1555-1560.

95.   Garra BS, Cespedes EI, Ophir J, Spratt SR, Zuurbier RA, Magnant CM, Pennanen MF. Elastography of breast lesions: initial clinical results. Radiology. 1997;202(1):79-86.

96.   Mitchell DG, Bjorgvinsson E, terMeulen D, Lane P, Greberman M, Friedman AC. Gastrografin versus dilute barium for colonic CT examination: a blind, randomized study. J Comput Assist Tomogr. 1985;9(3):451-453.

97.   Iannaccone R, Laghi A, Catalano C, Mangiapane F, Piacentini F, Passariello R. Feasibility of ultra-low-dose multislice CT colonography for the detection of colorectal lesions: preliminary experience. Eur Radiol. 2003;13(6):1297-1302.

98.   Awai K, Takada K, Onishi H, Hori S. Aortic and hepatic enhancement and tumor-to-liver contrast: analysis of the effect of different concentrations of contrast material at multidetector row helical CT. Radiology. 2002;224(3):757-763.

99.   Keberle M, Tschammler A, Hahn D. Single-bolus technique for spiral CT of laryngopharyngeal squamous cell carcinoma: comparison of different contrast material volumes, flow rates, and start delays. Radiology. 2002;224(1):171-176.

100.   Yamashita Y, Komohara Y, Takahashi M, Uchida M, Hayabuchi N, Shimizu T, Narabayashi I. Abdominal helical CT: evaluation of optimal doses of intravenous contrast material--a prospective randomized study. Radiology. 2000;216(3):718-723.

101.   Haage P, Schmitz-Rode T, Hubner D, Piroth W, Gunther RW. Reduction of contrast material dose and artifacts by a saline flush using a double power injector in helical CT of the thorax. Am J Roentgenol. 2000;174(4):1049-1053.

102.   Awai K, Hori S. Effect of contrast injection protocol with dose tailored to patient weight and fixed injection duration on aortic and hepatic enhancement at multidetector-row helical CT. Eur Radiol. 2003;13(9):2155-2160.

103.   Dorio PJ, Lee FT Jr, Henseler KP, Pilot M, Pozniak MA, Winter TC 3rd, Shock SA. Using a saline chaser to decrease contrast media in abdominal CT. Am J Roentgenol. 2003;180(4):929-934.

104.   Irie T, Kajitani M, Yamaguchi M, Itai Y. Contrast-enhanced CT with saline flush technique using two automated injectors: how much contrast medium does it save? J Comput Assist Tomogr. 2002;26(2):287-291.

105.   Sokiranski R, Elsner K, Welke M, Gorich J, Rilinger N, Fleiter T. A new method in the determination of individual delay time in bolus application in spiral CT. Rofo Fortschr Geb Rontgenstr Neuen Bildgeb Verfahr. 1997;166(6):550-553.

106.   Kirchner J, Kickuth R, Laufer U, Noack M, Liermann D. Optimized enhancement in helical CT: experiences with a real-time bolus tracking system in 628 patients. Clin Radiol. 2000;55(5):368-373.

107.   Wakoh M, Yamada M, Mori T, Shibuya H, Kobayashi N, Kuroyanagi K. Contrast-enhanced conventional CT in patients after surgery for malignant tumors: evaluation of the optimal method of the administration of the contrast medium. Bull Tokyo Dent Coll. 2000;41(3):99-107.

From FDG-PET to FDG-PET/CT Imaging

J. Czernin and C. Yap

PET imaging with F-18 deoxyglucose (FDG) diagnoses, stages and restages most cancers with a high diagnostic accuracy.[1,2] Treatment effects can be monitored early and with greater accuracy than with anatomic imaging modalities. FDG-PET provides prognostic information that is superior to that of conventional imaging.[3-5] The high diagnostic and prognostic accuracy of PET has led to its acceptance as a standard oncological imaging tool.

Nevertheless, several limitations of PET have led to the rapid acceptance of PET/CT imaging in the medical community. Foremost among these is its inability to localize accurately to anatomical structures areas of increased glycolytic activity. Whole body PET imaging is also time consuming. For instance, standard imaging protocols of the whole body require about 60 minutes for completion resulting in low patient throughput and inefficient use of the imaging equipment.

PET/CT is changing clinical molecular imaging. Comprehensive whole body examinations providing detailed anatomical and molecular information can now be consistently performed in 30 minutes or less. Initial studies suggest that the diagnostic accuracy of PET/CT imaging exceeds that of PET, CT and MRI alone.[6-11]

The following chapter provides a brief overview of the transformation from PET to PET/CT imaging and summarizes the current clinical experience with PET/CT imaging.

Marked increases in glucose metabolism to provide energy for rapidly proliferating cancer tissue has been known for more than 80 years. In the 1920's, the German biochemist Otto Warburg conducted animal experimental studies and found that the metabolism of cancer cells was predominantly one of glycolysis.[12] After confirming these findings in a variety of human cancer cells he established that tumor cells use ATP generated from glycolysis to accommodate for the energy requirements of rapidly replicating tissue. Glucose utilization of tumor cells is further increased because of activation of the hexose monophosphate pathway providing the carbon backbone for DNA and RNA synthesis in growing tumors.[13,14] Glucose transporter proteins in tumor cell membranes and expression of hexokinase are also up-regulated.[15] Thus, neoplastic degeneration and cell proliferation are associated with increased glucose utilization.

Fifty years after these fundamental discoveries, PET was introduced by Phelps and Hoffman in 1975.[16] Since then, the technology has matured and has revolutionized tumor imaging. Whole body PET scanners have now been available for clinical use for more than a decade. A prerequisite for the acceptance of PET was commercial availability of the positron emitter and glucose analogue ^{18}F-deoxyglucose (FDG). This has become reality through regional distribution centers that can deliver FDG to health care providers throughout the world.

FDG distributes throughout the body in proportion to glucose metabolism of tissues (Figure 1). Normal tissues that utilize large amounts of glucose as substrate for energy production exhibit increased glucose metabolic activity. These include for instance the brain, working muscles, mucous membranes and the liver. The renal excretion of FDG implies that considerable tracer activity accumulates in the renal collecting system and in the urinary bladder.

Glucose transporters facilitate FDG uptake in tumor cells and hexokinase subsequently phosphorylates FDG to FDG-6-phosphate.[17-19] FDG-6-phosphate[20] is not metabolized in the glycolytic pathway. It remains essentially trapped intracellularly because tumor cells do not contain significant amounts of glucose-6-phosphatase to reverse the phosphorylation.

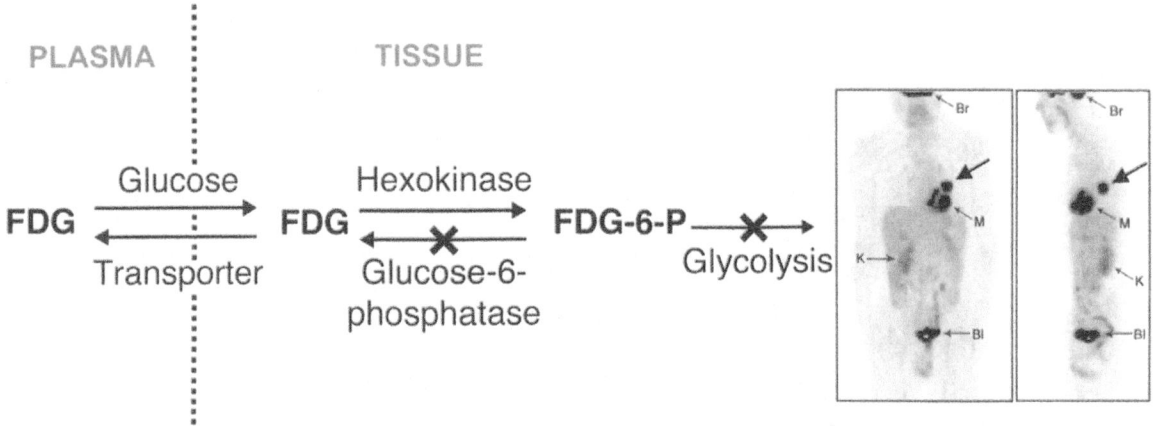

PLASMA   TISSUE

FDG $\xrightleftharpoons[\text{Transporter}]{\text{Glucose}}$ FDG $\xrightarrow[\text{Glucose-6-phosphatase}]{\text{Hexokinase}}$ FDG-6-P $\xrightarrow{\text{Glycolysis}}$

Figure 1. Uptake kinetics of FDG in a patient with non-small-cell lung cancer. FDG uptake is facilitated by glucose transporter I. The phosphorylated product FDG-6-phosphate (FDG-6-P) is not a substrate of the glycolytic pathway and glucose-6-phosphatase activity in tumor tissue is low. Thus, FDG-6-P is essentially trapped in tumor cells. FDG undergoes renal clearance resulting in tracer accumulation in kidneys (K) and bladder (Bl) FDG-PET images represent the distribution of FDG-6-P throughout the body. The inserted PET images show normal uptake of FDG in the lower brain portions (Br), normal myocardial tracer uptake (M) and markedly increased FDG uptake in the tumor (arrow).

The level of FDG uptake in tumor cells is a reliable marker of tumor cell glycolysis. Importantly, tumor cell glucose utilization is inversely related to the degree of tumor cell differentiation and linearly related to tumor cell proliferative activity (Figure 2).[21]

However, benign, and some well-differentiated tumors can also consume considerable amounts of glucose. In addition, inflammatory tissue exhibits increased rates of glucose metabolism due to glycolytic activity of inflammatory cells. The degree of glucose utilization varies between and within different cancers (Figure 3). This is due to differences in "aggressiveness" and differentiation of tumor cells,[22,23] but is also explained by certain morphological and functional tumor features. For instance, mucin-producing tumors exhibit low rates of glucose metabolic activity[24] and tumors largely composed of cystic components are not well imaged with FDG-PET. Similarly, malignancies lacking tumor bulk can be difficult to image with FDG-PET.

Physiological uptake and distribution patterns throughout the body also determine the usefulness of FDG-PET for imaging certain cancers. For instance, primary renal cell[25] or prostate cancers can be obscured by urine activity in the renal collecting system and the urinary bladder.

Some of these limitations will be overcome by the introduction of novel PET imaging probes that target tumor-specific processes. Several of these are currently being tested for their clinical usefulness in cancer patients. Among these are C-11 acetate and F-18 choline designed for imaging lipid synthesis that is markedly increased in prostate cancer.[26] Renal clear-

Tumor Proliferation and FDG Uptake

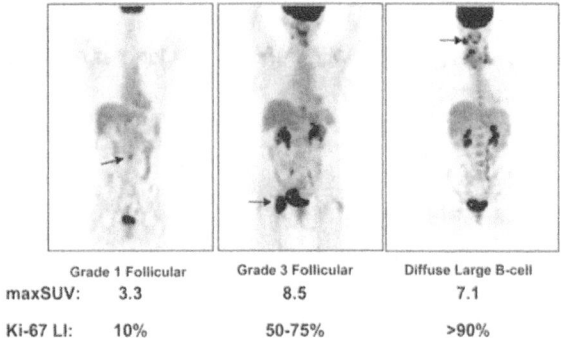

	Grade 1 Follicular	Grade 3 Follicular	Diffuse Large B-cell
maxSUV:	3.3	8.5	7.1
Ki-67 LI:	10%	50-75%	>90%

Figure 2. FDG uptake in cancer tissue is determined among other factors by tumor proliferation rates or aggressiveness. This is exemplified in three different lymphoma patients. Ki-67 labeling index (Ki-67 LI), an immuno-histochemical marker of tumor cell proliferation Is lowest in the patient with low grade lymphoma (arrow) shown in the left panel. This results in relatively low FDG standardized uptake value (SUV). The patients in the middle and right panels have high-grade lymphoma (arrows) with high Ki-67 LI and high SUV.

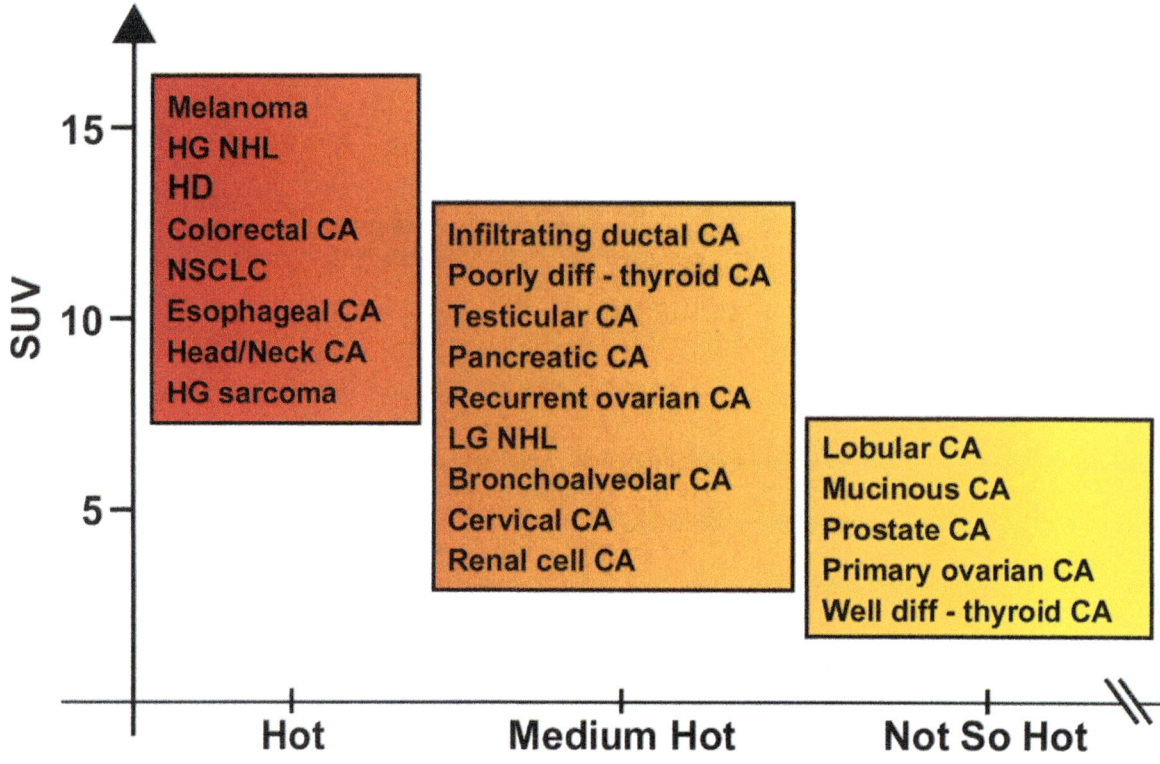

Figure 3. The degree of FDG uptake varies between different cancer types. Note that high grade (HG) tumors generally exhibit higher FDG uptake than low grade (LG) tumors. For instance, poorly differentiated (diff) thyroid cancer shows moderately or severely increased FDG uptake while well differentiated thyroid cancer is frequently low in FDG uptake. Functional features of tumors also determine FDG uptake. For instance, mucinous carcinoma (CA) generally exhibit very low FDG uptake.
Tumor morphology is also an important predictor FDG uptake. For instance, primary ovarian cancer frequently consists of large cystic portions resulting in poor FDG uptake.

Abbreviations: NHL: Non-Hodgkin Lymphoma; HD: Hodgkin's Disease.

ance of activity is eliminated in the case of C-11 acetate. Thus, the prostate bed can be visualized without contamination from bladder activity.

Initial studies with F-18 choline[27] suggest that this tracer detects primary and recurrent prostate cancer with a good diagnostic accuracy.

Shields et al.[28] used F-18 fluoro-thymidine (FLT) to image cell replication and proliferation of tumors in vivo. This tracer is retained in proliferating tissues through the enzyme thymidine kinase 1. The authors obtained high target to background images of tumor proliferation in human subjects.

In vivo imaging of gene expression has been accomplished in animal experimental studies.[29-31] This approach might in the future allow in vivo monitoring of gene therapy.

The understanding of the metabolism of tumor cells along with the development of PET[16] has resulted in the widespread clinical use of FDG-PET. The acceptance of FDG-PET as a clinical tool was however slow with many experts in nuclear medicine resisting this new technology for several reasons. Conventional nuclear medicine equipment and more importantly, the philosophy behind functional imaging needed to change, a process that took a long time. Radiologists had little interest in PET, a modality that was not considered financially viable. Availability of FDG was another problem since in the early years the production of positron emitting isotopes was largely limited to academic sites that had access to an on-site cyclotron.

Most importantly, the concept of molecular imaging had not been introduced.[32] Thus, the medical community had not realized the striking discrepancy between anatomical masses and tumor viability that can be encountered every day by comparing PET to CT images. PET was considered expensive, complicated, and images were thought to be difficult to interpret. Thus, most radiologists and oncologists relied on anatomic imaging for diagnosing, staging and re-staging of cancer. This includes computed tomography (CT), magnetic resonance imaging (MRI), and ultrasound (US). Because of their exquisite spatial resolution these technologies can detect very small "lesions". However, they cannot reliably distinguish between benign and malignant tumors or pre- and post-therapeutic anatomical alterations such as scarring, inflammation or necrosis and neoplastic processes.

In the late 1990's the published literature had so unequivocally demonstrated PET's high diagnostic and prognostic accuracy that molecular imaging simply could no longer be overlooked.[2,33,34] The emergence of regional distribution centers of molecular imaging probes that commercially produced FDG as well as the reduction in the costs of PET devices were other important milestones for making PET imaging clinically feasible. Finally, the Health Care Finance Administration (HCFA) acknowledged research data obtained in more than 20,000 patients[2] and approved FDG-PET for several important oncological indications (Table I).

As a consequence of its convincing clinical performance and improved reimbursement the volume of PET studies performed nationwide has doubled every year over the last 3 years. In 2004, more than one million PET studies will be performed in the United States.

Medicare Approved FDG PET Procedures

Oncology

Lung Cancer: Solitary Pulmonary Nodule (SPN)

G0125 Single Pulmonary Nodule
- Evidence of primary tumor by concurrent thoracic CT
- No negative PET scan in last 90 days

Lung Cancer: Non-Small Cell (NSCLC)		Melanoma: Excludes Initial Staging of Regional Nodes		Head and Neck Cancer: Excludes Thyroid & CNS	
G0210	Diagnosis	G0216	Diagnosis	G0223	Diagnosis
G0211	Staging	G0217	Staging	G0224	Staging
G0212	Restaging	G0218	Restaging	G0225	Restaging
		G0219	Non-covered Indications		

Colorectal Cancer		Lymphoma		Esophageal Cancer	
G0213	Diagnosis	G0220	Diagnosis	G0226	Diagnosis
G0214	Staging	G0221	Staging	G0227	Staging
G0215	Restaging	G0222	Restaging	G0228	Restaging

Breast Cancer: Excludes Initial Diagnosis and Initial Staging of Axillary Nodes

G0253 Staging/Restaging
- Local regional recurrence or distant metastases prior to or after course of treatment

G0254 Evaluation of Response to Treatment
- During course of treatment

Thyroid Cancer

TBA Staging
G0296 Restaging
- Postsurgical where I-131 is known to be insufficient or for follicular cell type when TG is rising and I-131 is negative

Table I. Abbreviations: G: Codes for Medicare billing; TBA: To be announced; CNS: Central Nervous System; TG: Thyroglobulin.

Why, if FDG-PET fulfills so many requirements for cancer imaging, would the concept of PET/CT imaging be so intriguing? First, the concept of merging anatomical with molecular image information is simple and makes clinical sense. Molecular imaging benefits from anatomical landmarks and anatomic imaging without molecular information is superficial and simplistic in its nature. PET/CT has introduced to radiologists the importance of molecular imaging and helps to conceptualize the inherent limitations of size criteria for defining anatomical abnormalities as malignant or benign. The molecular information provided by PET enables radiologists for the first time to clearly characterize anatomical abnormalities as malignant or benign. On the other hand, molecular imaging benefits from the anatomical framework provided by CT. Hyper-metabolic lesions can now be assigned to specific "normal" or "abnormal" anatomical structures.

Townsend, Beyer, Nutt and their co-workers[35] pioneered the concept of PET/CT imaging by fusing near simultaneously obtained molecular and anatomical images. This vision resulted in the first PET/CT system consisting of a half-ring PET and single-slice CT system that was installed at the University of Pittsburgh in 1999. Early studies conducted with this device in many patients with head and neck and a variety of other cancers proved the feasibility of PET/CT.[36] The subsequent widespread acceptance of this technology has, however, not been driven by clinical research evidence. Only a few conclusive clinical studies have thus far been published to validate the clinical role of this rather expensive cancer imaging modality.

PET/CT reduces image acquisition times resulting in increased patient throughput.[37] Conventional PET utilized a transmission scan for photon attenuation correction using an external radiation source.[38] Completion of this transmission scan required 3- to 4-minutes/bed-position and thus up to 30 minutes for a whole body PET study. Differently, PET/CT imaging utilizes the whole body CT data for attenuation correction. Depending upon the number of CT detectors attenuation correction can now be performed within seconds to slightly more than a minute. Thus the whole body imaging time can be reduced by 50%. Such short imaging protocols have advantages. First, almost all patients can be studied in the "arms up" position thereby avoiding CT "beam hardening" artifacts. Secondly, shorter imaging times

are likely to reduce patient motion that can create problems for image fusion. Thirdly, short imaging protocols permit high utilization of the expensive equipment, i.e., patient throughput for any PET/CT system is at least 50% higher than for conventional PET systems. Fourth, shorter image acquisition protocols are convenient for patients. Even the addition of high resolution and contrast CT studies results in image acquisition times of less than 1 hour. Finally, cancer patients can now undergo a comprehensive anatomic and molecular work-up conveniently in a single study.

Beyond these procedural issues there are obvious clinical advantages of PET/CT over PET alone. PET/CT allows the localization of molecular alterations of cancer tissue, a task that is difficult to accomplish with PET alone. For instance, the level of mediastinal lymph node involvement in lung cancer patients cannot be determined reliably with PET alone. Appropriate localization of hypermetabolic foci to chest wall vs. lung, lung base vs. liver, neck vs. superior mediastinum and others might also have some impact on patient management. Exact lesion localization with PET/CT can also reduce the number of false positive and false negative PET findings as recently reported by Yap et al.[39] The impact of improved lesion localization on patient management remains to be elucidated.[6] It is however evident that patients for whom surgical or radiation treatment is contemplated need accurate localization of lesions, which requires exact anatomical information.

Clinical data are emerging that demonstrate an incremental value of PET/CT over PET alone in a variety of cancers. In a large study that included more than 200 patients with a variety of cancers PET/CT characterized 10% of equivocal PET lesions as definitely benign and classified 5% of equivocal lesions as definitely malignant. The authors concluded that PET/CT had an impact on both diagnostic and therapeutic aspects of patient management.[8]

A recent prospective study published in the New England Journal of Medicine[6] reported the diagnostic accuracy of integrated PET /CT in patients with non-small cell lung cancer. This study included 50 patients with non-small cell lung cancer and the staging accuracy of PET/CT was compared to visually correlated PET and CT as well as PET and CT alone. PET/CT had a significantly lower number of incorrectly assigned tumor stages than CT or PET alone, and the accuracy of PET/CT was superior to that of "visual" image fusion. Differently, with regards to lymph nodes, PET alone had the lowest number of incorrectly assigned stages. As expected the number of equivocal nodes by PET alone was higher than that for integrated PET/CT. PET/CT provided additional "important" information in 41% of the patients including localization of lymph nodes (n=9), precise evaluation of chest wall infiltration (n=3), correct differentiation between tumor and inflammation (n=7) and localization of distant metastases in 2 patients. Surprisingly, the accuracy of PET alone for staging of lung cancer appeared to be considerably lower than previously reported. This is likely explained by the introduction of an additional category for classifying metabolic lesions termed "correct classification but equivocal". Importantly, this study did not address prospectively whether the "additional important information" led to "important" changes in patient management. More and larger clinical trials will be required to establish possible advantages of PET/CT over PET and CT alone for each type of cancer.

Antoch et al.[40] reported a less dramatic impact of PET/CT on the lung cancer stage as derived from PET. PET/CT and PET staged mediastinal lymph nodes with a similar accuracy (93% versus 89%) but PET/CT resulted in treatment changes in 15% of the 27 patients.

In another study, 45 patients with colorectal cancer were imaged with PET/CT. PET/CT resulted in significantly improved reader conference and, more importantly, in an improved staging and restaging accuracy from 78% to 89%.[41] The same group, however, pointed to some limitations of PET/CT and reported significant mis-registration of lesions between PET and CT in six of 300 patients (2%).[42]

We have recently analyzed PET/CT studies obtained in more than 70 patients with breast cancer and 100 patients with lymphoma. Both studies (unpublished data) suggest that PET/CT changes the stage derived from PET in 5-15% of the patients. Recently published data in lymphoma patients appear to confirm that PET/CT impacts lymphoma staging only to a small degree.[43] In a study of 27 lymphoma patients PET/CT improved lesion localization, but did not significantly affect patient stage.

A large number of abstracts yet few published full research studies examined the incremental value of PET/CT over PET alone for staging and restaging of cancer. These preliminary data suggest increments in diagnostic and staging accuracy, reductions in the number of false positive and false negative findings and an increased reader confidence in PET findings.

Because PET can distinguish cancer tissue from necrosis PET/CT might result in improved radiation therapy planning. CT masses can consist of various tissue types such as inflammation, necrosis, scar and viable tumor. Exact localization of viable tumor components with FDG-PET can affect radiation target volumes and might alter radiation doses. Whether PET/CT-based radiation planning will improve outcome or quality of life of cancer patients is unknown and will be difficult to establish. This is because many end-stage cancer patients receive palliative radiation treatment and the aggressiveness of the underlying malignancy might outweigh any benefits of a more targeted radiation treatment. Moreover, large areas of "necrosis" appearing as hypometabolic tumor masses might contain isolated island of tumor cells which would remain untreated if the radiation target only includes viable, i.e., hyper-metabolic, tumor sections. For the same reasons, PET/CT is increasingly considered useful for biopsy planning.

In summary, dual modality PET/CT imaging has several advantages. It affords localization of molecular abnormalities to anatomical structures and reduces image acquisition times by 50% or more. The diagnostic accuracy of PET/CT appears to be superior to that of PET alone. More studies are needed to determine which specific cancer types benefit most from combined PET/CT imaging. The emergence of PET/CT requires a new look at training and educational requirements for nuclear medicine specialists, radiologists and technologists.

Nuclear medicine physicians need to be trained in cross-sectional anatomy while radiologists need to become familiar with molecular imaging. Cross training programs between X-ray and nuclear medicine technologists also need to be established.

Extensive discussions are underway to design PET/CT combinations that stand on their own as the cancer imaging modality of choice. How many CT detectors are necessary to provide a comprehensive metabolic and anatomic evaluation of cancer patients? Does the combination with PET really provide the best utilization of 16-slice CT scanners? Should 16 slice CT be reserved for cardiac applications because a comprehensive cardiac work-up including myocardial perfusion, coronary calcification, wall motion and non-invasive coronary angiography can be provided in one examination? Differing opinions have also been voiced regarding the optimal imaging protocols. One school of thought believes that CT image data should only be used for attenuation correction of PET and for localizing hypermetabolic lesions while others demand that the most elaborate contrast and high-resolution CT studies should be performed. Can "ultra fast" PET imaging protocols be established without compromising diagnostic quality to further reduce whole body PET/CT imaging times?

Many of these debates have not resulted in a consensus. However, sales of PET/CT have eclipsed those of stand-alone PET systems and all PET will be PET/CT in the near future. Training requirements for radiologists and nuclear medicine specialists will change and molecular imaging will emerge as the most powerful diagnostic modality in oncology.

References

1. Czernin J, Phelps ME. Positron emission tomography scanning: current and future applications. Annu Rev Med. 2002;53:89-112.
2. Gambhir SS, Czernin J, Schwimmer J, Silverman DH, Coleman RE, Phelps ME. A tabulated summary of the FDG PET literature. J Nucl Med. 2001;42(5 Suppl):1S-93S.
3. Jerusalem G, Beguin Y, Fasotte MF, Najjar F, Paulus P, Rigo P, Fillet G. Whole-body positron emission tomograpohy using 18F-fluorodeoxyglucose for posttreatment evaluation in Hodgkin's disease and non-Hodgkin's lymphoma has higher diagnostic and prognostic value than classical computed tomography scan imaging. Blood. 1999;94(2):429-433.
4. Spaepen K, Stroobants S, Dupont P, Van Steenweghen S, Thomas J, Vandenberghe P, Vanuytsel L, Bormans G, Balzarini J, De Wolf-Peeters C, Mortelmans L, Verhoef G. Prognostic value of positron emission tomoraphy (PET) with fluorine-18 fluorodeoxyglucose ([18F]FDG) after first-line chemotherapy in non-Hodgkin's lymphoma: is [18F]FDG-PET a valid alternative to conventional diagnostic methods? J Clin Oncol. 2001;19(2):414-419.
5. Vranjesevic D, Filmont JE, Meta J, Silverman DH, Phelps ME, Rao J, Valk PE, Czernin J. Whole-body 18F-FDG PET and conventional imaging for predicting outcome in previously treated breast cancer patients. J Nucl Med. 2002;43(3):325-329.
6. Lardinois D, Weder W, Hany TE, Kamel EM, Korom S, Seifert B, von Schulthess GK, Steinert HC. Staging of non–small-cell lung cancer with integrated positron-emission tomography and computed tomography. N Engl J Med. 2003;348(25):2500-2507.
7. Bar-Shalom R, Keidar Z, Guralnik L, Yefremov N, Sachs J, Israel O. Added value of fused PET/CT imaging with FDG in diagnostic imaging and management of cancer patients. J Nucl Med. 2002;43(5 Suppl):32P-33P.
8. Bar-Shalom R, Yefremov N, Guralnik L, Gaitini D, Frenkel A, Kuten A, Altman H, Keidar Z, Israel O. Clinical performance of PET/CT in evaluation of cancer: additional value for diagnostic imaging and patient management. J Nucl Med. 2003;44(8):1200-1209.
9. Antoch G, Freudenberg LS, Nemat AT, Beyer T, Bockisch A, Debatin JF. Preoperative staging of non-small cell lung cancer with dual-modality PET/CT imaging: a comparison with PET and CT. J Nucl Med. 2003;44(5 Suppl):172P.
10. Cohade C, Mourtzikos KA, Pannu HK, Leal JP, Bristow RE, Wahl RL. Direct comparison of PET and PET/CT in the detection of recurrent ovarian cancer. J Nucl Med. 2003;44(5 Suppl):129 P-130P.
11. Antoch G, Vogt FM, Freudenberg LS, Nazaradeh F, Goehde SC, Barkhausen J, Dahmen G, Bockisch A, Debatin JF, Ruehm SG. Whole-body dual-modality PET/CT and whole-body MRI for tumor staging in oncology. JAMA. 2003;290(24):3199-3206.
12. Warburg O, Posener K, Negelein E. VIII. The metabolism of cancer cells. Biochem Zeitschr. 1924;152:129-169.
13. Weber G. Enzymology of cancer cells (Part 1). N Engl J Med. 1977;296(9):486-492.
14. Weber G. Enzymology of cancer cells (Part 2). N Engl J Med. 1977;296(10):541-551.
15. Flier JS, Mueckler MJM, Usher P, Lodish HF. Elevated levels of glucose transport and transporter messenger RNA are induced by ras and src oncogenes. Science. 1987;235(4795):1492-1495.
16. Phelps ME, Hoffman EJ, Mullani NA, Ter-Pogossian MM. Application of annihilation coincidence detection to transaxial reconstruction tomography. J Nucl Med. 1975;16(3):210-224.
17. Zhao S, Kuge Y, Tsukamoto E, Mochizuki T, Kato T, Hikosaka K, Nakada K, Hosokawa M, Kohanawa M, Tamaki N. Fluorodeoxyglucose uptake and glucose transporter expression in experimental inflammatory lesions and malignant tumours: effects of insulin and glucose loading. Nucl Med Commun. 2002;23(6):545-550.
18. Pedersen MW, Holm S, Lund EL, Hojgaard L, Kristjansen PE. Coregulation of glucose uptake and vascular endothelial growth factor (VEGF) in two small-cell lung cancer (SCLC) sublines in vivo and in vitro. Neoplasia. 2001;3(1):80-87.
19. Brown RS, Leung JY, Fisher SJ, Frey KA, Ethier SP, Wahl RL. Intratumoral distribution of tritiated-FDG in breast carcinoma: correlation between Glut-1 expression and FDG uptake. J Nucl Med. 1996;37(6):1042-1047.
20. Bos R, van Der Hoeven JJ, van Der Wall E, van Der Groep P, van Diest PJ, Comans EF, Joshi U, Semenza GL, Hoekstra OS, Lammertsma AA, Molthoff CF. Biologic correlates of 18fluorodeoxyglucose uptake in human breast cancer measured by positron emission tomography. J Clin Oncol. 2002;20(2):379-387.
21. Buck AK, Halter G, Schirrmeister H, Kotzerke J, Wurziger I, Glatting G, Mattfeldt T, Neumaier B, Reske SN, Hetzel M. Imaging proliferation in lung tumors with PET: 18F-FLT versus 18F-FDG. J Nucl Med. 2003;44(9):1426-1431.

22. Adams S, Baum R, Stuckensen T, Bitter K, Hör G. Prospective comparison of 18F-FDG PET with conventional imaging modalities (CT, MRI, US) in lymph node staging of head and neck cancer. Eur J Nucl Med. 1998;25(9):1255-1260.

23. Rodriguez M, Rehn S, Ahlstrom H, Sundström C, Glimelius B. Predicting malignancy grade with PET in non-Hodgkin's lymphoma. J Nucl Med. 1995;36(10):1790-1796.

24. Yap CS, Valk P, Ariannejad M, Seltzer MA, Phelps ME, Gambhir SS, Czernin J. FDG-PET influences the clinical management of lymphoma patients. J Nucl Med. 2000;41(5 Suppl):70P.

25. Safaei A, Figlin R, Hoh CK, Silverman DH, Seltzer M, Phelps ME, Czernin J. The usefulness of F-18 deoxyglucose whole-body positron emission tomography (PET) for re-staging of renal cell cancer. Clin Nephrol. 2002;57(1):56-62.

26. Seltzer MA, Barbaric Z, Belldegrun A, Naitoh J, Dorey F, Phelps ME, Gambhir SS, Hoh CK. Comparison of helical computerized tomography, positron emission tomography and monoclonal antibody scans for evaluation of lymph node metastases in patients with prostate specific antigen relapse after treatment for localized prostate cancer. J Urol. 1999;162(4):1322-1328.

27. DeGrado TR, Coleman RE, Wang S, Baldwin SW, Orr MD, Robertson CN, Polascik TJ, Price DT. Synthesis and evaluation of 18F-labeled choline as an oncologic tracer for positron emission tomography: initial findings in prostate cancer. Cancer Res. 2001;61(1):110-117.

28. Shields AF, Grierson JR, Dohmen BM, Machulla HJ, Stayanoff JC, Lawhorn-Crews JM, Obradovich JE, Muzik O, Mangner TJ. Imaging proliferation in vivo with [F-18]FLT and positron emission tomography. Nat Med. 1998;4(11):1334-1336.

29. Tjuvajev JG, Chen SH, Joshi A, Joshi R, Guo ZS, Balatoni J, Ballon D, Koutcher J, Finn R, Woo SL, Blasberg RG. Imaging adenoviral-mediated herpes virus thymidine kinase gene transfer and expression in vivo. Cancer Res. 1999;59(20):5186-5193.

30. Gambhir SS, Barrio JR, Wu L, Iyer M, Namavari M, Satyamurthy N, Bauer E, Parrish C, MacLaren DC, Borghei AR, Green LA, Sharfstein S, Berk AJ, Cherry SR, Phelps ME, Herschman HR. Imaging of adenoviral-directed herpes simplex virus type 1 thymidine kinase reporter gene expression in mice with radiolabeled ganciclovir. J Nucl Med. 1998;39(11):2003-2011.

31. MacLaren DC, Toyokuni T, Cherry SR, Barrio JR, Phelps ME, Herschman HR, Gambhir SS. PET imaging of transgene expression. Biol Psychiatry. 2000;48(5):337-348.

32. Phelps ME. Positron emission tomography provides molecular imaging of biological processes. Proc Natl Acad Sci U S A. 2000;97(16):9226-9233.

33. Conti PS, Lilien DL, Hawley K, Keppler J, Grafton ST, Bading JR. PET and [18F]-FDG in oncology: a clinical update. Nucl Med Biol. 1996;23(6):717-735.

34. Hoh CK, Schiepers C, Seltzer MA, Gambhir SS, Silverman DH, Czernin J, Maddahi J, Phelps ME. PET in oncology: will it replace the other modalities? Semin Nucl Med. 1997;27(2):94-106.

35. Beyer T, Townsend DW, Brun T, Kinahan PE, Charron M, Roddy R, Jerin J, Young J, Byars L, Nutt R. A combined PET/CT scanner for clinical oncology. J Nucl Med. 2000;41(8):1369-1379.

36. Kluetz PG, Meltzer CC, Villemagne VL, Kinahan PE, Chander S, Martinelli MA, Townsend DW. Combined PET/CT imaging in oncology: impact on patient management. Clin Positron Imaging. 2000;3(6):223-230.

37. Halpern B, Dahlbom M, Vranjesevic D, Ratib O, Schiepers C, Silverman DH, Waldherr C, Quon A, Czernin J. LSO-PET/CT whole body imaging in 7 minutes: is it feasible? J Nucl Med. 2003;44(5 Suppl):380P-381P.

38. Dahlbom M, Hoffman EJ, Hoh CK, Schiepers C, Rosenqvist G, Hawkins RA, Phelps ME. Whole-body positron emission tomography: part I. Methods and performance characteristics. J Nucl Med. 1992;33(6):1191-1199.

39. Yap C, Quon A, Schiepers C, Dahlbom M, Ratib O, Czernin J. Additional Value of PET CT over PET for Cancer Staging and Lesion Localization. Radiology. 2003;229(Suppl):487.

40. Antoch G, Stattaus J, Nemat AT, Marnitz S, Beyer T, Kuehl H, Bockisch A, Debatin JF, Freudenberg LS. Non-small cell lung cancer: dual-modality PET/CT in preoperative staging. Radiology. 2003;229:526-533.

41. Cohade C, Osman M, Leal J, Wahl RL. Direct comparison of 18F-FDG PET and PET/CT in patients with colorectal carcinoma. J Nucl Med. 2003;44(11):1797-1803.

42. Osman MM, Cohade C, Nakamoto Y, Marshall LT, Leal JP, Wahl RL. Clinically significant inaccurate localization of lesions with PET/CT: frequency in 300 patients. J Nucl Med. 2003;44(2):240-243.

43. Freudenberg LS, Antoch G, Schutt P, Beyer T, Jentzen W, Muller SP, Gorges R, Nowrousian MR, Bockisch A, Debatin JF. FDG-PET/CT in re-staging of patients with lymphoma. Eur J Nucl Med Mol Imaging. 2003;In Press.

Normal Pattern and Common Pitfalls of FDG-PET Image Interpretation

M. Seltzer, C. Schiepers

Appropriate interpretation of PET and PET/CT images requires knowledge of normal glucose metabolic activity and it's variants throughout the body.

The following section introduces in detail expected and sometimes surprising norm variants as well as pitfalls for PET image interpretation.

The standard "whole body" PET scan for most oncology applications includes the neck, chest, abdomen, and pelvis (Figure 1). If a patient has a known or suspected site of malignancy in the head or in the lower extremities, the imaging field is expanded to include these regions. For melanoma patients, the entire body (top of head to bottom of feet) is routinely scanned so as to include all soft tissue and skeletal sites in the body. For the specific purpose of detecting brain metastases, a gadolinium-enhanced brain MRI should be the imaging modality of choice, as metastatic lesions can be missed by PET due to the relatively high glucose metabolic activity of cortical gray matter (typically 2.5 times the mean liver activity).

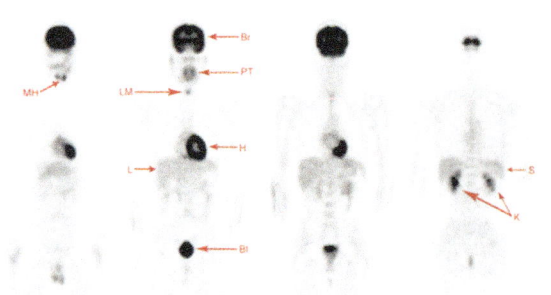

Figure 1. Normal whole body PET scan (coronal) from top of head to mid thighs. Br=brain, PT=pharyngeal tonsil, MH=Myelohyoid muscles, LM=Laryngeal muscles, H=heart, L=liver, S=spleen, K=kidney, Bl=bladder.

Head and Neck

Normal structures that typically exhibit a moderate degree of glucose metabolic activity include the lymphoid tissues of the palatine and pharyngeal tonsils, the salivary glands, and the myelohyoid muscles (Figures 2 and 3). A variable degree of activity is commonly seen in the laryngeal muscles. The muscles of mastication can be prominently seen in patients who have been eating or chewing gum within several hours of the tracer injection (Figure 4). In a small percentage of patients, diffusely increased thyroid activity is seen which could represent a clinical or subclinical presentation of a thyroiditis or

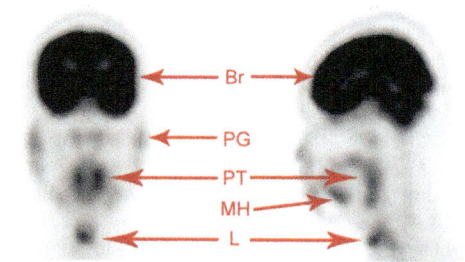

Figure 2. Normal head and neck metabolic anatomy (Left: coronal; right: sagittal). Br=brain, PG=Parotid gland, PT=pharyngeal tonsil, MH=myelohyoid muscles, L=laryngeal muscles.

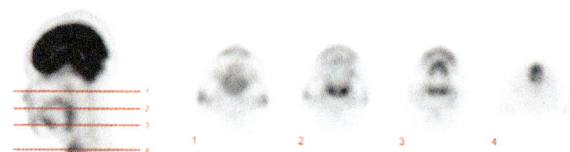

Figure 3. Corresponding transaxial image slices through the parotid glands, pharyngeal tonsils, myelohyoid muscles/sublingual glands, and vocal cords. Normal metabolic activity in the palatine and pharyngeal tonsils, myelohyoid muscles, parotid and sublingual glands, gingival mucosa, and vocal cords.

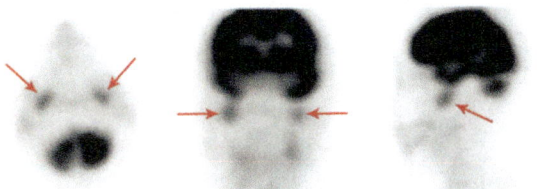

Figure 4. Pterygoid muscle activity (arrows) in a patient who was chewing gum just prior to FDG injection.

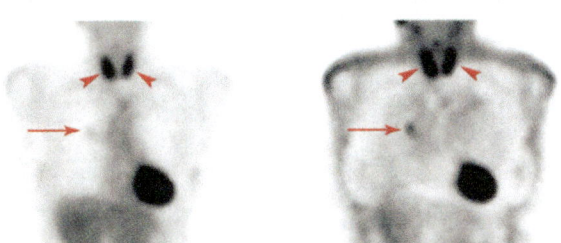

Figure 5. Diffuse thyroid activity (arrowheads) in a patient with known Hashimoto's thyroiditis and a recurrent lung cancer lesion in the right upper lobe. The non-attenuation corrected image (right) better shows the lesion in the medial portion of the right upper lung (arrows).

Graves' disease (Figure 5); this finding should be correlated with thyroid function tests.

Chest

The lungs normally have no significant metabolic activity (less than adjacent axillary soft tissue activity). The mediastinal blood pool activity is approximately 25% lower than the liver and similar in intensity to normal bone marrow activity. Areas of atelectasis and scarring can appear to have mildly increased activity relative to normal lung tissue (Figure 6). Asymptomatic granulomatous disease occasionally presents with markedly increased metabolic activity in the lungs and/or lymph nodes. Sarcoidosis, coccidiomycosis, histoplasmosis, and mycobacterial infection are common sources of benign inflammatory conditions seen on PET that can be indistinguishable from malignancy (Figure 7). Diffusely increased activity might be related to pleural effusion (Figure 8).

Breast tissue activity is normally less than mediastinal blood pool activity but can have a variable degree of intensity depending on the patient's age and hormonal factors (Figure 9). Normal thymus

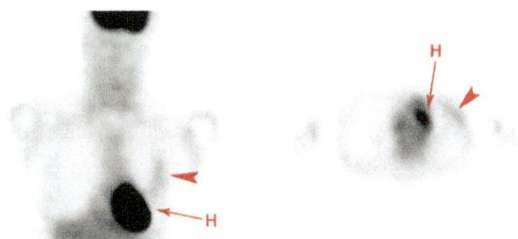

Figure 6. Diffuse activity in the anterior left lung which corresponds to an area of atelectasis and scarring in the lingula (arrowhead). H=heart.

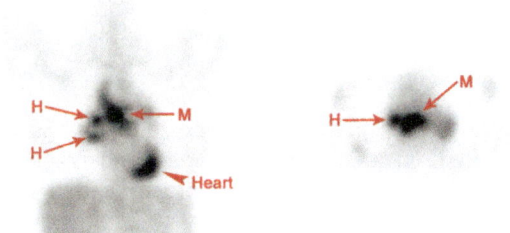

Figure 7. Metabolically active mediastinal (M) and hilar (H) adenopathy which was biopsy proven to be sarcoidosis.

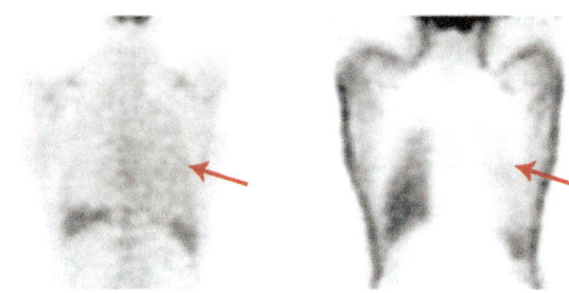

Figure 8. Mild diffusely increased metabolic activity on attenuation corrected image (left) which represents a large benign pleural effusion (arrow). On non-corrected image (right) this appears as a large area of absent activity.

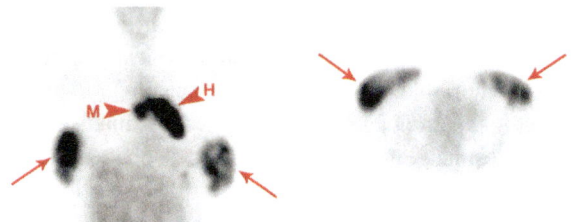

Figure 9. Intense breast activity (arrow) due to breast feeding in a 31 year old woman with newly diagnosed Hodgkin's lymphoma in the hilum (H) and mediastinum (M) (arrowhead).

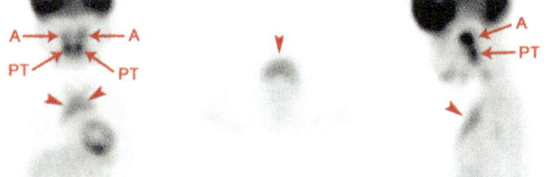

Figure 10. Normal thymus (arrowhead), pharyngeal tonsillar (PT), and adenoid (A) activity in a 7-year-old boy being evaluated for recurrent lymphoma.

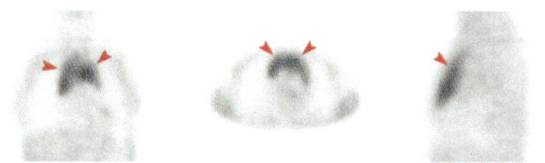

Figure 11. Benign thymic hyperplasia (biopsy proven after PET) in a 24-year-old woman who presented with progressive shortness of breath and a large anterior mediastinal mass.

activity is always seen in pre-pubertal children. Reactive thymus hyperplasia can be seen with varying degrees of intensity in young to middle aged adults who have recently received chemotherapy (typically within the first few months post-chemotherapy; Figures 10 and 11).

Abdomen

The liver and spleen exhibit a moderate degree of glycolytic activity. The adrenals are normally not seen on PET. Benign adrenal adenomas typically have activity equal to or less than the liver. Renally excreted activity pooling focally in the ureter can mimic a retroperitoneal lymph node metastasis. Diaphragmatic and intercostal muscle activity can be seen in patients who are hyperventilating or are hiccupping near the time of tracer injection (Figure 12). Focal physiologic bowel activity is most commonly seen in the cecal region but can appear elsewhere in the small and large bowel without clinical symptoms or identifiable abnormalities on anatomic imaging. Benign pathologic sources of focally intense gastrointestinal activity include gastroesophageal reflux (Figure 12), gastritis (Figure 13), diverticulitis, inflammatory bowel disease, abscess and hiatal hernia (Figure 14).

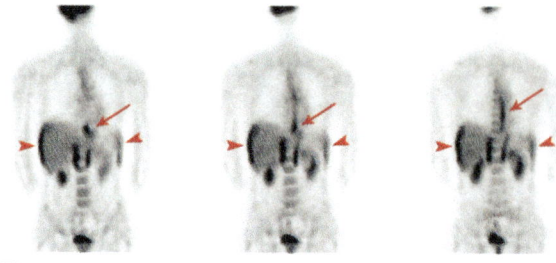

Figure 12. Reflux esophagitis (arrow) and diaphragmatic muscle activity (arrowhead) due to chronic hiccupping.

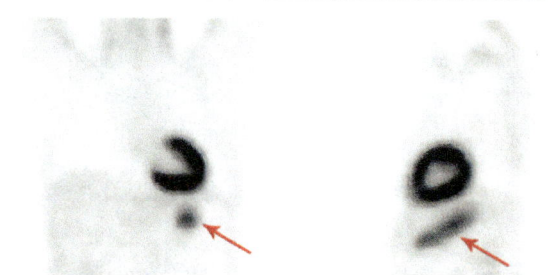

Figure 13. Endoscopically proven gastritis (arrow).

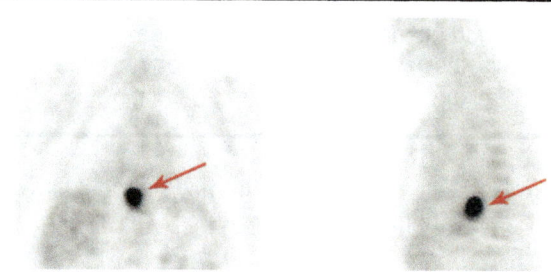

Figure 14. Large hiatal hernia with inflammation (arrow).

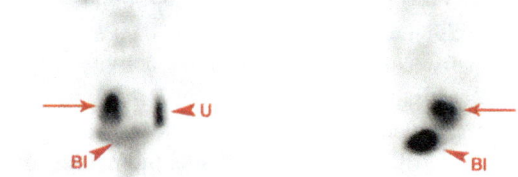

Figure 15. Large uterine fibroid (arrow) in the right pelvis and normal urine activity pooling in the left distal ureter (U) and bladder (Bl) (arrowhead).

Figure 16. Normal left testicular activity and absent right testicular activity (arrow) due to recent right inguinal orchiectomy.

Pelvis

Benign uterine fibroids have a variable degree of metabolic activity (typically heterogeneous or solid in appearance; Figure 15). The suspicion of a benign fibroid should be confirmed by ultrasound and/or MRI. A variable degree of physiologic bowel wall activity is frequently seen in both the small and large bowel. In men, physiologic testicular activity is commonly seen (Figure 16). The prostate is normally indistinguishable from adjacent perineal blood pool activity.

Skeleton

Benign healing fractures can have focally increased metabolic activity that can mimic a metastatic lesion (Figures 17 and 18). These lesions should be correlated with anatomic imaging (CT or MRI) in order to further characterize them as likely benign or malignant. Increased activity and also be

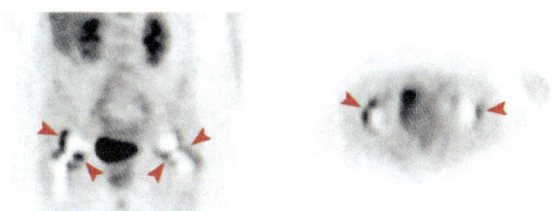

Figure 19. Non-specific activity (arrowhead) adjacent to the proximal femoral component of bilateral hip prostheses (placed 8 years ago). The patient was asymptomatic and had a recent bone scan which showed no evidence for loosening or infection.

present surrounding prosthetic devices (Figure 19). Diffusely increased bone marrow activity in the axial and proximal appendicular skeleton is commonly seen on post-chemotherapy PET scans due to ongoing or recent therapy with colony stimulating factors (erythropoietin and granulocyte colony stimulating factor; Figure 20). Diffuse splenic activity is occa-

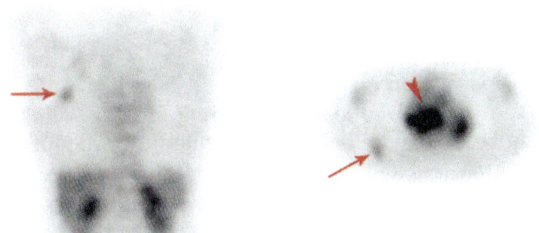

Figure 17. Right posterior upper rib fracture (arrow) confirmed by thin-section CT scan. Transaxial image also shows bulky mediastinal lymph node (arrowhead) activity which was proven by biopsy to be sarcoidosis.

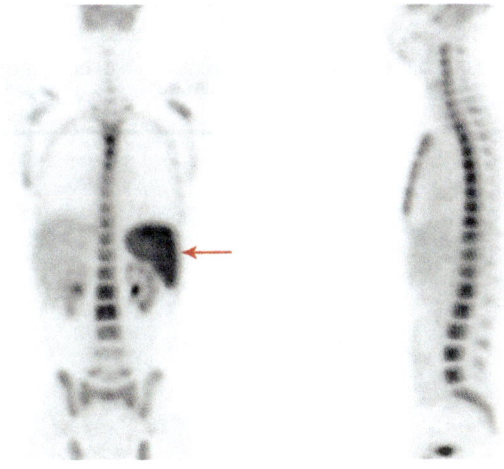

Figure 20. Diffuse bone marrow and splenic (arrow) hyperplasia due to recent treatment with granulocyte colony stimulating factor. Recovering bone marrow after chemotherapy has an identical appearance.

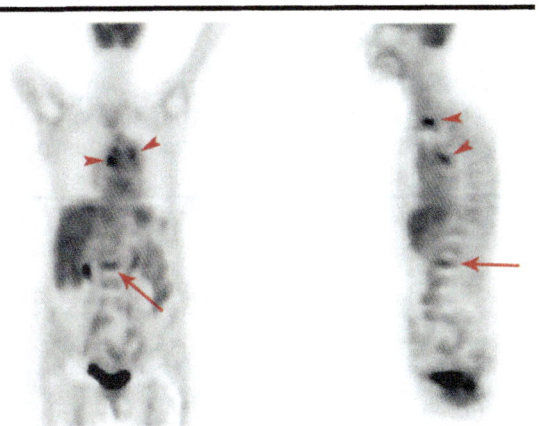

Figure 18. Lumbar spine compression fracture (arrow) in a patient with mediastinal lymph node metastases (arrowhead) due to lung cancer. MRI demonstrated a benign appearing L3 compression fracture.

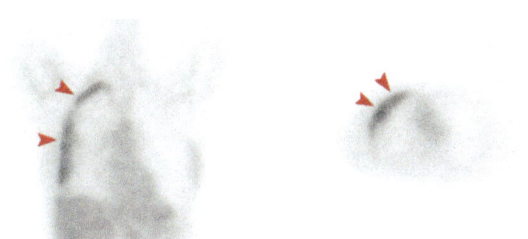

Figure 21. Radiation induced pleural inflammation (arrowhead): scan performed one week after completing radiation therapy to the right breast, axilla, and supraclavicular regions.

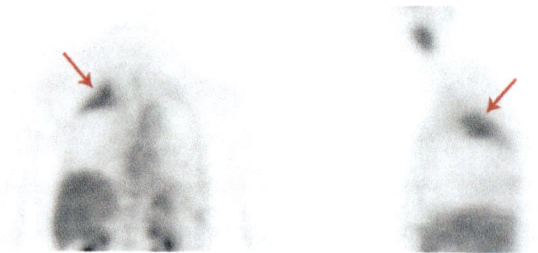

Figure 22. Radiation induced pneumonitis in the left upper lobe (arrow): scan performed 1 month after completing radiation therapy to the right supraclavicular region.

---

sionally seen as a response to therapy with granulocyte colony stimulating factor (Figure 20).

Treatment Effects

Post-surgical and post-radiation induced inflammatory changes are usually easily recognizable but can potentially mask the presence of malignancy in the previously treated field (Figures 21 and 22). These changes typically persist for several months post-therapy.

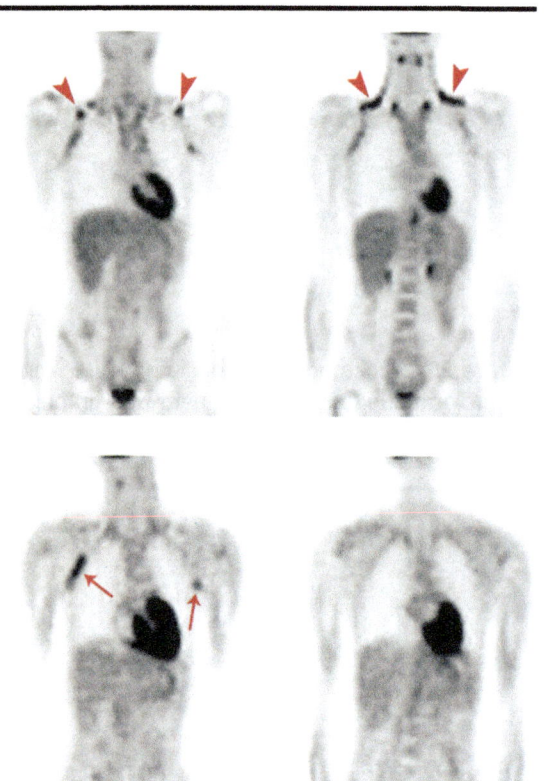

Figure 23. Initial staging exam in a 17-year-old boy with biopsy proven Hodgkin's lymphoma in the right

axilla. Top: a pattern of multifocal skeletal muscle and/or brown fat uptake is suggested in the periclavicular, mediastinal, and paraspinal (cervical and lower thoracic) regions (arrowhead). Bottom: repeat scan one day later with alprazolam premedication shows near complete resolution of the previously noted multifocal pattern. There remains focally intense activity in the right axilla and there is a solitary intense focus in the left axilla which represents a site of previously unsuspected lymphoma (arrow).

Brown Fat and Muscle

FDG accumulation in skeletal muscle and/or brown fat can occur with variable degrees of intensity in multiple sites of the body —- most commonly seen in the neck, mediastinum, and paraspinal locations (Figure 23). This pattern is usually easily recognizable but in some cases can mask or mimic the presence of a malignant process. Pre-medication with a muscle relaxant such as alprazolam is an effective method of suppressing both skeletal muscle and brown fat activity.

Non-Attenuation Corrected Images

Review of non-attenuation corrected images can be extremely helpful, particularly for identifying small lesions within the lungs or lesions near peripheral interfaces such as the lung/mediastinum, lung/chest wall, and lung/liver (Figures 24 and 25).

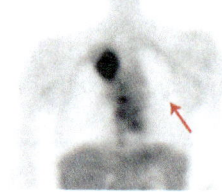 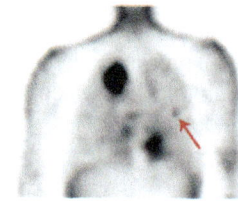

Figure 24. Right upper lobe cancer with an 8 mm diameter metastatic lesion in the left lower lobe (arrow) which is better seen on non-attenuation corrected images.

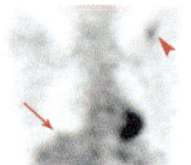 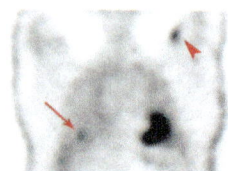

Figure 25. Solitary pulmonary nodule of 1.5 cm diameter (arrow) in the right lung base (subsequently biopsy confirmed adenocarcinoma) which is better seen on non-attenuation corrected image (right). Focal activity in the left shoulder (arrowhead) most likely represents a benign musculoskeletal inflammatory process such as tendonitis or bursitis.

Summary

Proper PET image interpretation requires a knowledge of the normal biodistribution of FDG throughout the body, and of the variable degree of FDG uptake that can occur in a variety of benign processes as exemplified in this chapter. In many cases, the pattern of FDG uptake can strongly suggest a benign versus malignant process. In other cases, the pattern is entirely non-specific and the abnormalities seen on PET must be compared to findings on anatomic imaging tests such as CT or MRI in order to further characterize them as likely malignant or benign.

Suggested Reading

Vesselle HJ, Miraldi FD. FDG PET of the retroperitoneum: normal anatomy, variants, pathologic conditions, and strategies to avoid diagnostic pitfalls. Radiographics. 1998;18(4):805-823.

Shreve PD, Anzai Y, Wahl RL. Pitfalls in oncologic diagnosis with FDG PET imaging: physiologic and benign variants. Radiographics. 1999;19(1):61-77.

Heller MT, Meltzer CC, Fukui MB, Rosen CA, Chander S, Martinelli MA, Townsend DW. Superphysiologic FDG uptake in the non-paralyzed vocal cord. Resolution of a false-positive PET result with combined PET-CT imaging. Clin Positron Imaging. 2000;3(5):207-211.

Pitman AG, Binns DS, Ciavarella F, Hicks RJ. Inadvertent 2-deoxy-2-[18F]fluoro-D-glucose lymphoscintigraphy: a potential pitfall characterized by hybrid PET-CT. Mol Imaging Biol. 2002;4(4):276-278.

Hany TF, Heuberger J, von Schulthess GK. Iatrogenic FDG foci in the lungs: a pitfall of PET image interpretation. Eur Radiol. 2003;13(9):2122-2127.

Chapter 1

PET/CT Image Artifacts

Cases:

Chapter 1

PET/CT Image Artifacts

The merging of PET and CT into one system promises to improve the management of cancer patients as outlined in the previous chapters. Several terms are used to describe such systems: combined gantry, hybrid scanner, in-line system, integrated systems or mechanical image fusion systems.

The individual components of integrated PET/CT systems can introduce artifacts when images are combined and fused. Theoretically, the number of artifacts introduced by one component could be reduced with integrated PET/CT systems, because one of the two modalities might be able to resolve a problem introduced by the other. Since the two systems are integrated and heavily dependent on each other, specific problems arise in addition to the well-known artifacts and normal variants of the individual imaging systems.

Table 1 lists an overview of the types of artifacts that may be distinguished related to source.

ARTIFACTS AND VARIANTS RELATED TO COMBINED PET/CT IMAGING	
1 Technology related:	System or imaging modality dependent
2 Patient related:	Motion, moving structures (stomach, bowel) or pulsing organs (heart, lung)
3 Operator related:	Imaging protocol dependent, i.e. timing of contrast injection, FDG uptake interval
4 Algorithm related:	Type of image reconstruction used, e.g. filtered backprojection vs. iteratiove reconstruction methods, segmentation protocols, attenuation correction methods

The technology, i.e. detectors, radiation source, electronics, etc., determines spatial and temporal resolution of the modalities. Bed motion control, pitch, etc. have an effect on the longitudinal axis sampling and determine the z-axis resolution in CT. The combination together with the final reconstruction software determines the three dimensional spatial resolution of the system. The hardware electronics determine temporal resolution of the PET acquisition.

Motion and movement artifacts are difficult to resolve and are due to involuntary and uncontrollable movement of internal organs, as well as preventable shift and sliding because of patient discomfort during scanning. Artifacts induced by respiration are inevitable and cannot be circumvented when patients are imaged over an extended period of time.

The following Table 2 categorizes artifacts topographically.

TOPOGRAPHICAL DISCUSSION OF ARTIFACTS AND VARIANTS

Head
- Attenuation artifacts due to dentures and fillings in the oral cavity

Neck
- Rotation in the cervical spine between CT and PET
- Tense striated muscles
- Activated brown fat
- Vocal cords and thyroid gland variations
- Pharyngeal muscles

Chest
- Breathing
- Segmentation problems due to shift between CT and PET acquisition
- Attenuation artifacts due to moving diaphragm and liver dome
- Foreign body such as pacemaker, AED, catheter

Abdomen
- Movement of internal organs and bowel
- Oral and intra-venous contrast artifacts
- GI tract mucosal activity

Pelvis
- Empty or full bladder
- Uterine myomas
- Pelvic inflammatory diseases

Skeleton
- Bone marrow activation or expansion related to chemotherapy
- Osteo-arthritis
- Healing fractures
- Degenerative changes

Discussion of the normal variation in FDG uptake in the human body are presented in chapter 7 and basic knowledge of the normal FDG distribution is a prerequisite. Thus, normal variants can be recognized and pitfalls identified. Recognition of PET, CT and PET/CT artifacts is of critical importance for the appropriate interpretation of combined PET/CT studies. The selected literature listed below provides deeper insights into the nature and origin of artifacts encountered when reviewing PET/CT images.

Suggested Reading

Beyer T, Townsend DW, Brun T, Kinahan PE, Charron M, Roddy R, Jerin J, Young J, Byars L, Nutt R. A combined PET/CT scanner for clinical oncology. J Nucl Med. 2000;41(8):1369-1379.

Skalski J, Wahl RL, Meyer CR. Comparison of mutual information-based warping accuracy for fusing body CT and PET by 2 methods: CT mapped onto PET emission scan versus CT mapped onto PET transmission scan. J Nucl Med. 2002;43(9):1184-1187.

Antoch G, Freudenberg LS, Egelhof T, Stattaus J, Jentzen W, Debatin JF, Bockisch A. Focal tracer uptake: a potential artifact in contrast-enhanced dual-modality PET/CT scans. J Nucl Med. 2002;43(10):1339-1342.

Bujenovic S, Mannting F, Chakrabarti R, Ladnier D. Artifactual 2-deoxy-2-[18F]fluoro-D-glucose localization surrounding metallic objects in a PET/CT scanner using CT-based attenuation correction. Mol Imaging Biol. 2003;5(1):20-22.

Cohade C, Osman M, Nakamoto Y, Marshall LT, Links JM, Fishman EK, Wahl RL. Initial experience with oral contrast in PET/CT: phantom and clinical studies. J Nucl Med. 2003;44(3):412-416.

Goerres GW, Burger C, Kamel E, Seifert B, Kaim AH, Buck A, Buehler TC, von Schulthess GK. Respiration-induced attenuation artifact at PET/CT: technical considerations. Radiology. 2003;226(3):906-910.

Goerres GW, Burger C, Schwitter MR, Heidelberg TN, Seifert B, von Schulthess GK. PET/CT of the abdomen: optimizing the patient breathing pattern. Eur Radiol. 2003;13(4):734-739.

Kamel EM, Burger C, Buck A, von Schulthess GK, Goerres GW. Impact of metallic dental implants on CT-based attenuation correction in a combined PET/CT scanner. Eur Radiol. 2003;13(4):724-728.

Osman MM, Cohade C, Nakamoto Y, Wahl RL. Respiratory motion artifacts on PET emission images obtained using CT attenuation correction on PET-CT. Eur J Nucl Med Mol Imaging. 2003;30(4):603-606.

Koh DM, Cook GJ, Husband JE. New horizons in oncologic imaging. N Engl J Med. 2003;348(25):2487-2488.

Cohade C, Wahl RL. Applications of positron emission tomography/computed tomography image fusion in clinical positron emission tomography-clinical use, interpretation methods, diagnostic improvements. Semin Nucl Med. 2003;33(3):228-237.

Kinahan PE, Hasegawa BH, Beyer T. X-ray-based attenuation correction for positron emission tomography/computed tomography scanners. Semin Nucl Med. 2003;33(3):166-179.

Slomka PJ, Dey D, Przetak C, Aladl UE, Baum RP. Automated 3-dimensional registration of stand-alone 18F-FDG whole-body PET with CT. J Nucl Med. 2003;44(7):1156-1167.

Townsend DW, Beyer T, Blodgett TM. PET/CT scanners: a hardware approach to image fusion. Semin Nucl Med. 2003;33(3):193-204.

Nehmeh SA, Erdi YE, Kalaigian H, Kolbert KS, Pan T, Yeung H, Squire O, Sinha A, Larson SM, Humm JL. Correction for oral contrast artifacts in CT attenuation-corrected PET images obtained by combined PET/CT. J Nucl Med. 2003;44(12):1940-1944.

Cardiac Pacemaker

Clinical History

A 66-year-old patient with T-cell lymphoma is evaluated 3 months after chemotherapy. A cardiac pacemaker had been placed several years prior to this study.

PET/CT indication: Restaging.

Findings

Normal study except for increased FDG uptake in the left supraclavicular region on attenuation-corrected images but not on uncorrected images.

Teaching Point

Metallic implants such as cardiac pacemakers result in inappropriate attenuation correction and "pseudo-increase" of FGD uptake when CT data are used for attenuation correction. Uncorrected PET images demonstrate a "hypometabolic" area due to photon attenuation by the pacemaker device. Thus, in order to differentiate between artifacts and true increased FDG uptake, both corrected and uncorrected images need to be reviewed in patients with metallic implants.

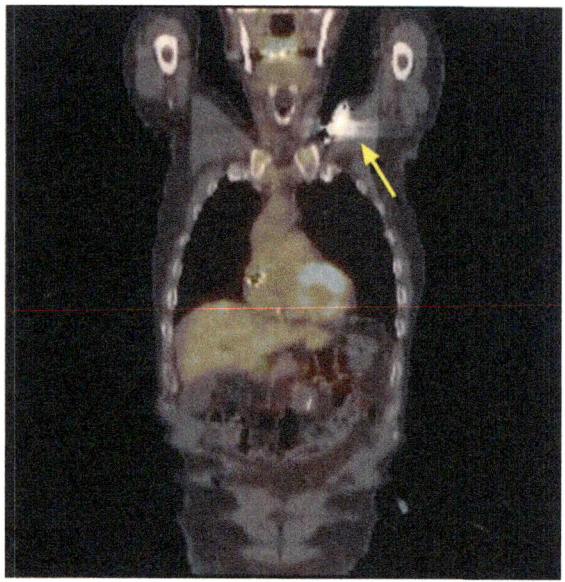

Image 1. Fused coronal image showing the attenuation artifact induced by the metallic pacemaker resulting in "pseudo-increase" of FDG uptake (arrow).

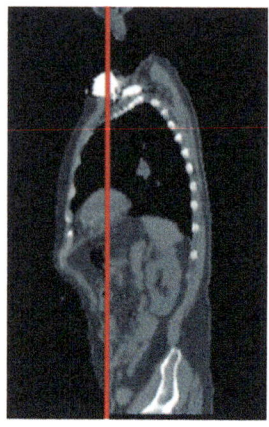

Image 1 (coronal)

Localizer

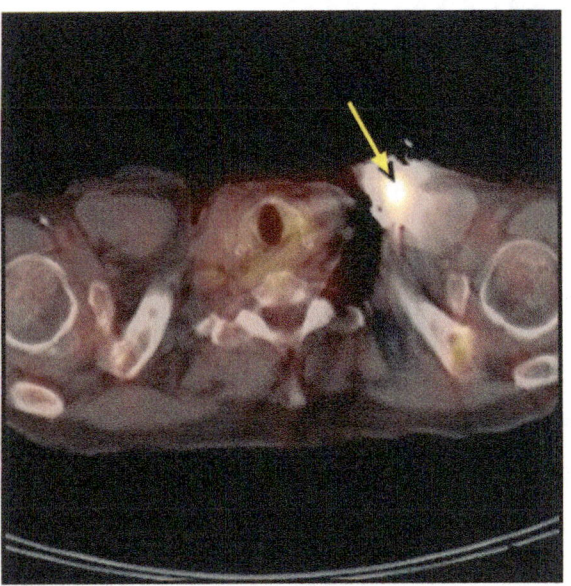

Image 2 (axial)

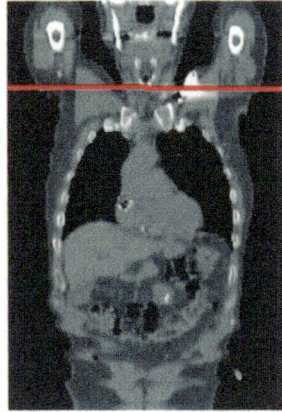

Localizer

Image 2. Axial image showing the "pseudo-increase" in FDG uptake induced by the attenuation artifact from the metallic pacemaker.

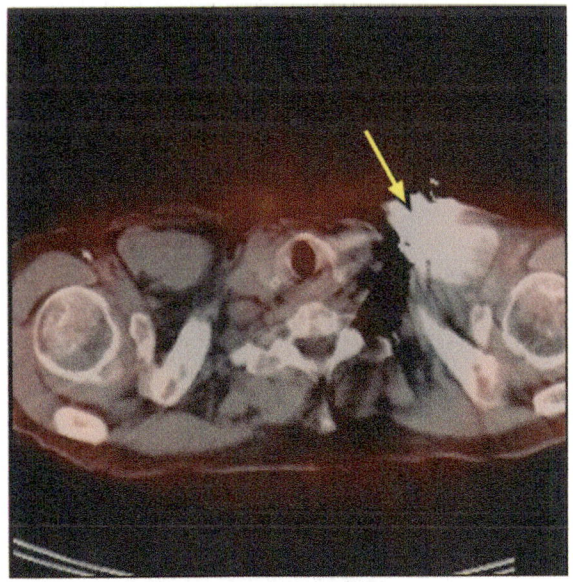

Image 3 (axial)

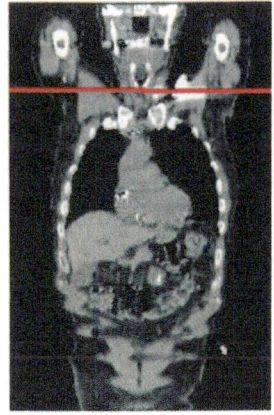

Localizer

Image 3. Absent FDG uptake in the pacemaker area on the fused uncorrected image.

Hip Prosthesis

Clinical History

81-year-old female with breast cancer and left hip prosthesis.

PET/CT indication: Restaging.

Findings

Pseudo-increase in FDG uptake is noted in the region of the left hip on corrected images. This is due to inappropriate attenuation correction in the region of the metallic implant. Uncorrected images revealed normal glucose metabolic activity.

Teaching Point

For many reasons, both corrected and uncorrected PET images should be reviewed. This is particularly important in patients with metallic implants and in whom CT data are used for attenuation correction. In these patients, inappropriate attenuation correction results in pseudo-FDG uptake.

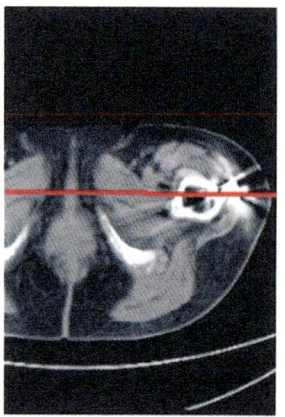

Image 1. Fused coronal image with "pseudo FDG uptake" in the region of the left hip prosthesis.

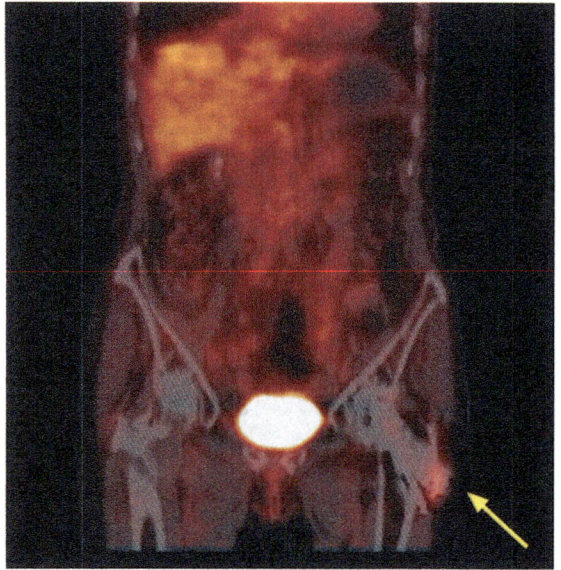

Image 1 (coronal)

Localizer

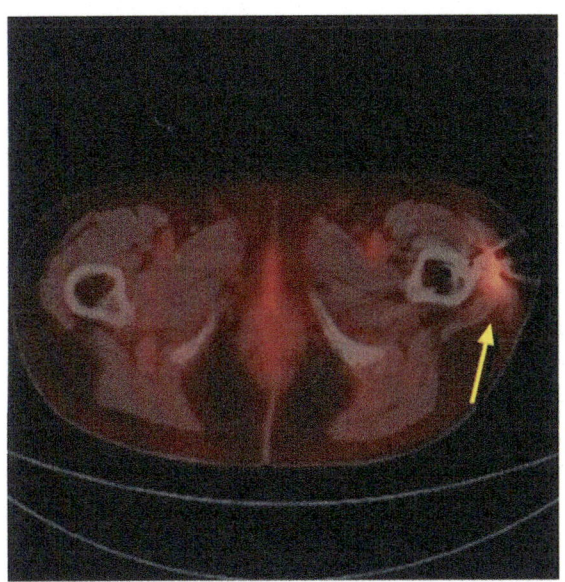

Image 2 (axial)

Image 2. Fused axial image demonstrating the "pseudo-FDG uptake". Uncorrected image revealed normal glucose metabolic activity (image not shown here). Corresponding axial CT image demonstrated an artifact induced by metal.

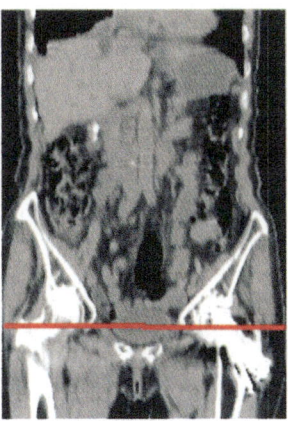

Localizer

Image 3. Corresponding axial CT image demonstrating an artifact induced by metal.

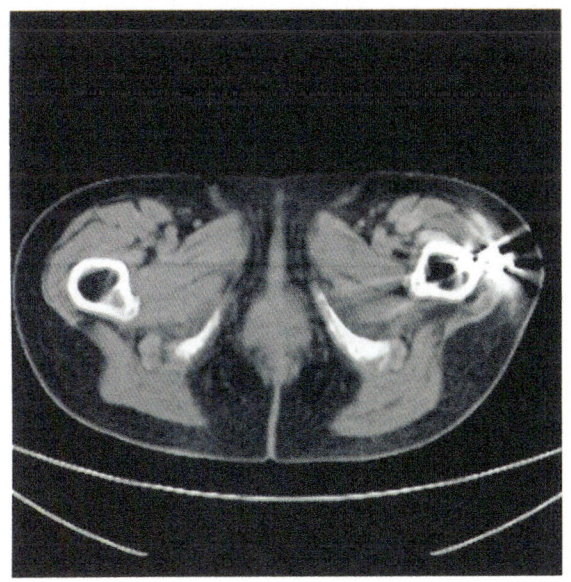

Image 3 (axial)

Dental Artifact

Clinical History

75-year old patient with head and neck cancer.

PET/CT indication: Restaging after treatment

Findings

Increased uptake is present in the region of maxilla and mandible on CT corrected PET images. Uncorrected images exhibit normal FDG distribution in this region.
No abnormalities consistent with residual cancer are identified.

Teaching Point

Metallic objects result in over-correction for photon attenuation with subsequent generation of "pseudo-FDG" uptake. This pitfall is easily avoided by inspecting uncorrected PET mages in all patients.

Image 1. Axial image depicting pseudo-FDG uptake due to metallic dental implant (arrows)

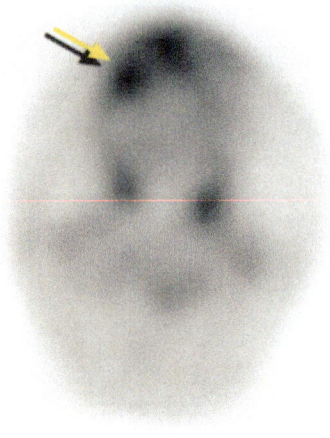

Image 1 (axial)

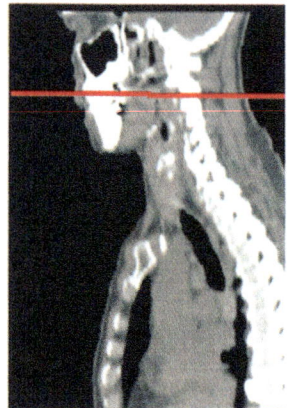

Localizer

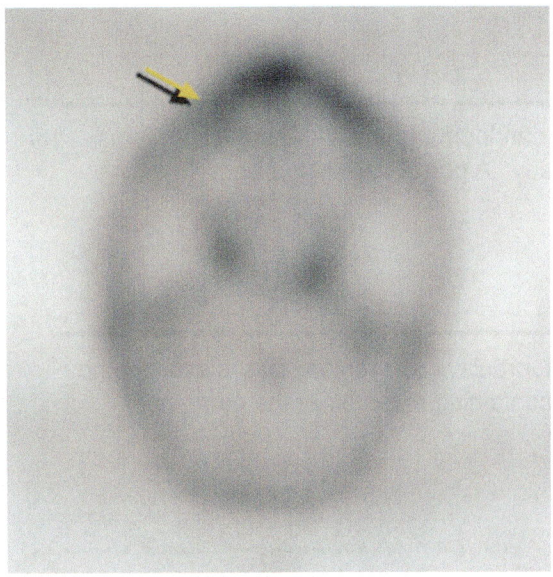

Image 2. Axial Image depicting pseudo-FDG uptake due to artifacts metallic dental implant (arrow)

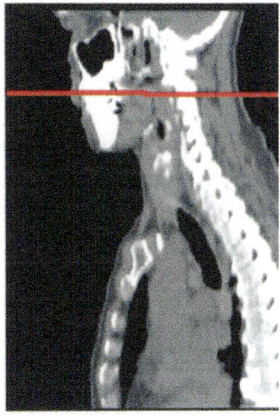

Image 2 (axial)   **Localizer**

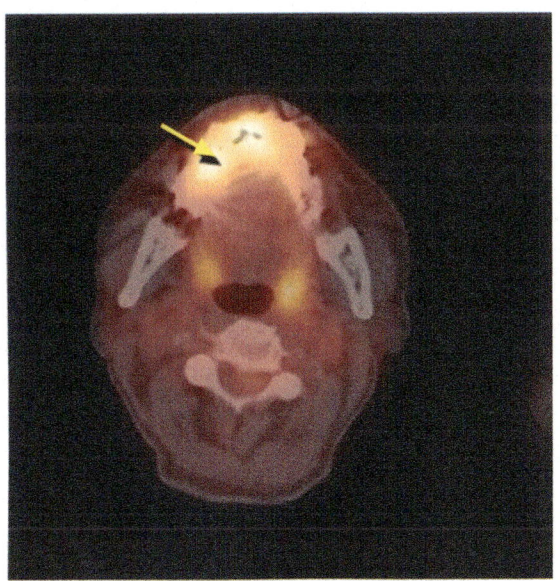

Image 3. Fused axial image of non-attenuation corrected FDG-PET without artifactual FDG uptake.

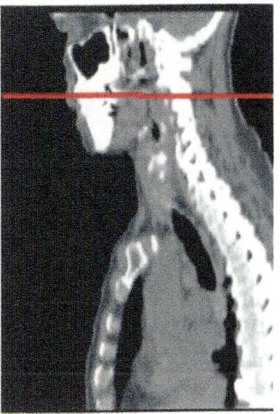

Image 3 (axial)   **Localizer**

Permanent Central Intravenous Line Artifact

Clinical History

78-year-old male with history of non-small cell lung carcinoma of the left upper lobe, status post left upper lobectomy, radiation and chemotherapy. A port-A-cath is in place.

PET/CT indication: Restaging.

Findings

Focus of mildly increased FDG uptake in the right supraclavicular region. This is explained by over-correction for photon attenuation in the metal-containing reservoir of the permanent intravenous line (Port-A-Cath).

Teaching Point

Metallic implants such as metal-containing reservoirs can result in inappropriate attenuation correction and "pseudo-increase" of FDG uptake when CT data are used for attenuation correction. Uncorrected PET images demonstrate a "hypometabolic" area due to photon attenuation by the device. Thus, in order to differentiate between artifacts and true increased FDG uptake, both corrected and uncorrected images need to be reviewed in patients with metallic implants.

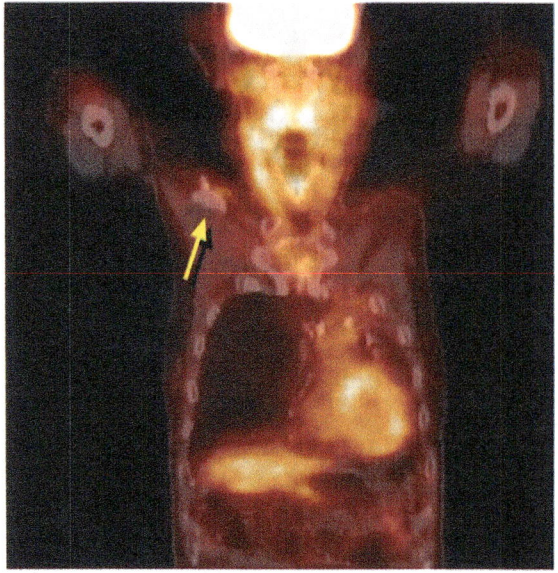

Image 1 (coronal)

Image 1. Fused coronal image showing the localization of the reservoir generating "pseudo FDG uptake" artifact.

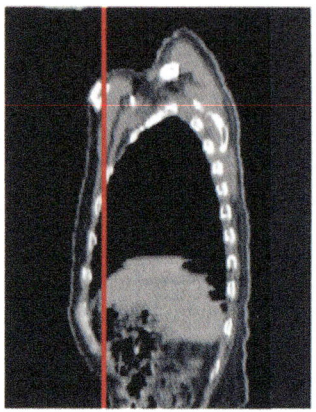

Localizer

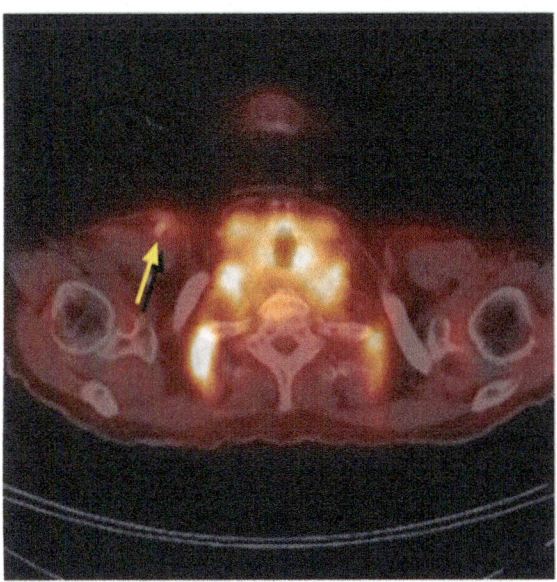

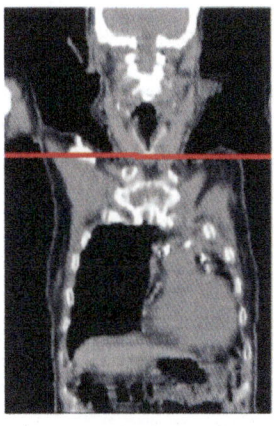

Images 2. Fused attenuation corrected axial image demonstrating mild "pseudo FDG uptake" in the region of the reservoir.

Image 2 (axial)　　　　　**Localizer**

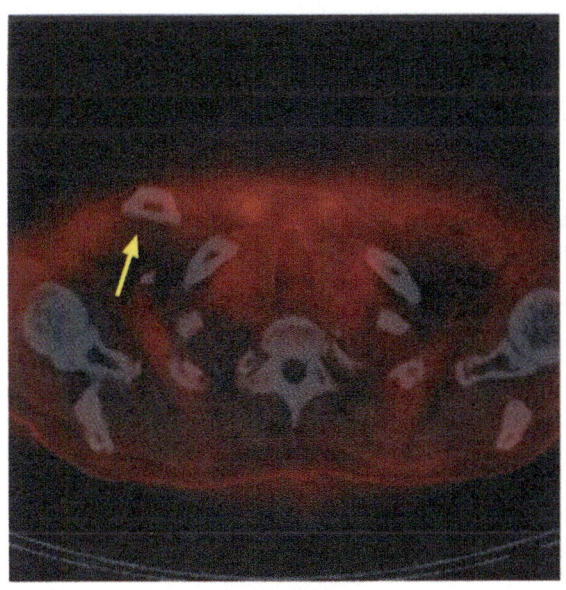

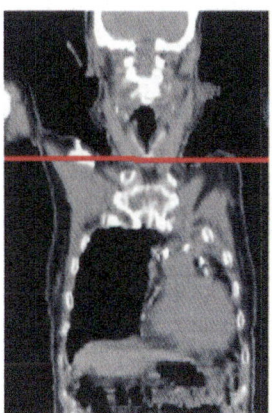

Image 3. Fused axial image of non-attenuation corrected FDG-PET showing the absence of FDG uptake in the region of the reservoir.

Image 3 (axial)　　　　　**Localizer**

Respiratory Motion Artifact

Clinical History

68-year-old male with history of Non-Hodgkin's Lymphoma status post left nephrectomy and chemotherapy.

PET/CT indication: Restaging.

Findings

Increased FDG uptake in lymph nodes posterior to the right main stem bronchus and in the AP window are consistent with infection or an inflammatory process. Liver "mushroom" artifact due to respiratory motion is noted.

Teaching Point

The "mushroom artifact" results in incorrect attenuation correction from CT images acquired during respiratory motion and thus inducing an artifact on PET images at the liver-lung interface. Review of uncorrected PET images will help to avoid misinterpretation.

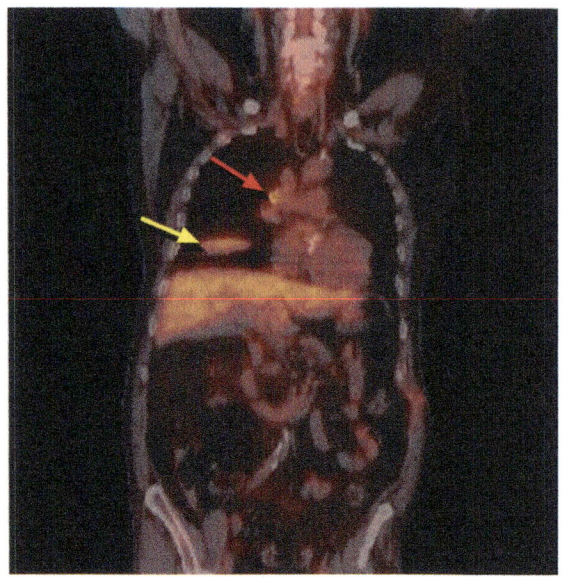

Image 1 (coronal)

Image 1. Fused coronal images depicting the mushroom artifact (yellow arrow) and focally increased activity in the right mediastinum (red arrow)

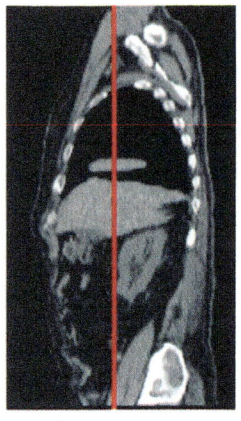

Localizer

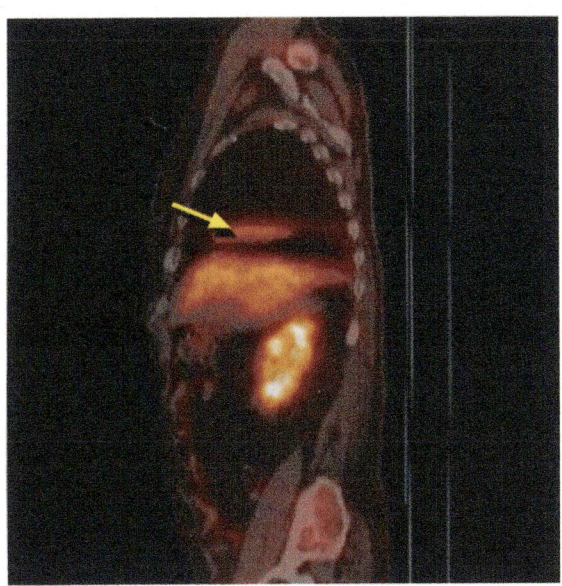

Image 2. Fused sagittal image of attenuation-corrected PET depicting the respiratory "mushroom" artifact (arrow).

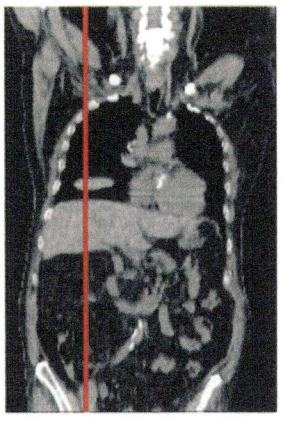

Image 2 (sagittal)

Localizer

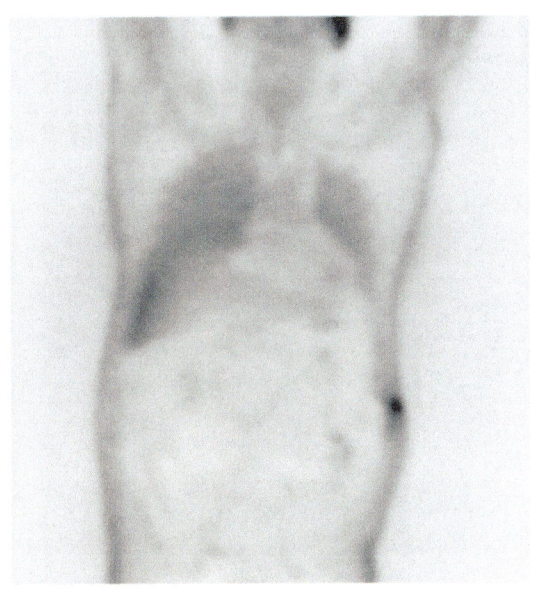

Image 3. Coronal image of uncorrected PET depicting the absence of respiratory "mushroom" artifact.

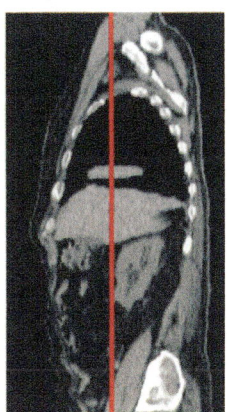

Image 3 (coronal)

Localizer

Chapter 2

Physiological Variants

Cases:

Chapter 2

Physiological Variants

Several interesting physiological variants have been identified with PET/CT imaging. Foremost among these is the identification of brown fat as FDG-avid tissue. Brown fat is heat-producing tissue that occurs more frequently in young patients and the degree of glucose metabolic activity appears to be related to temperature. FDG uptake in brown fat occurs most frequently in the supra-clavicular region but can also be seen as perivascular fat in the mediastinum. Prior to PET/CT increased uptake was always attributed to FDG uptake in striated muscle. More detailed information is provided in chapter 7.

Suggested Reading

Hany TF, Gharehpapagh E, Kamel EM, Buck A, Himms-Hagen J, von Schulthess GK. Brown adipose tissue: a factor to consider in symmetrical tracer uptake in the neck and upper chest region. Eur J Nucl Med Mol Imaging. 2002;29(10):1393-1398.

Cohade C, Osman M, Pannu HK, Wahl RL. Uptake in supra-clavicular area fat ("USA-Fat"): description on 18F-FDG PET/CT. J Nucl Med. 2003;44(2):170-176.

Cohade C, Mourtzikos KA, Wahl RL. "USA-Fat": prevalence is related to ambient outdoor temperature-evaluation with 18F-FDG PET/CT. J Nucl Med. 2003;44(8):1267-1270.

Yeung HW, Grewal RK, Gonen M, Schoder H, Larson SM. Patterns of 18F-FDG uptake in adipose tissue and muscle: a potential source of false-positives for PET. J Nucl Med. 2003;44(11):1789-1796.

Brown Fat

Clinical History

12-year-old male patient who underwent thyroidectomy with radical neck dissection followed by multiple radio-iodine treatments for thyroid cancer.

PET/CT indication: Restaging.

Findings

Several foci of intense FDG uptake are located in the bilateral supraclavicular region. Co-registration with CT revealed that the increased FDG uptake was localized to fat.

Teaching Point

Brown fat, present in children and more frequently in young female adults can complicate the interpretation of FDG-PET studies. Brown fat produces heat and exhibits increased rates of glucose metabolic activity. Interestingly, brown fat activity was markedly reduced after mild sedation. The reasons for this phenomenon are not completely understood.

Image 1. Coronal fused PET/CT image demonstrating intense glucose metabolic activity of the brain, supraclavicular region (arrows) and renal collecting system.

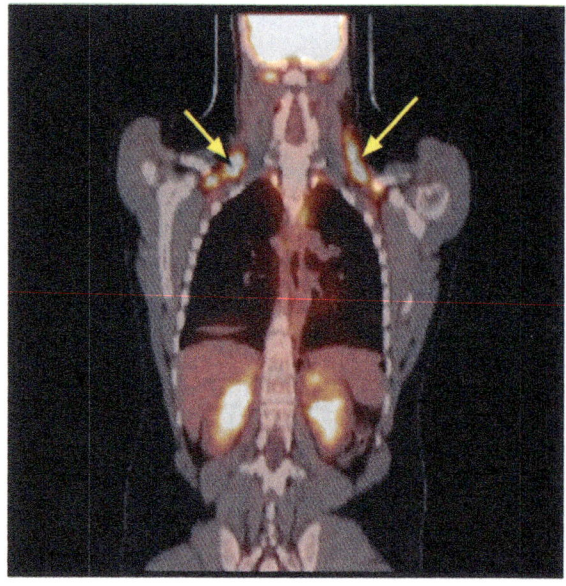

Image 1 (coronal)

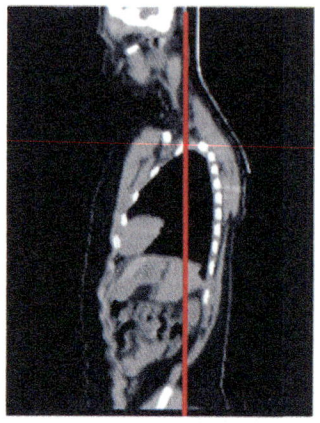

Localizer

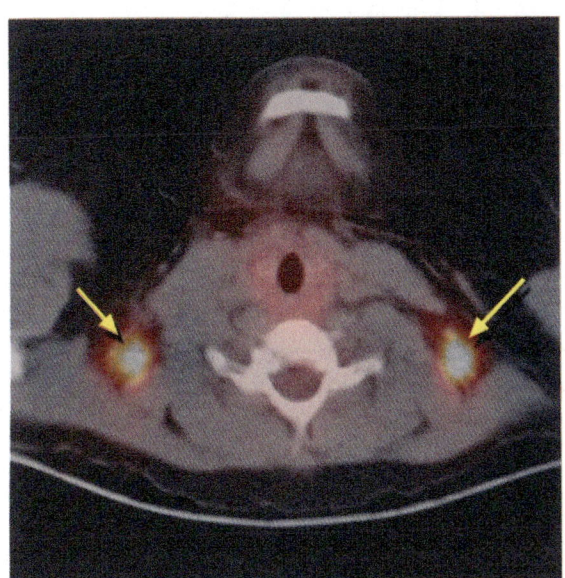

Image 2. Fused axial image with intense glucose metabolic activity localized to brown fat (see arrows).

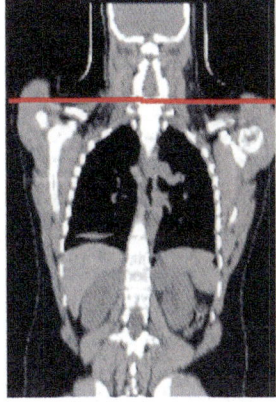

Image 2 (axial)

Localizer

Vocal Cord Activity

Clinical History

59-year-old female with a history of left ocular lymphoma.

PET/CT indication: Restaging.

Findings

No evidence for FDG avid lymphoma. The increased FDG uptake in the neck is due to vocal cord activity.

Teaching Point

Head and neck lymphomas as well as other head and neck cancer pose a diagnostic dilemma for PET, CT and MRI alone. This is due to the complex anatomy of this region as well as asymmetric glucose metabolic activity after surgery or radiation. In the current study, PET/CT ruled out tumor recurrence. Increased FDG uptake was related to normal vocal cord activity.

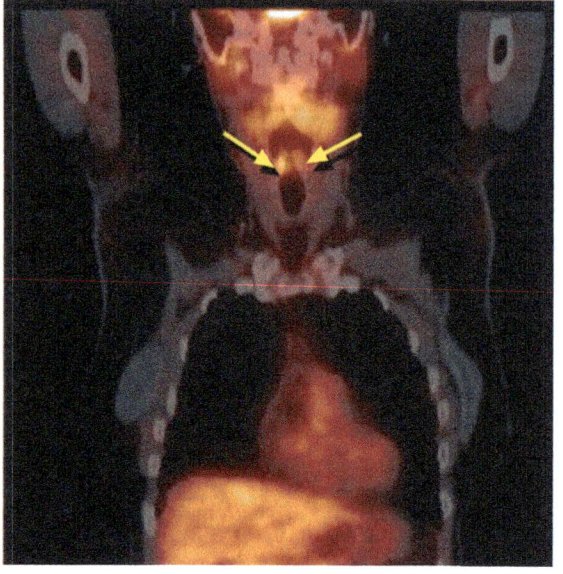

Image 1. Fused coronal image demonstrating increased metabolic activity of the vocal cords.

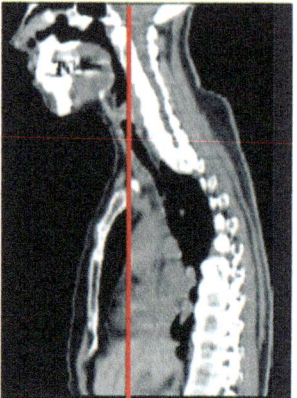

Image 1 (coronal)

Localizer

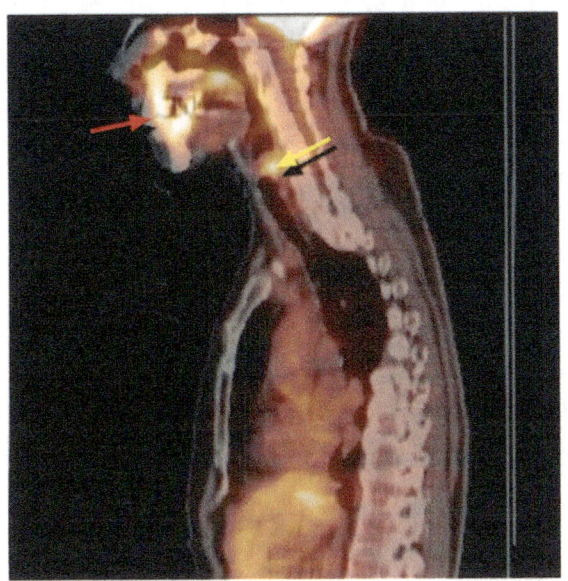

Image 2 (sagittal)

Image 2. Fused sagittal image depicting artifactually increased FDG uptake corresponding to dental work (red arrow). This is explained by over-correction for photon attenuation resulting in "pseudo-FDG-uptake". Physiologically increased FDG uptake in the region of the vocal cords is indicated by the yellow arrow.

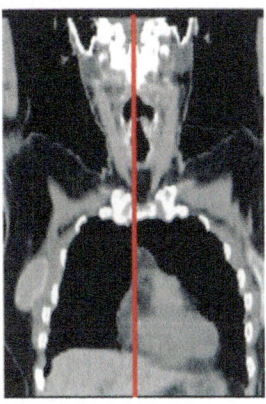

Localizer

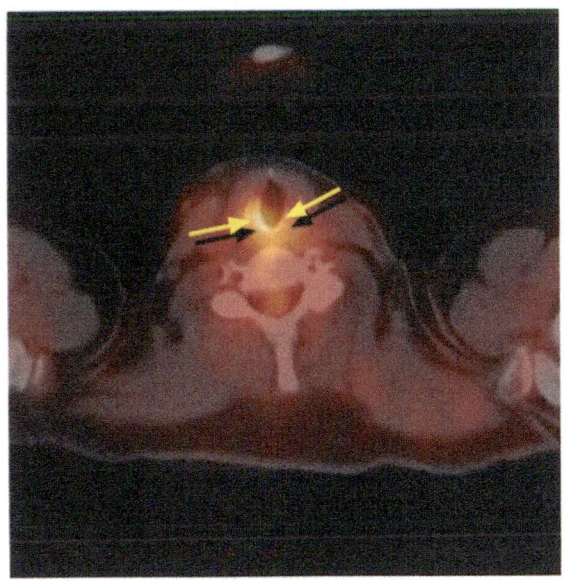

Image 3 (axial)

Image 3. Fused axial image with increased glycolytic activity related to physiologically increased vocal cord activity (arrows).

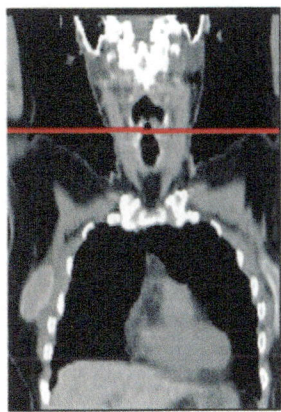

Localizer

Rebound Thymic Hyperplasia

Clinical History

15-year-old female with history of right leg amputation secondary to osteosarcoma. The patient was subsequently treated with chemotherapy and interferon.

PET/CT indication: Restaging.

Findings

An inverse v-shaped structure of hypermetabolic activity is located in the anterior mediastinum. This most likely represents rebound thymic hyperplasia after chemotherapy.

Teaching Point

Thymic activity is frequently observed in healthy young patients but also occasionally in some older patients after chemotherapy. Thymic activity most frequently presents as an inverted v-shaped structure of hypermetabolic activity of mild-to-moderate intensity. In the current case, rebound thymic hyperplasia after chemotherapy most likely accounted for the hypermetabolism.

Image 1. Fused coronal image demonstrating moderately increased glycolytic activity in the anterior mediastinum.

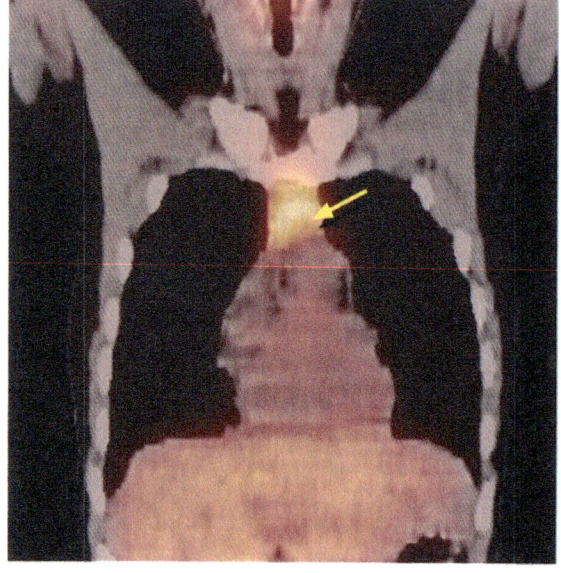

Image 1 (coronal)

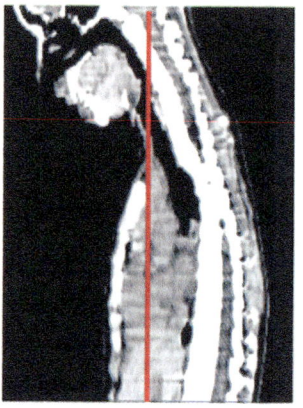

Localizer

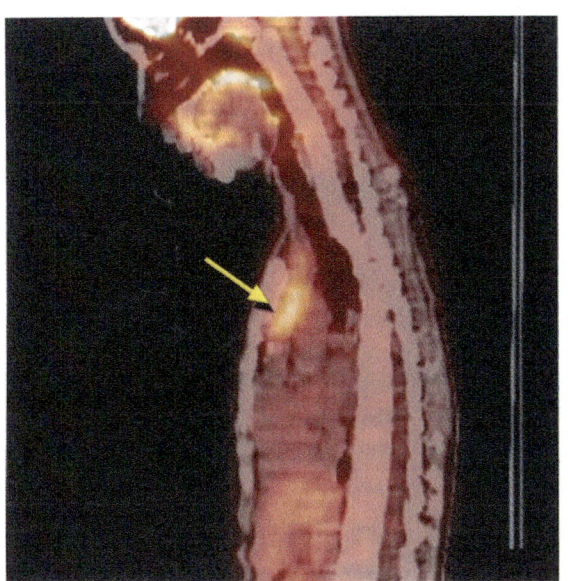

Image 2. Fused sagittal image with retrosternal hypermetabolic activity.

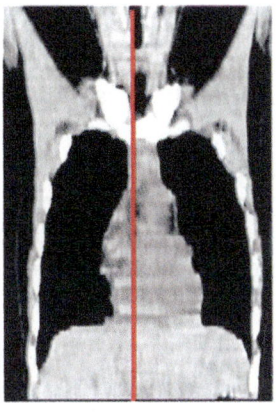

Image 2 (sagittal)

Localizer

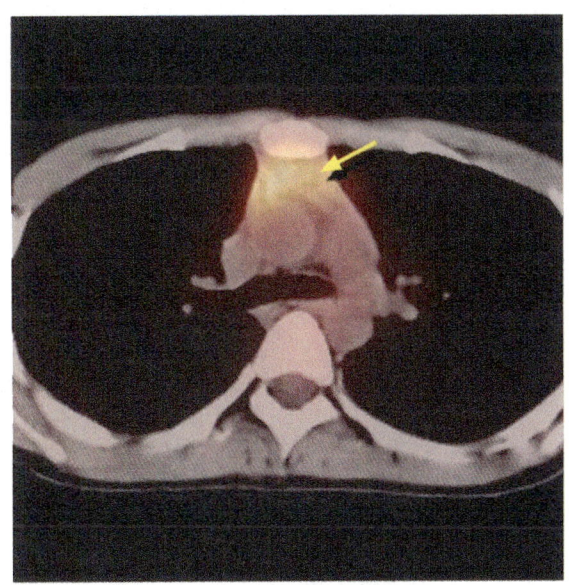

Image 3. Mild anterior mediastinal activity (arrow) is seen on fused axial image. Review of CT images did not reveal lymphadenopathy. The finding is consistent with rebound thymic hyperplasia.

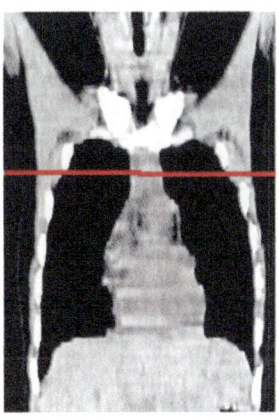

Image 3 (axial)

Localizer

Blood Pool Activity

Clinical History

A 47-year-old female patient with breast cancer and liver mass on CT. The study was performed 2 months after the last cycle of chemotherapy.

PET/CT indication: Treatment monitoring.

Findings

Prominent mediastinal FDG accumulation subsequently identified as blood pool activity. Hypodense liver mass identified on CT that does not exhibit increased glycolytic activity.

Teaching Points

1. Increased blood pool activity in the mediastinum present on PET images might be interpreted as abnormal. Based on our experience with PET/CT increased blood pool activity can frequently have the appearance of focal hypermetabolism.

2. The discrepancy between the CT liver mass and normal PET findings underscores the need for molecular imaging for treatment monitoring.

Image 1. Fused coronal image demonstrating mildly increased glucose metabolic activity in the aortic arch (arrow).

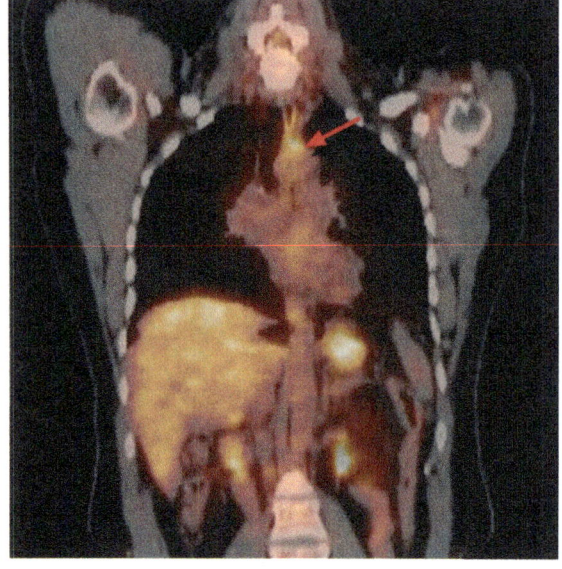

Image 1 (coronal)

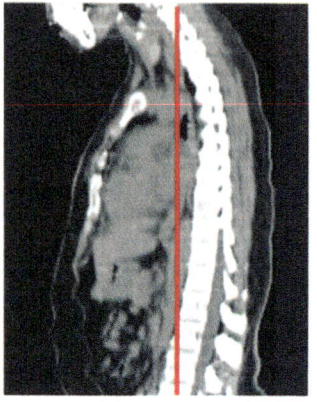

Localizer

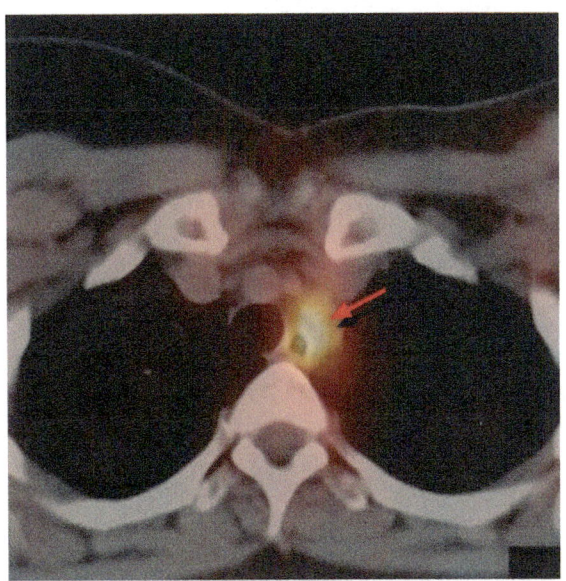

Image 2 (axial)

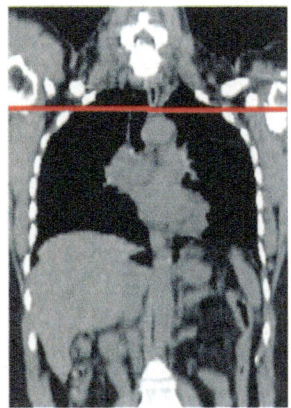

Localizer

Image 2. FDG uptake in the mediastinum is not associated with any abnormal structure and is consistent with blood pool activity.

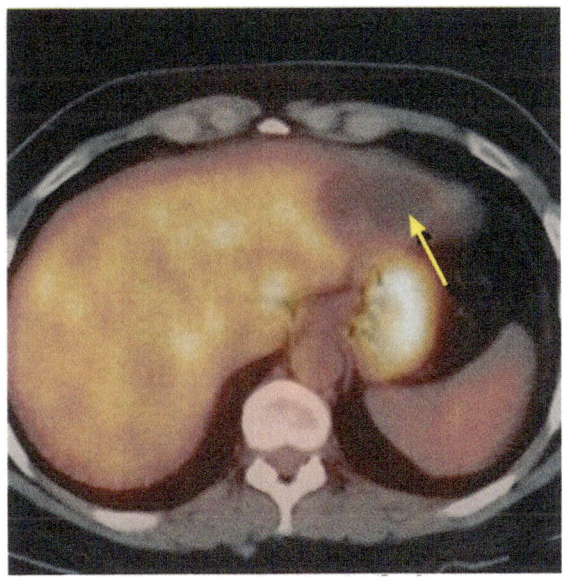

Image 3 (axial)

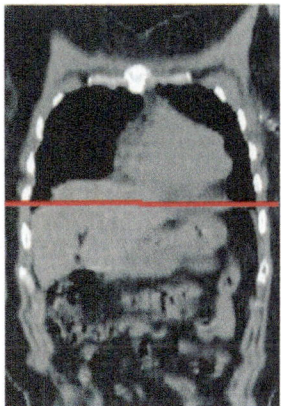

Localizer

Image 3. Fused axial image demonstrating hypodense liver mass without increased glycolytic activity. Thus, the liver lesion is likely benign.

Thyroid Uptake

Clinical History

65-year-old female patient with a history of breast cancer.

PET/CT indication: Restaging.

Findings

Incidental finding of an enlarged thyroid with markedly increased FDG uptake.

Teaching Point

Increased glucose metabolic activity in the thyroid occurs in about 4% of all patients undergoing whole body PET/CT. In our population this occurs almost exclusively in women. The underlying mechanisms have not been elucidated and the finding might represent a normal variant rather than an abnormality.

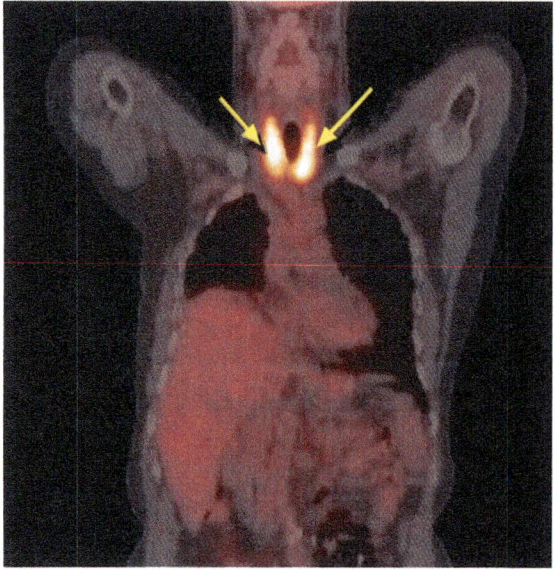

Image 1. Fused coronal image demonstrating markedly increased FDG uptake in both lobes of the thyroid (arrows).

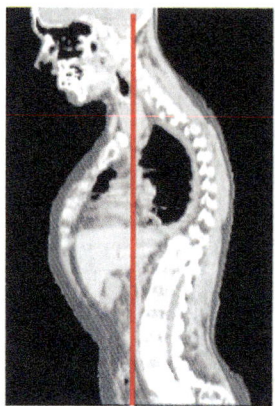

Image 1 (coronal)

Localizer

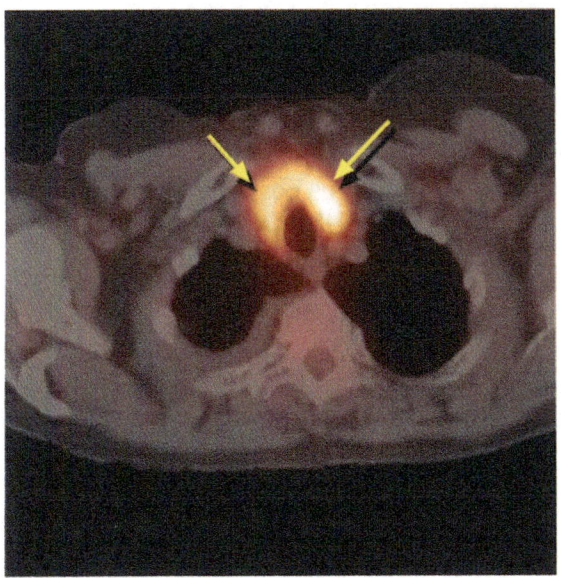

Image 2. Fused axial image depicting hypermetabolic thyroid (arrows).

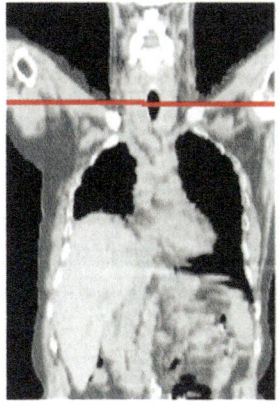

Image 2 (axial) **Localizer**

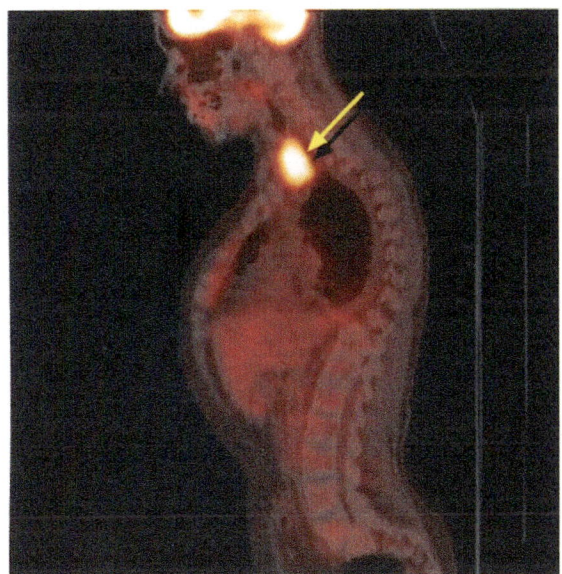

Image 3. Increased FDG uptake in the thyroid depicted on fused sagittal image (arrow).

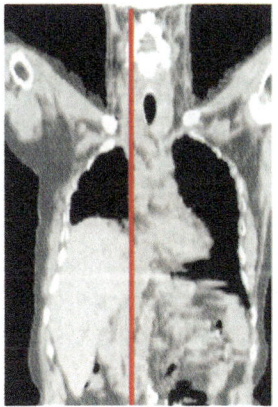

Image 3 (sagittal) **Localizer**

Post-Surgically Altered Anatomy

Clinical History

72-year-old male with history of esophageal carcinoma who is status post esophagectomy and gastric pull-through. Patient underwent recent balloon dilatation of the proximal esophagus.

PET/CT indication: Restaging.

Findings

A nodular structure along the posterior wall of the esophagus is hypermetabolic and concerning for malignancy. Differential diagnosis includes post-dilatation inflammation.

Teaching Point

In this patient with history of gastric pull through surgery PET alone cannot localize the area of hypermetabolism. Gastric stump activity displaced into the chest can result in false positive PET findings.

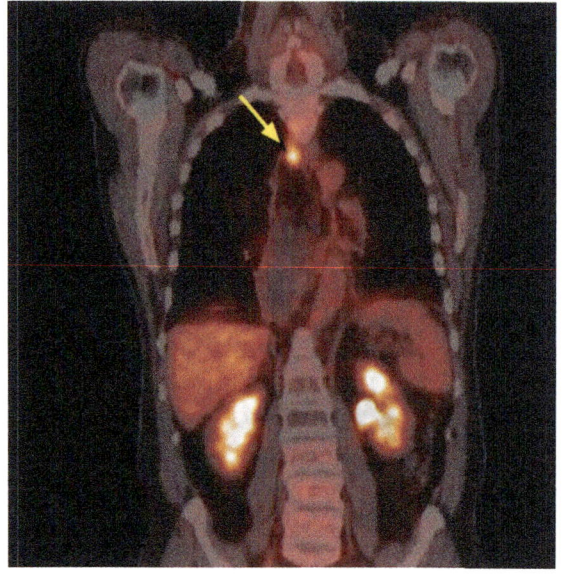

Image 1. Fused coronal image with focus of increased FDG uptake in the upper mediastinum (arrow).

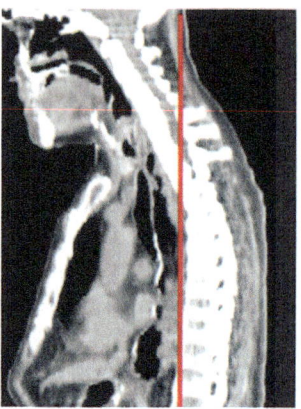

Image 1 (coronal)

Localizer

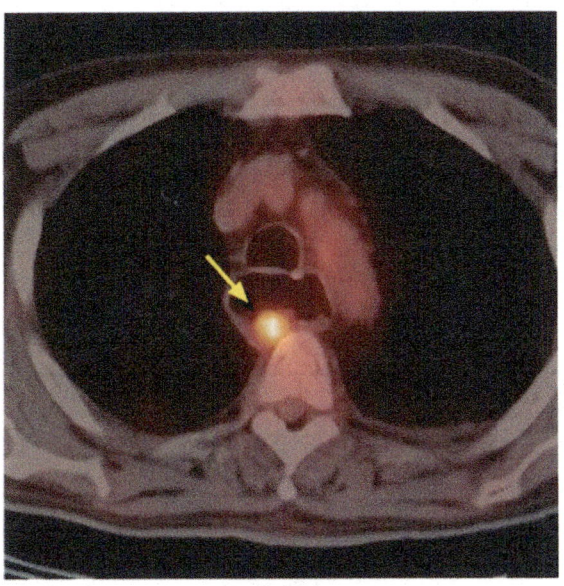

Image 2 (axial)

Image 2. The focus of increased FDG uptake was localized in the posterior aspect of the proximal esophagus (arrow) as shown on fused axial image.

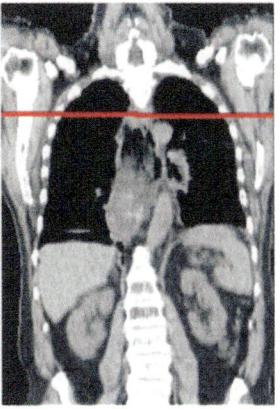

Localizer

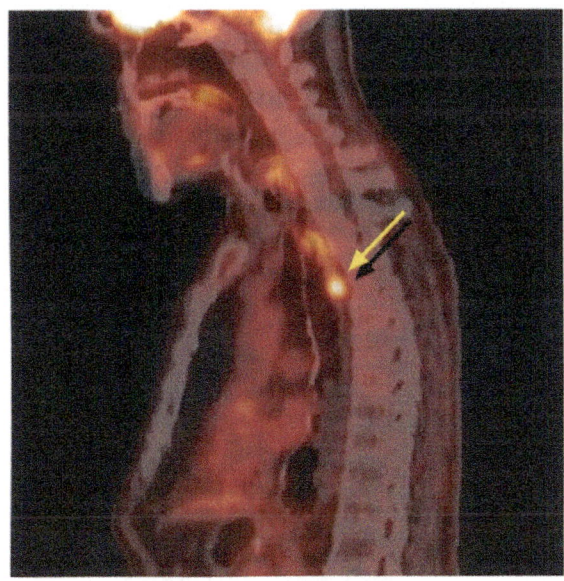

Image 3 (sagittal)

Image 3. Fused sagittal images revealed additional linearly increased FDG uptake along the esophageal wall (arrow). This might be consistent with inflammatory changes after dilation of post-surgical stricture.

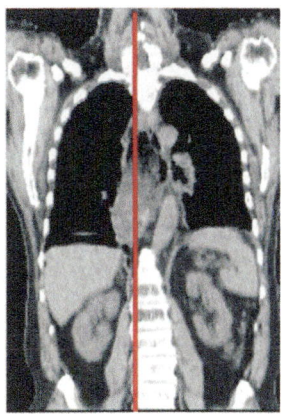

Localizer

Post-Surgical Variant

Clinical History

13-year-old patient with history of liver transplantation and Hodgkin's disease for which he received radiation treatment and chemotherapy several years ago.

PET/CT indication: Restaging.

Findings

Normal whole body PET scan with no evidence of disease recurrence.

Teaching Point

Increased FDG uptake was noted in the in the right infra-diaphragmatic region and the right renal fossa. CT revealed that anatomic changes due to liver transplantation accounted for the unusual localization of FDG hypermetabolism. Abnormal anatomy in post-surgical patients can render interpretation of PET images difficult. In this case the kidney is displaced posteriorly and upwards. In addition, the bowel activity is also shifted posteriorly and laterally.

Image 1. Coronal PET image with markedly increased FDG uptake in the right upper abdomen (arrow).

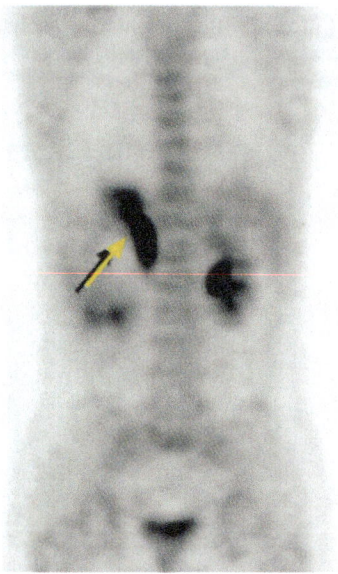

Image 1 (coronal)

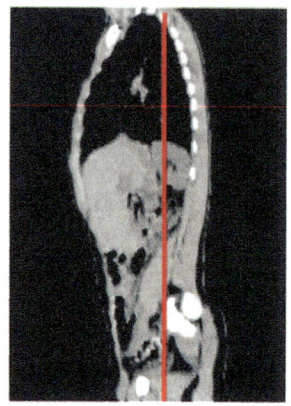

Localizer

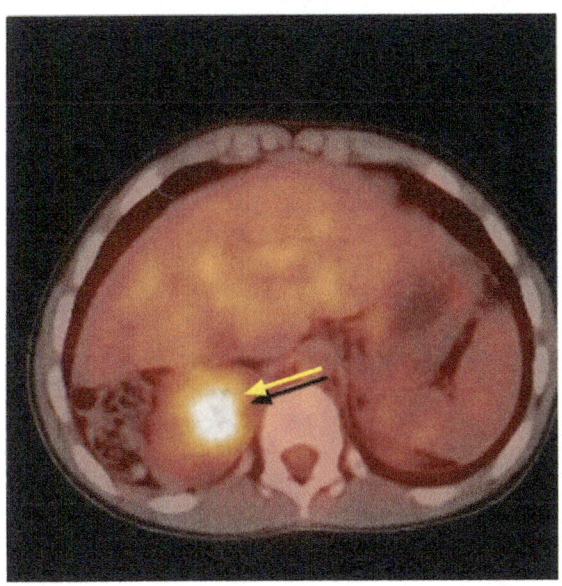

Image 2. Fused axial image showing FDG activity in the pelvis of atypically elevated right kidney (arrow).

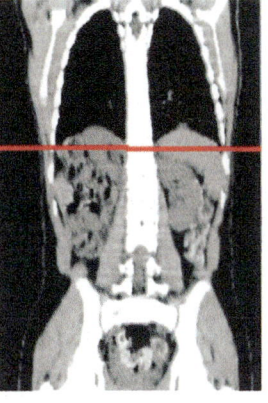

Image 2 (axial)

Localizer

Image 3. Fused axial Image showing normal bowel activity in the area behind the transplanted liver.

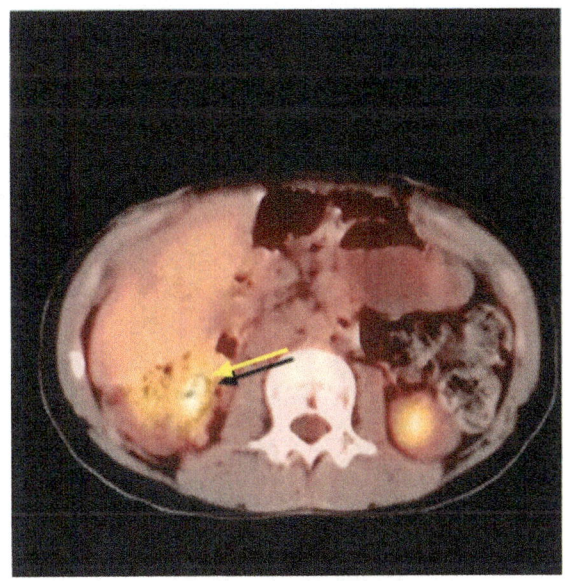

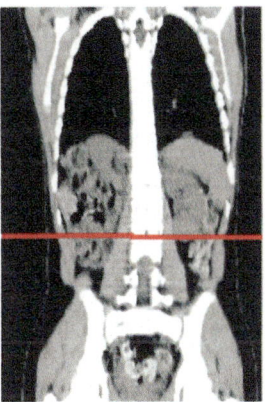

Image 3 (axial)

Localizer

Pancreatic Mass

Clinical History

51-year-old male with incidental finding of pancreatic mass on abdominal CT

PET/CT indication: Lesion characterization.

Findings

Normal whole body PET/CT study without hypermetabolic activity corresponding to the pancreatic mass.
Incidental note is made of prominent bilateral vocal cord activity.

Teaching Point

1. FDG-PET/CT is useful for discriminating malignant from benign pancreatic masses.

2. Prominent physiologic vocal cord activity can be misinterpreted as head and neck pathology.

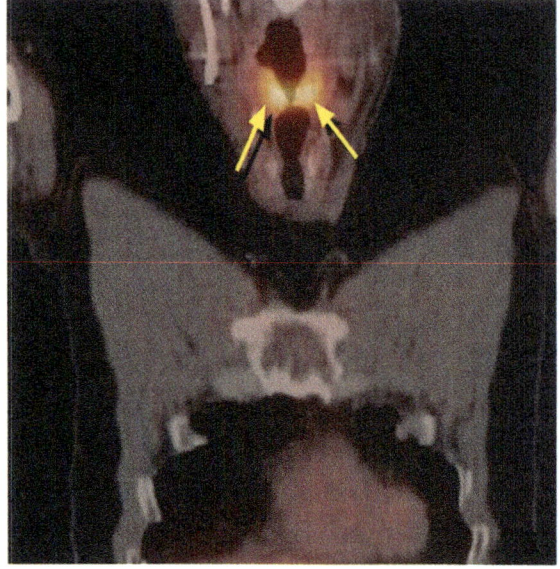

Image 1. Fused coronal image demonstrating the prominent vocal cord activity (arrows).

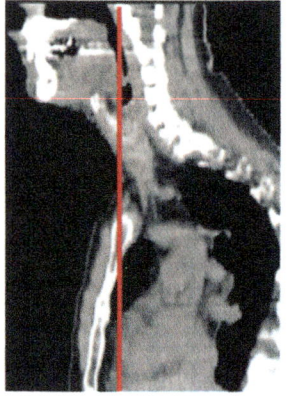

Image 1 (coronal)

Localizer

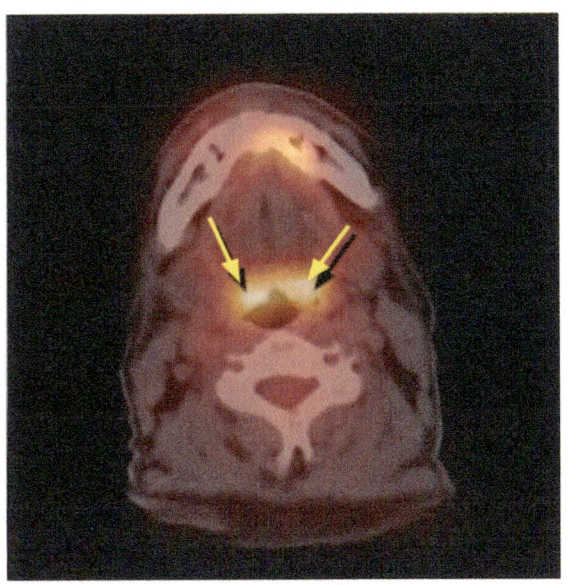

Image 2. Fused axial image depicting the prominent vocal cord activity (arrow).

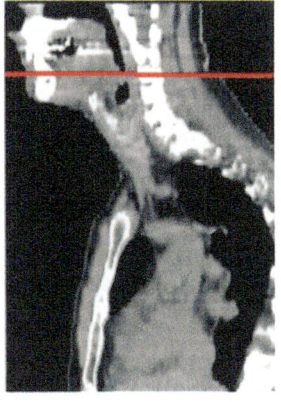

Image 2 (axial)

Localizer

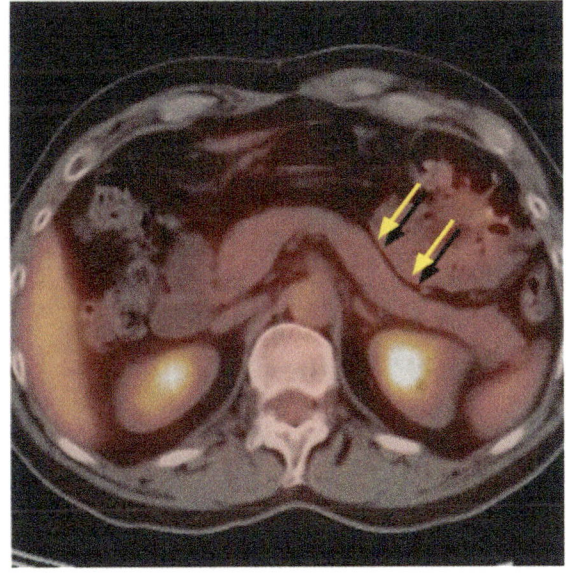

Image 3. Fused axial image showing the elongated yet normal pancreas (arrows).

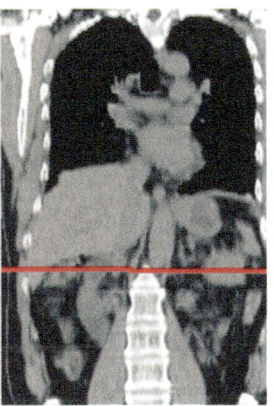

Image 3 (axial)

Localizer

Chapter 3

Anatomical Masses vs. Viable Tumor

Cases:

Chapter 3

Anatomical Masses vs. Viable Tumor

The extent of tumor viability by FDG-PET differs significantly from size of tumors as determined by CT. This discrepancy has important implications for biopsy and radiation planning. PET/CT allows a targeted approach to these interventions. Molecular PET imaging with FDG is the only non-invasive tool that permits to differentiate viable tumor from benign anatomical masses. The identification of viable tumor will gain considerable importance in the planning of biopsies and radiation treatment. It is hoped that a PET based approach to these interventions will result in higher diagnostic accuracy of biopsies and in more accurate delineation of the radiation target.

Suggested Reading

Hain SF, Curran KM, Beggs AD, Fogelman I, O'Doherty MJ, Maisey MN. FDG-PET as a "metabolic biopsy" tool in thoracic lesions with indeterminate biopsy. Eur J Nucl Med. 2001;28(9):1336-1340.

Brahme A. Biologically optimized 3-dimensional in vivo predictive assay-based radiation therapy using positron emission tomography-computerized tomography imaging. Acta Oncol. 2003;42(2):123-136.

Jang S, Greskovich JF, Milla BA, Zhang Y, Nelson AD, Devlin AL, Faulhaber PF. Effects of PET/CT image registration on radiation treatment planning in lung cancer. Int J Radiat Oncol Biol Phys. 2003;57(2 Suppl):S414-S415.

Ciernik IF, Dizendorf E, Baumert BG, Reiner B, Burger C, Davis JB, Lutolf UM, Steinert HC, Von Schulthess GK. Radiation treatment planning with an integrated positron emission and computer tomography (PET/CT): a feasibility study. Int J Radiat Oncol Biol Phys. 2003;57(3):853-863.

Bradley JD, Perez CA, Dehdashti F, Siegel BA. Implementing biologic target volumes in radiation treatment planning for non-small cell lung cancr. J Nucl Med. 2004;45(Suppl 1):96S-101S.

Eccentric Tumor Viability

Clinical History

63-year-old patient with newly detected lung mass.

PET/CT indication: Tissue characterization.

Findings

Right upper lobe mass exhibits eccentric glucose metabolic activity in the postero-medial aspect. The remainder of the mass is hypometabolic suggesting tumor necrosis.

Teaching Point

The case underscores the fundamental discrepancy between anatomical mass and viable tumor. The assessment of tumor viability is important for guiding biopsy and radiation planning.

Image 1. Fused coronal PET/CT image with right upper lobe mass that exhibits an eccentric rim of viable tumor (arrow).

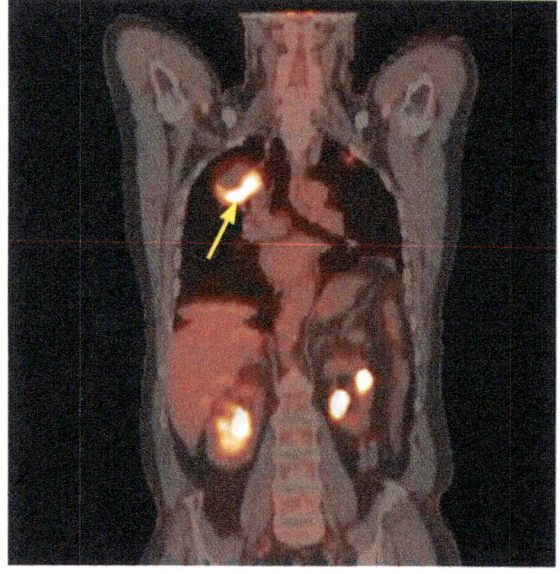

Image 1 (coronal)

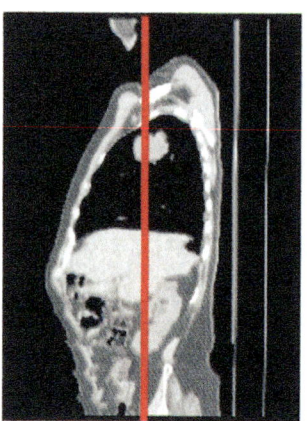

Localizer

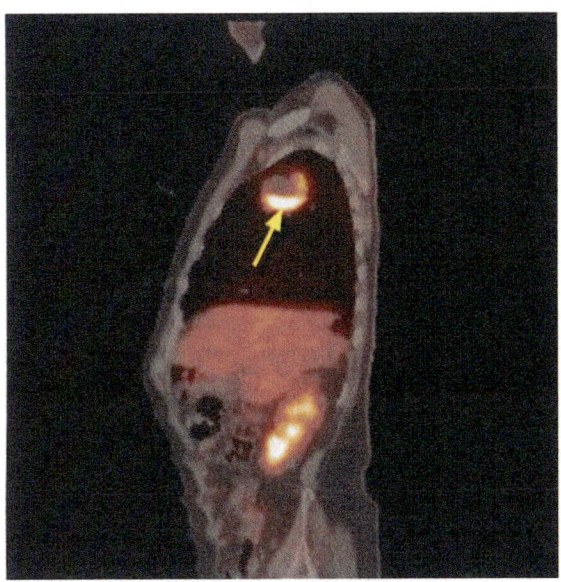

Image 2. Fused sagittal image of the eccentric tumor lesion (arrow).

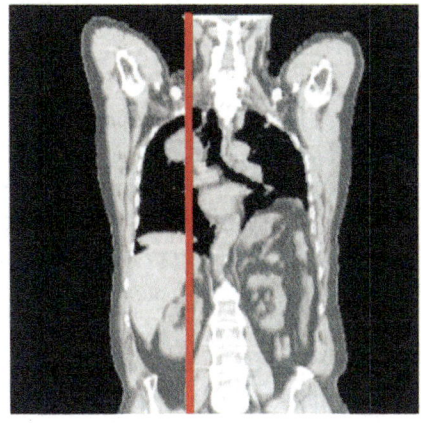

Image 2 (sagittal)   **Localizer**

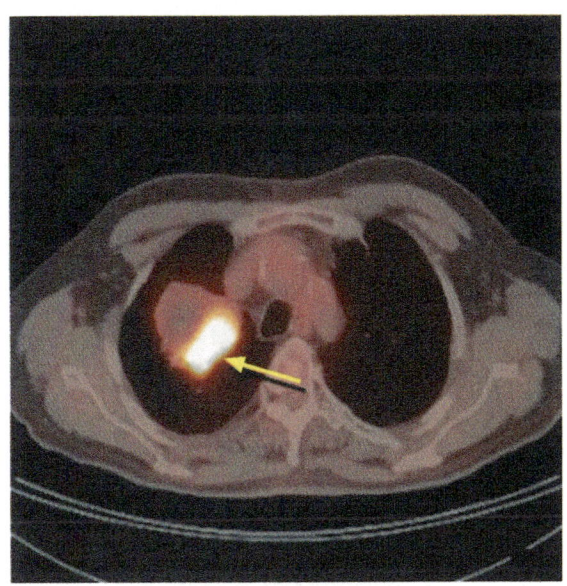

Image 3. The viable portion of the tumor encompasses the postero-medial aspect of the mass as shown on this axial image (arrow). Note the implications for biopsy planning.

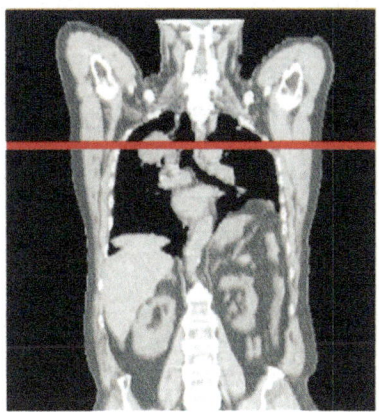

Image 3 (axial)   **Localizer**

Tumor Viability

Clinical History

62-year-old male with pulmonary malignancy and colon cancer.

PET/CT indication: Restaging.

Findings

Large and complex mass in the left upper lobe of the lung demonstrating peripheral hyper-metabolic activity. This is consistent with the patient's known adenocarcinoma. The central photopenia suggests central necrosis of this tumor.

No evidence for metastatic disease.

Teaching Point

Note the eccentric hypermetabolic rim. Assessment of tumor viability is important to avoid sampling errors during biopsy.

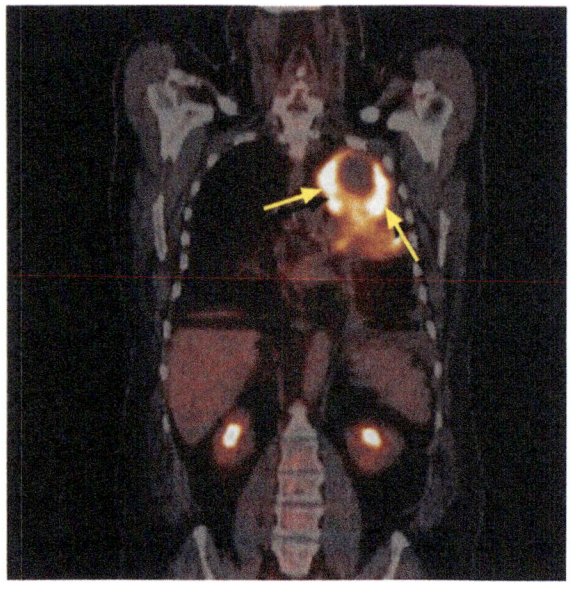

Image 1 (coronal)

Image 1. Fused coronal image with hypermetabolic area surrounding central ametabolic core suggesting central necrosis with surrounding rim of viable tumor (arrow).

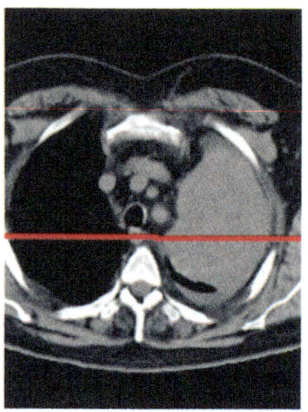

Localizer

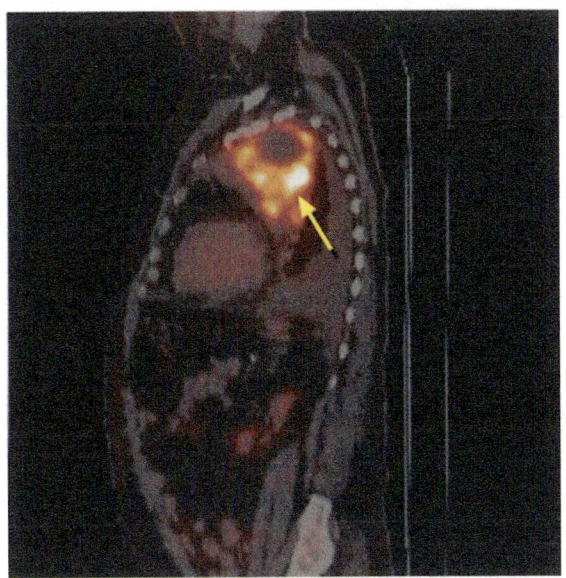

Image 2 (sagittal)

Image 2. Fused sagittal image assigns the most intense hyper-metabolic area to the inferior aspect of the mass (arrow).

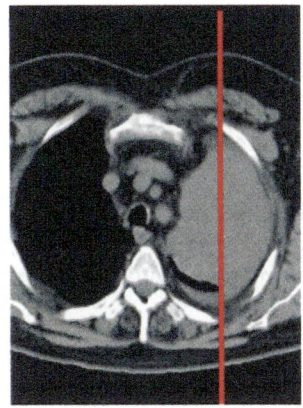

Localizer

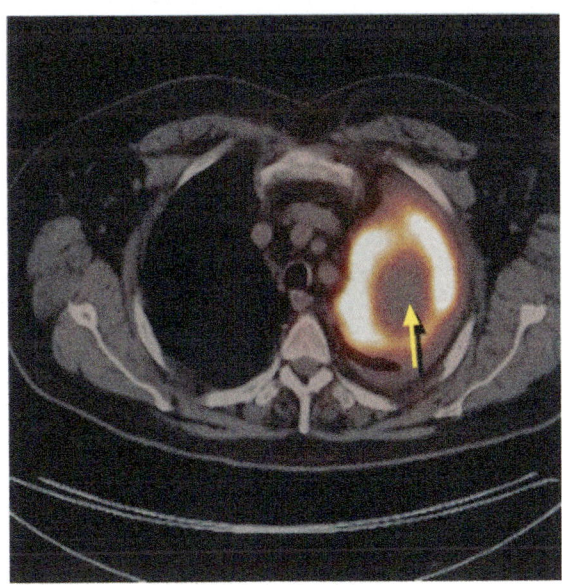

Image 3 (axial)

Image 3. Fused axial image shows the metabolic activity distribution in the tumor mass and identifies areas that are not suitable for biopsy (arrow).

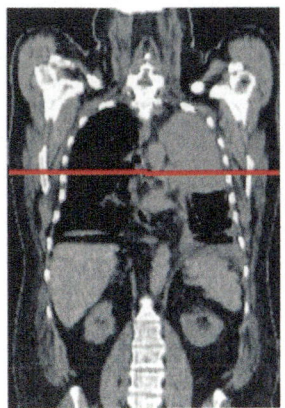

Localizer

Liver Cyst

Clinical History

73-year-old female with lung cancer and a well rounded liver lesion on CT.

PET/CT indication: Tissue characterization.

Findings

A small a-metabolic area in the dome of the liver measuring 2.5 cm x 3 cm is consistent with a liver cyst.

Teaching Point

Molecular PET imaging is the best imaging tool for differentiating malignant from benign diseases.

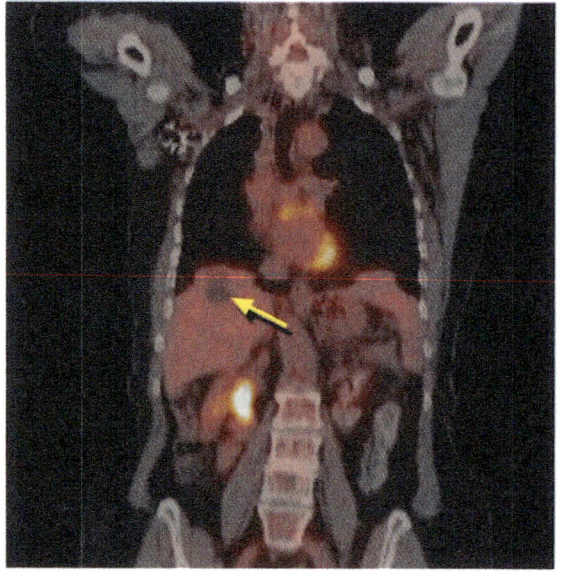

Image 1. Fused coronal images with rounded liver lesion (arrow) that does not exhibit glycolytic activity.

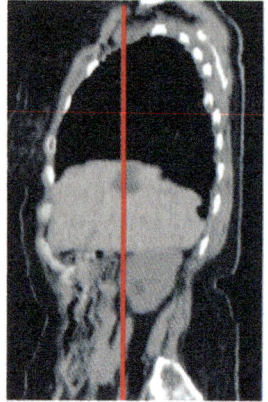

Image 1 (coronal)

Localizer

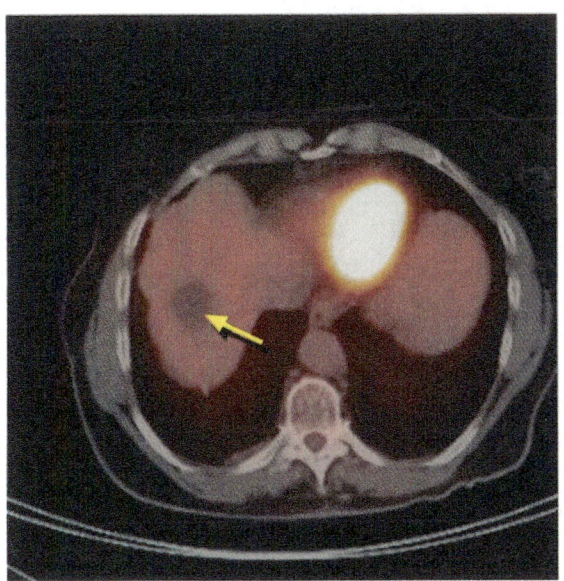

Image 2. Fused axial images demonstrating the liver cyst without metabolic activity.

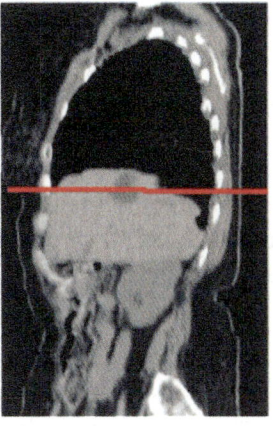

Image 2 (axial)

Localizer

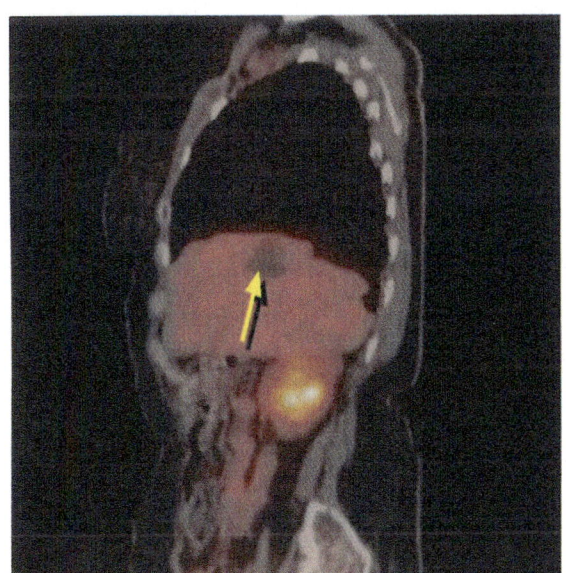

Image 3. Fused sagittal images depicting the liver cyst (arrow).

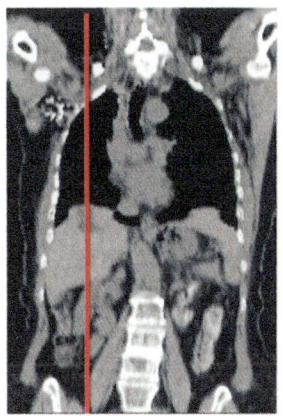

Image 3 (sagittal)

Localizer

Tumor Viability

Clinical History

71-year-old woman with breast cancer who is status post left mastectomy and radiation therapy.

PET/CT indication: Restaging.

Findings

CT demonstrates sclerotic changes of the T7 vertebral body corresponding to a vertebral lesion described on a prior bone scan. This lesion demonstrates no increased metabolic activity.
Multiple hypodense liver lesions do not exhibit increased FDG uptake.

Teaching Point

FDG-PET is ideally suited to characterize anatomic abnormalities as malignant or benign. In this case, a sclerotic bone lesion unchanged for several months on anatomic images and on bone scan remained negative for metastasis by FDG-PET. Similarly, multiple hypodense liver lesions without FDG uptake are consistent with cysts.

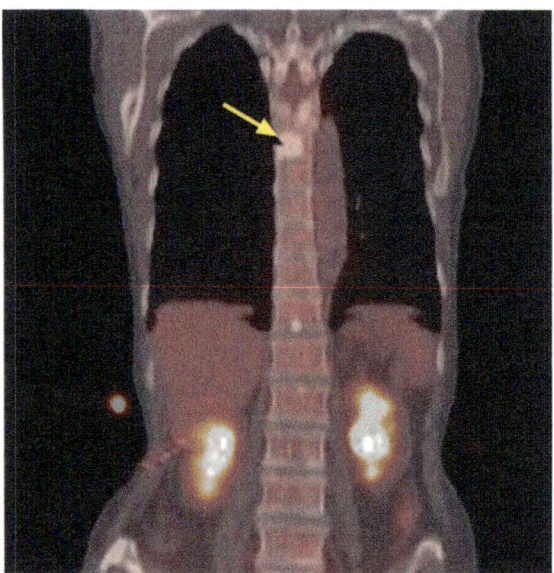

Image 1. Fused coronal image with sclerotic lesion at the level of T7 without increased FDG uptake (arrow) consistent with benign disease.

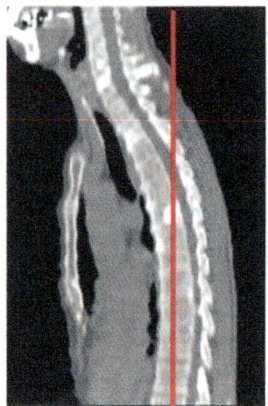

Image 1 (coronal)

Localizer

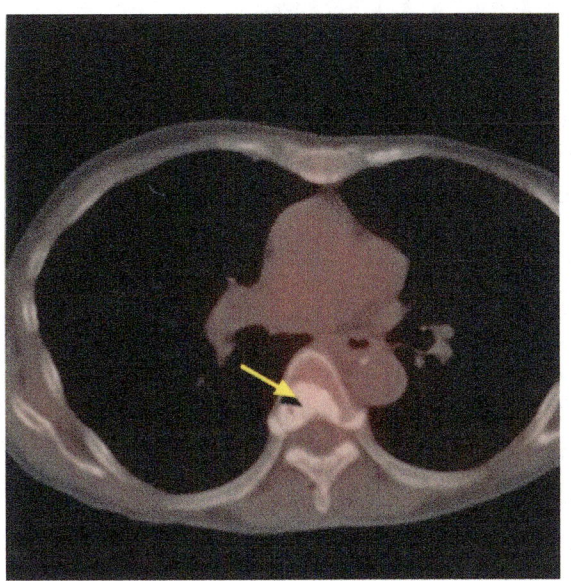

Image 2 (axial)

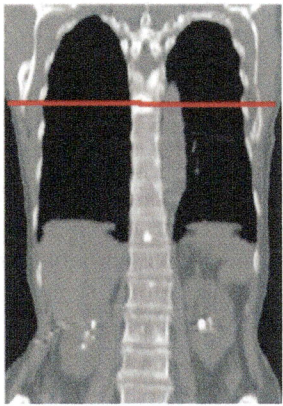

Localizer

Image 2. Fused axial image depicting the sclerotic T7 lesion (arrow).

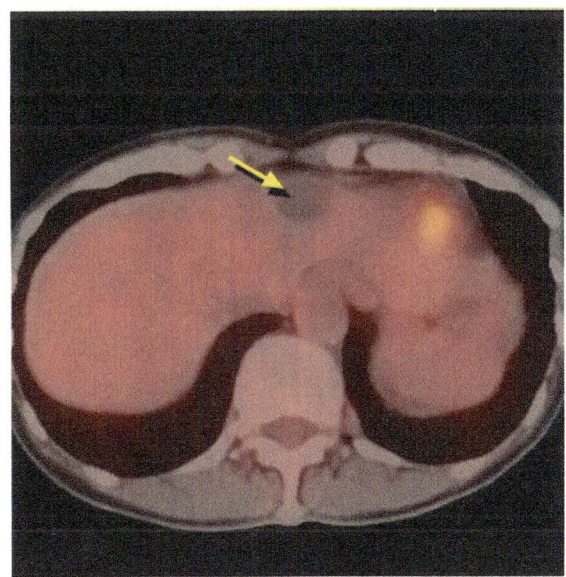

Image 3 (axial)

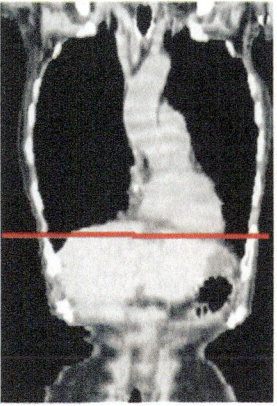

Localizer

Image 3. Fused axial image depicting hypodense liver lesion without FDG uptake (arrow). This is consistent with a liver cyst.

Tumor Necrosis

Clinical History

71-year-old male with history of colon cancer who is status post radiofrequency ablation of liver metastases.

PET/CT indication: Restaging.

Findings

Several hypodense lesions seen on CT in the lateral aspect of the right liver lobe do not exhibit increased glucose metabolic and are consistent with post-ablation necrosis.

Teaching Point

Treatment monitoring is best accomplished with molecular PET imaging. As shown in this example, extensive anatomical abnormalities can represent scar, necrosis or inflammation rather than residual tumor.

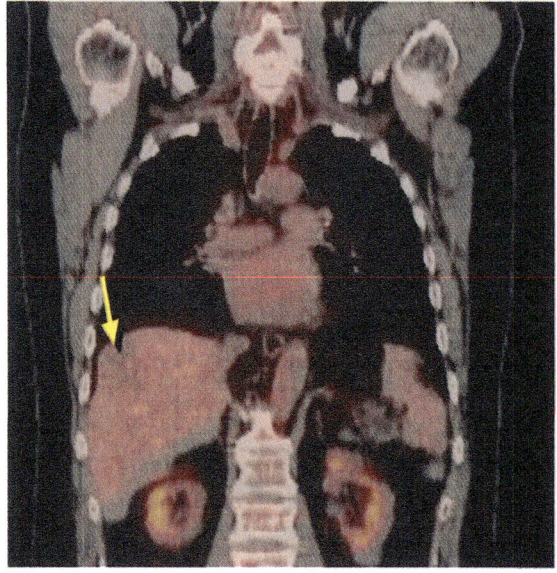

Image 1 (coronal)

Image 1. Fused coronal image demonstrating large hypodense liver lesion without FDG uptake in the right lobe of the liver (arrow) consistent with post-radiofrequency ablation necrosis.

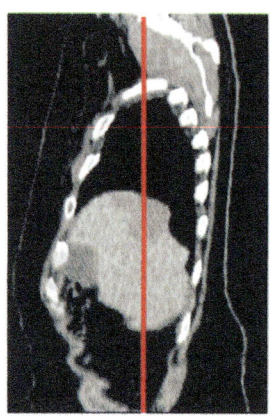

Localizer

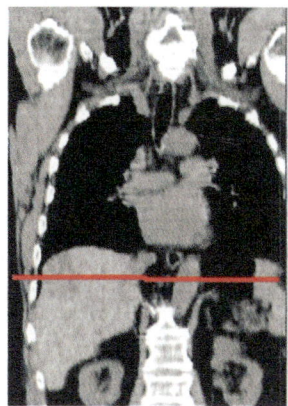

Image 2. Fused axial image of the hypodense liver mass located in the right liver lobe (arrow) without metabolic activity (arrow).

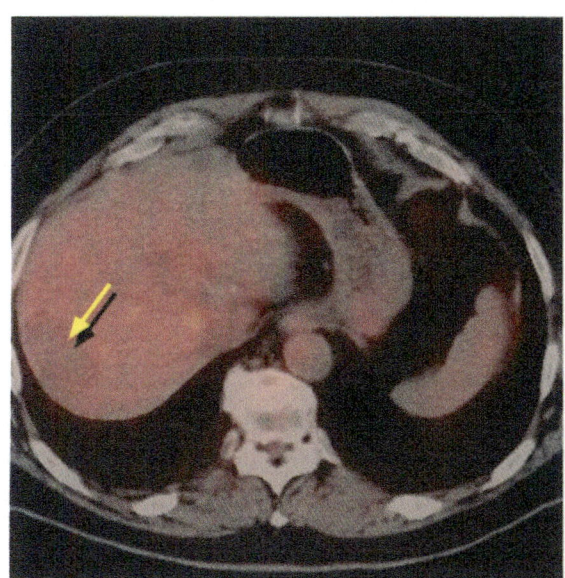

Image 2 (axial)

Localizer

Partially Necrotic Nasopharyngeal Carcinoma Metastasis

Clinical History

66-year-old male patient with newly diagnosed left pharyngeal carcinoma.

PET/CT indication: Staging.

Findings

A hypermetabolic focus corresponding to a well-circumscribed 3.5 x 3.0 x 4.0 cm mass posterior to the left submandibular salivary gland is consistent with metastatic lymph node involvement.

Teaching Point

The discrepancy between viable tumor by FDG and an anatomic mass by CT is evident in this example. Note the relatively small area of viable tumor relative to the large anatomical mass. This discrepancy has implications for biopsy and radiation planning.

Image 1. Axial PET image at the level of the mandible. Arrow denotes large metastatic lymph node.

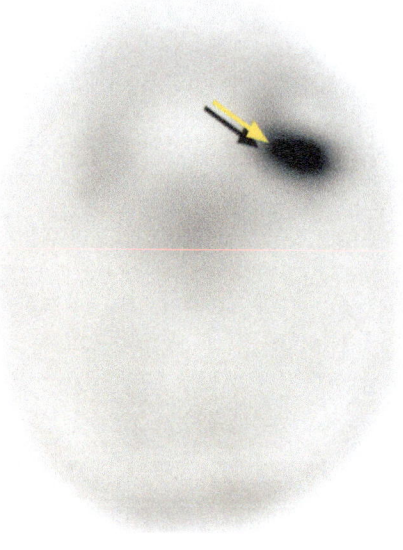

Image 1 (axial)

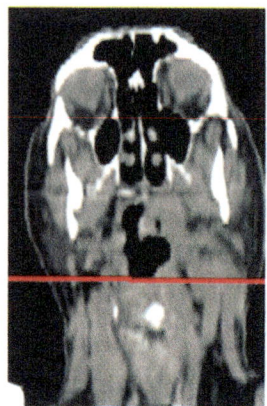

Localizer

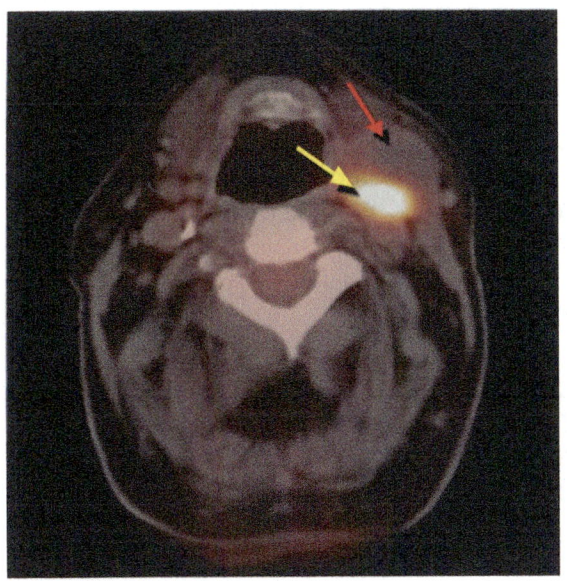

Image 2 (axial)

Image 2. Axial PET/CT image at the level of the mandible. The red arrow shows ametabolic, necrotic component of the mass while the yellow arrow indicates the viable portion of the markedly enlarged lymph node.

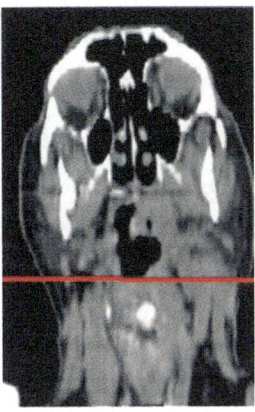

Localizer

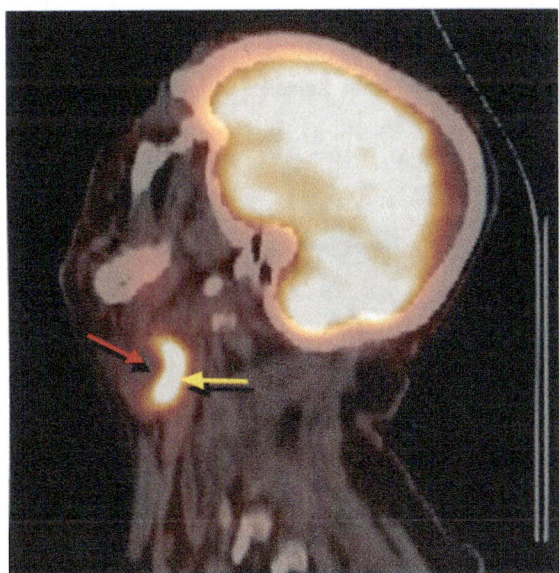

Image 3 (sagittal)

Image 3. Fused sagittal image showing metabolic activity of the metastatic tumoral mass, necrotic anterior part (red arrow) and posterior metabolically active tumor (yellow arrow).

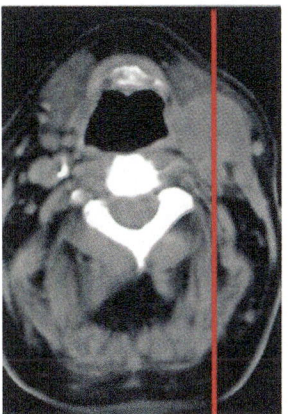

Localizer

Partially Necrotic Lung Metastasis of Glioblastoma Multiforme

Clinical History

40-year-old man with a history of glioblastoma multiforme who underwent surgical resection, chemotherapy and radiation therapy. A CT scan of the chest, obtained at an outside facility, revealed a right lower lobe mass.

PET/CT indication: Characterization of pulmonary mass.

Findings

There is a large mass in the right lower lobe of the lung, which demonstrates increased peripheral metabolic activity and a central photopenic area consistent with a tumor with central necrosis; this is suggestive of metastatic disease. However, second primary tumor cannot be ruled out.

Histological Verification: High-grade malignant neoplasm composed of giant and spindle cells with extensive necrosis (the neoplasm is identical to the patient's previously-resected right frontal brain lesion).

Teaching Point

PET provided guidance for the biopsy by identifying the viable components of this partially necrotic malignancy.

Image 1. Coronal PET image depicting the right lower lung tumor that exhibits peripheral FDG uptake (arrow).

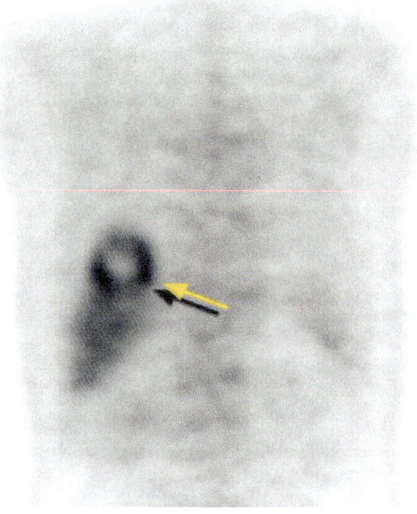

Image 1 (coronal)

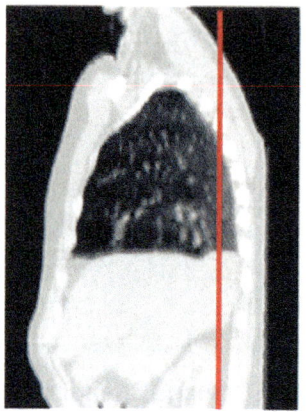

Localizer

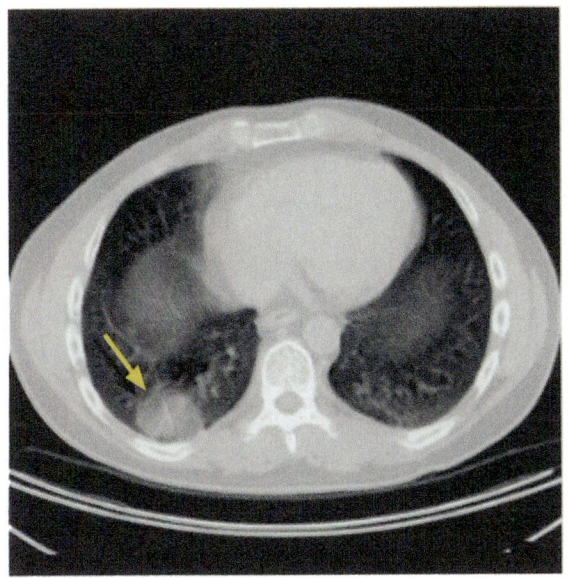

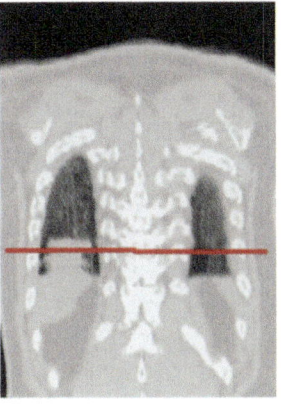

Image 2. Axial CT demonstrating the posterior right lower lobe mass (arrow). Differentiation between viable and non-viable tumor segments is not possible with CT.

Image 2 (axial)

Localizer

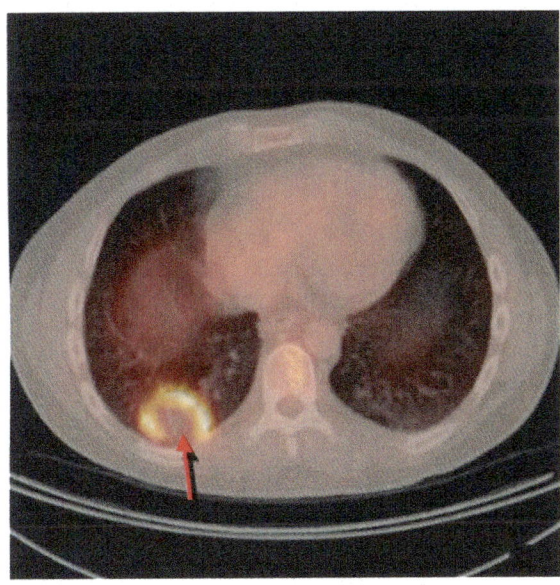

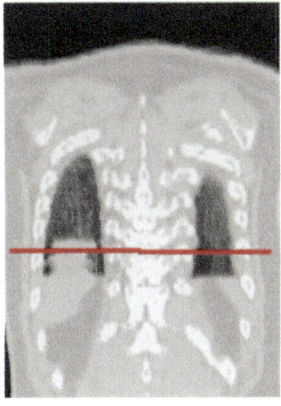

Image 3. Fused axial image demonstrating that the hypermetabolic rim is inhomogeneous (arrow). The arrow points to the hypometabolic segment of the rim corresponding to the necrotic part of the tumor.

Image 3 (axial)

Localizer

Chapter 4

Cancers of Head and Neck

Cases:

Chapter 4

Cancers of the Head and Neck

Head and neck cancers comprise about 5% of all cancers worldwide. Because of the complex normal head and neck anatomy, which is further altered after surgical or radiation treatment, PET imaging of glycolysis has contributed to the diagnostic work-up of these patients. However, physiological muscle activity, vocal cord and normal thyroid activity can render the interpretation of molecular images difficult. PET/CT has helped to overcome some of these difficulties and it was this indication for which the usefulness of PET/CT was first tested and established using the prototype PET/CT at the University of Pittsburg.

Key Indications: Staging and Restaging

Suggested Reading

Rege S, Maass A, Chaiken L, Hoh CK, Choi Y, Lufkin R, Anzai Y, Juillard G, Maddahi J, Phelps ME. Use of positron emission tomography with fluorodeoxyglucose in patients with extracranial head and neck cancers. Cancer. 1994;73(12):3047-3058.

Grünwald F, Menzel C, Bender H, Palmedo H, Willkomm P, Ruhlmann J, Franckson T, Biersack HJ. Comparison of 18FDG-PET with 131Iodine and 99mTc-sestamibi scintigraphy in differentiated thyroid cancer. Thyroid. 1997;7(3):327-335.

Lowe VJ, Dunphy FR, Varvares M, Kim H, Wittry M, Dunphy CH, Dunleavy T, McDonough E, Minster J, Fletcher JW, Boyd JH. Evaluation of chemotherapy response in patients with advanced head and neck cancer using [F-18] fluorodeoxyglucose positron emission tomography. Head Neck. 1997;19(8):666-674.

Altenvoerde G, Lerch H, Kuwert T, Matheja P, Schäfers M, Schober O. Positron emission tomography with F-18-deoxyglucose in patients with differentiated thyroid carcinoma, elevated thyroglobulin levels, and negative iodine scans. Langenbecks Arch Surg. 1998;383(2):160-163.

Schlüter B, Grimm-Riepe C, Beyer W, Lübeck M, Schirren-Bumann K, Clausen M. Histological verification of positive fluorine-18 fluorodexoyglucose findings in patients with differentiated thyroid cancer. Langenbecks Arch Surg. 1998;383(2):187-189.

Adam S, Baum RP, Stuckensen T, Bitter K, Hör G. Prospective comparison of 18F-FDG PET with conventional imaging modalities (CT, MRI, US) in lymph node staging of head and neck cancer. Eur J Nucl Med. 1998;25(9):1255-1260.

Wang W, Macapinlac H, Larson SM, Yeh SD, Akhurst T, Finn RD, Rosai J, Robbins RJ. [18F]-2-fluoro-2-deoxy-D-glucose positron emission tomography localizes residual thyroid cancer in patients with negative diagnostic 131I whole body scans and elevated serum thyroglobulin levels. J Clin Endocrinol Metab. 1999;84(7):2291-2302.

Conti PS, Durski JM, Bacqai F, Grafton ST, Singer PA. Imaging of locally recurrent and metastatic thyroid cancer with positron emission tomography. Thyroid. 1999;9(8):797-804.

Lowe VJ, Kim H, Boyd JH, Eisenbeis JF, Dunphy FR, Fletcher JW. Primary and recurrent early stage laryngeal cancer: preliminary results of 2-[fluorine 18]fluoro-2-deoxy-D-glucose PET imaging. Radiology. 1999;212(3):799-802.

Grünwald F, Kälicke T, Feine U, Lietzenmayer R, Scheidhauer K, Dietlein M, Schober O, Lerch H, Brandt-Mainz K, Burchert W, Hiltermann G, Cremerius U, Biersack HJ. Fluorine-18 fluorodeoxyglucose positron emission tomography in thyroid cancer: results of a multicentre study. Eur J Nucl Med. 1999;26(12):1547-1552.

Hubner KF, Thie JA, Smith GT, Chan AC, Fernandez PS, McCoy JM. Clinical utility of FDG-PET in detecting head and neck tumors: a comparison of diagnostic methods and modalities. Clin Positron Imaging. 2000;3(1):7-16.

Lowe VJ, Boyd JH, Dunphy FR, Kim H, Dunleavy T, Collins BT, Martin D, Stack BC Jr, Hollenbeak C, Fletcher JW. Surveillance for recurrent head and neck cancer using positron emission tomography. J Clin Oncol. 2000;18(3):651-658.

Squamous Cell Carcinoma of the Tongue

Clinical History

76-year-old female with Non-Hodgkin's lymphoma and squamous cell carcinoma of the tongue. The patient is status post right hemi-glossectomy with right supra-hyoid neck dissection and status post radiation and chemotherapy.

PET/CT indication: Restaging.

Findings

A small retro-mandibular focus of abnormally increased glycolysis on the right side is suspicious for residual or recurrent disease.

Increased glycolytic activity localized to a rib is consistent with metastatic disease.

Teaching Point

PET/CT allowed correct lesion localization in the head and neck region and left rib.

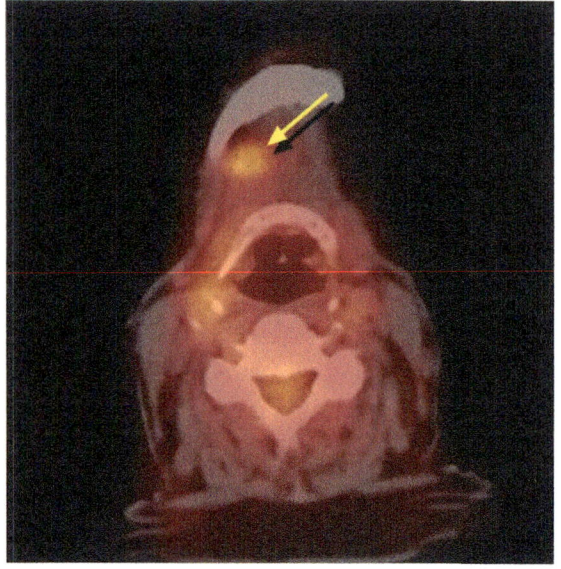

Image 1. (axial)

Image 1. Fused axial image of the head/neck region at the level of the mandible. The increased retro-mandibular FDG uptake corresponds to an enlarged lymph node on CT. Corresponding CT image revealed retro-mandibular mass.

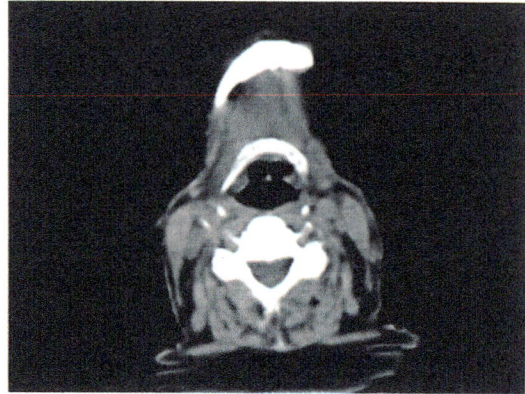

CT Image

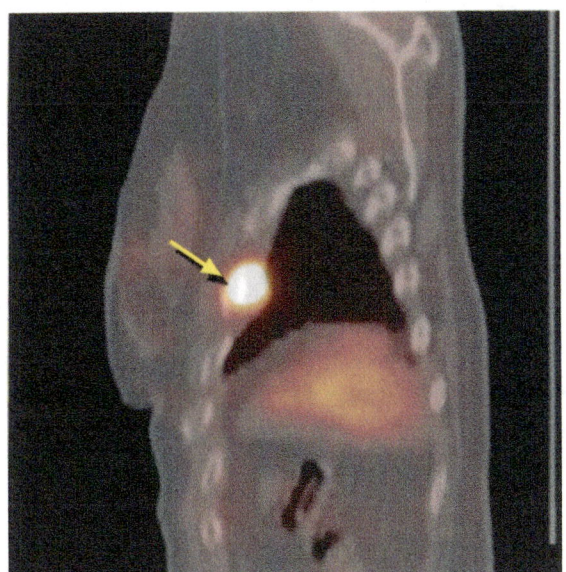

Image 2 (sagittal)

Image 2. Increased glycolytic activity localized to a lytic rib lesion shown on fused sagittal image.

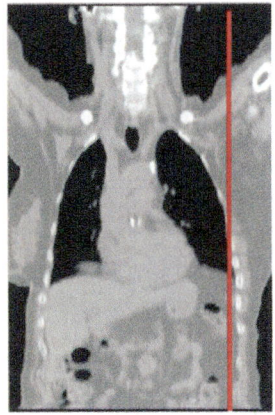

Localizer

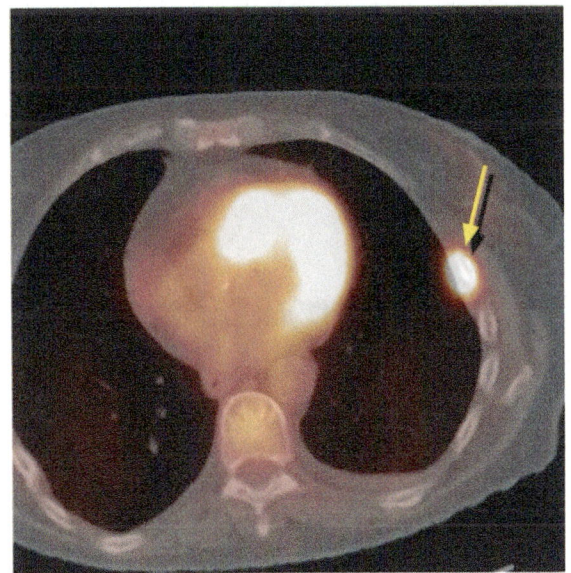

Image 3 (axial)

Image 3. Fused axial image depicting the same rib lesion.

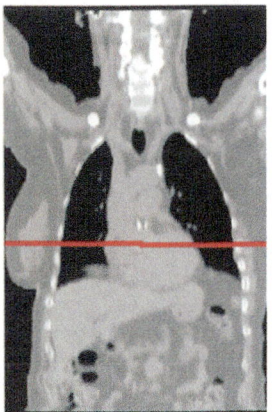

Localizer

Thyroid Cancer

Clinical History

38-year-old male with medullary thyroid carcinoma. Following thyroidectomy the patient presented with rising serum calcitonin levels.

PET/CT indication: Restaging.

Findings

A focus of mildly increased glycolytic activity was suspicious for metastatic spread to the right lower neck. CT localized the activity to a sub-centimeter lymph node.

Teaching Point

PET was equivocal for recurrent disease. CT was negative by size criteria. A 7-mm lymph node had mildly increased FDG uptake and was identified as site of recurrence by biopsy. Thus, sub-centimeter lesions by CT can harbor cancer. On the other hand, glycolytic activity was only mildly increased which might have been due to unspecific neck muscle activity. The co-registration of PET and CT resulted in the correct identification of the site of recurrence.

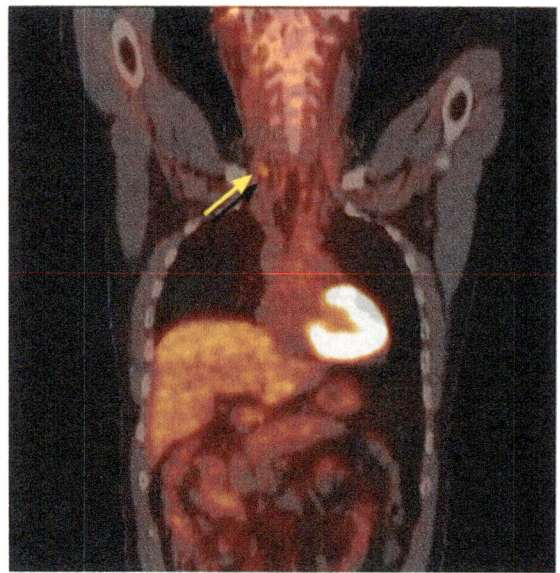

Image 1 (coronal)

Image 1. Small focus of mildly increased FDG uptake in the right neck (arrow). This was mildly suspicious for recurrent disease by PET alone. However, the activity was located in a small lymph node (7 mm) that was subsequently biopsied and found to be positive for recurrent medullary carcinoma.

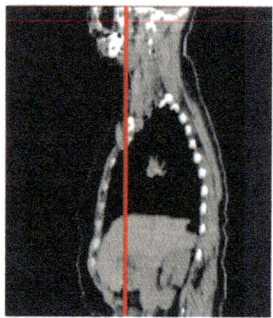

Localizer

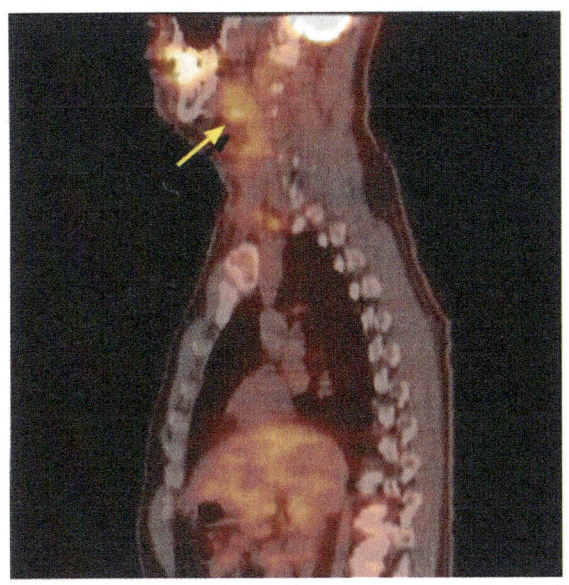

Image 2 (sagittal)

Image 2. Fused sagittal image reveals small right-sided lymph node consistent with site of recurrence (arrow).

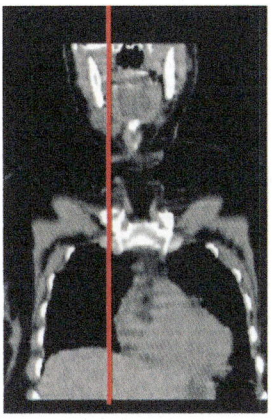

Localizer

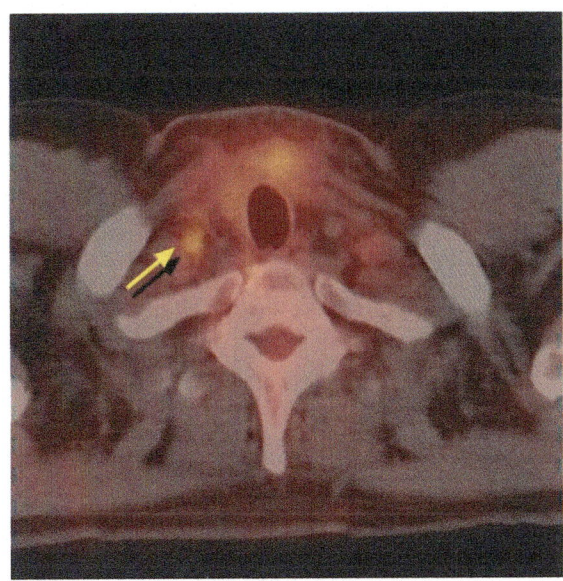

Image 3 (axial)

Image 3. Fused axial image reveals small right-sided lymph node consistent with site of recurrence (arrow).

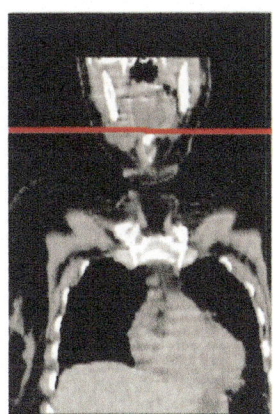

Localizer

Neuroendocrine Tumor

Clinical History

Patient is a 39-year-old male with history of neuroendocrine tumor of the right ethmoid sinus.

PET/CT indication: Staging.

Findings

A mass exhibiting markedly increased glucose metabolic activity seen in the right ethmoid sinus extending into the right frontal sinus and into the right medial orbit. PET/CT demonstrates penetration of the cribriform plate.

Teaching Point

PET can identify the area of viable tumor but cannot determine the level of bone invasion. PET/CT revealed tumor invasion into the cribriform plate.

Image 1. Sagittal fused image showing the sino-nasal hypermetabolic mass. Note the erosion of the cribriform plate (arrow).

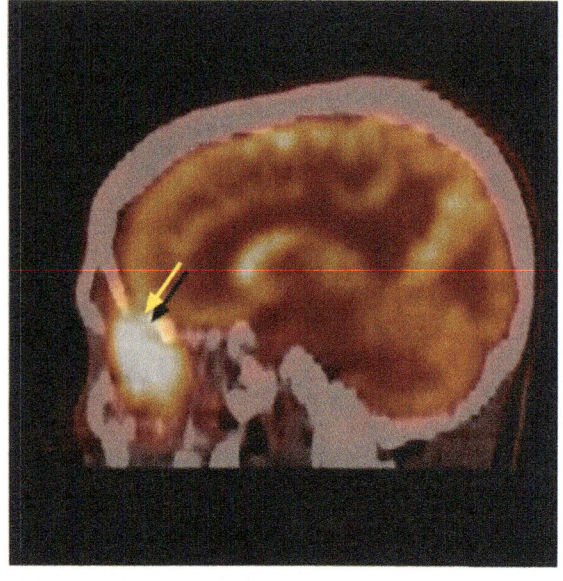

Image 1 (sagittal)

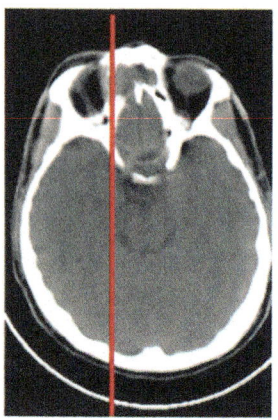

Localizer

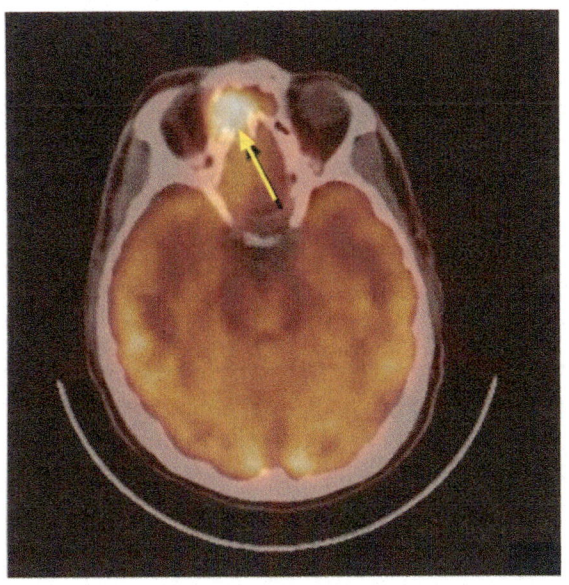

Image 2 (axial)

Image 2. Fused axial image demonstrating bone erosion (arrow).

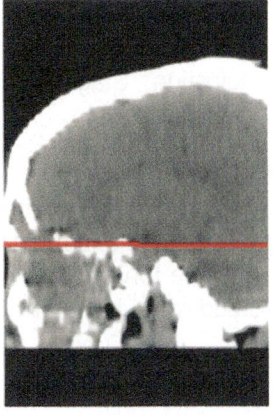

Localizer

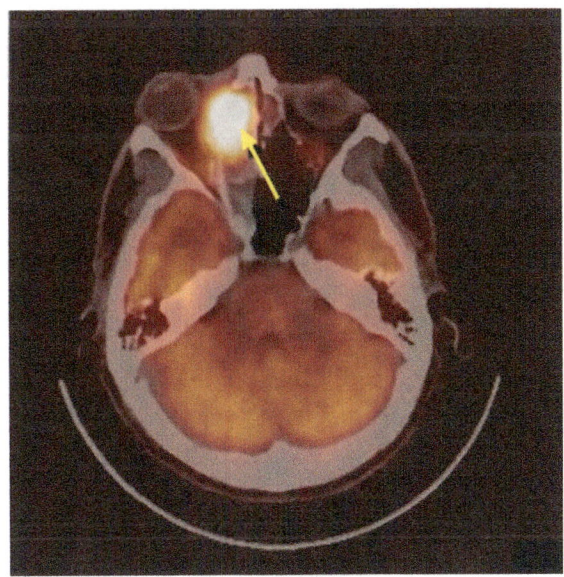

Image 3 (axial)

Image 3. Large right-sided sino-nasal hypermetabolic tumor depicted on this fused axial image.

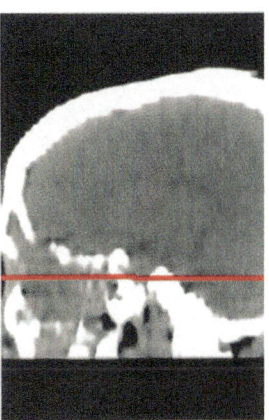

Localizer

Tonsillar Squamous Cell Carcinoma

Clinical History

55-year-old male patient with recently diagnosed squamous cell carcinoma of the right tonsil.

PET/CT indication: Staging.

Findings

A large focus of increased FDG uptake is present in the region of the right tonsil, which corresponds to a tonsillar mass on CT images. This is consistent with the known primary tumor. No additional foci of increased tracer activity are seen to suggest metastatic disease.

Teaching Point

CT demonstrates a right tonsillar mass. Fused PET/CT images showed intensely increased FDG uptake consistent with primary malignancy. CT and PET were concordantly true negative for lymph node involvement.

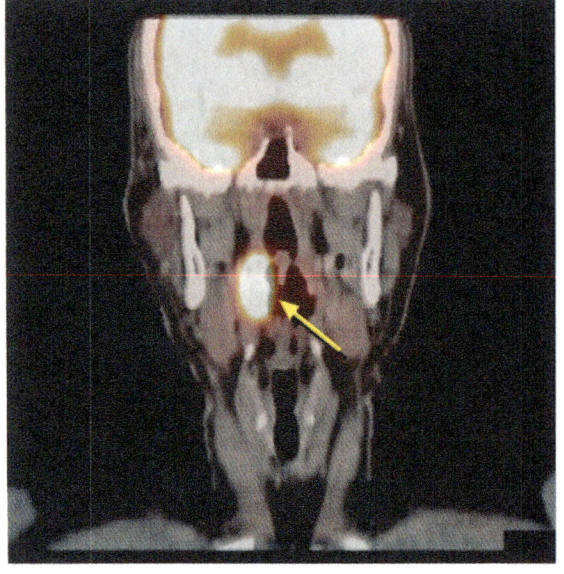

Image 1 (coronal)

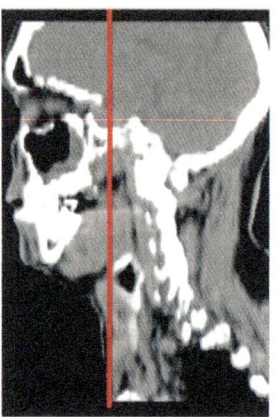

Localizer

Image 1. Fused coronal image of the head and neck region showing increased FDG uptake corresponding to a right tonsillar mass (arrow).

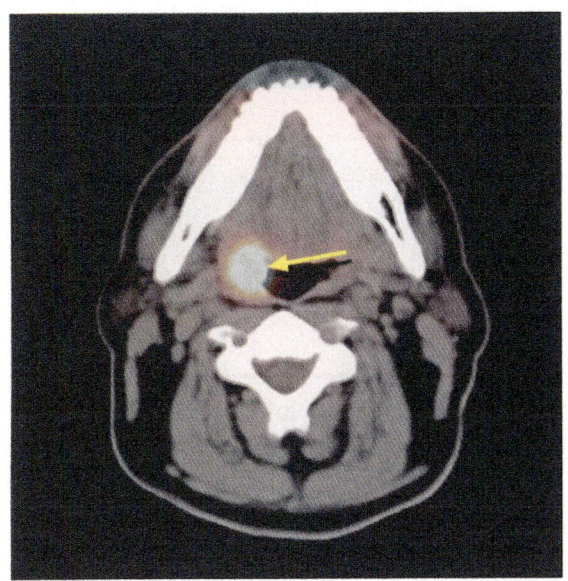

Image 2 (axial)

Image 2. Fused axial image showing increased FDG uptake in the right tonsillar mass (arrow). No enlarged lymph nodes were present.

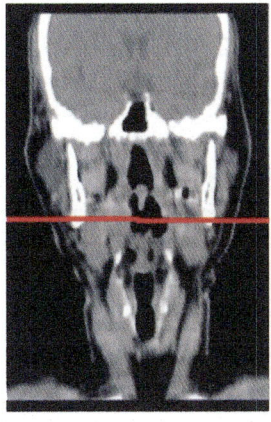

Localizer

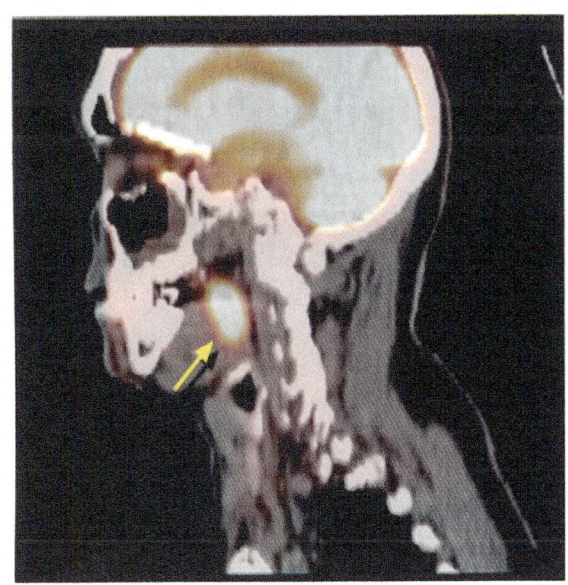

Image 2 (sagittal)

Image 3. Fused sagittal image showing increased FDG uptake in the the right tonsillar mass (arrow).

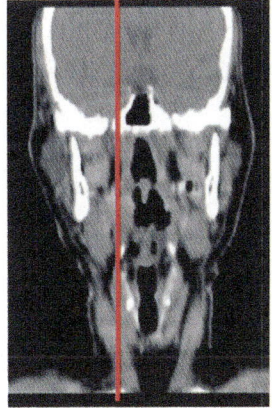

Localizer

Salivary Duct Carcinoma

Clinical History

60-year-old male patient with left neck mass that increased in size over one year. A recent biopsy suggested squamous cell carcinoma.

PET/CT indication: Staging.

Findings

Large irregular bulky hypermetabolic mass involving the soft tissue of left neck including the parotid. Extensive involvement of the cervical lymph node chain is also noted.

Pathology verification: Biopsy: Salivary duct carcinoma

Teaching Point

This patient was in renal failure and intravenous contrast was contraindicated. Intravenous contrast might not be required for diagnosing and staging of head and neck cancers in some patients. In these cases FDG can serve as a molecular "contrast agent."

Image 1. Large left-sided hypermetabolic mass with bulky lymph node involvement (arrow) is shown on this fused coronal image of the head and neck.

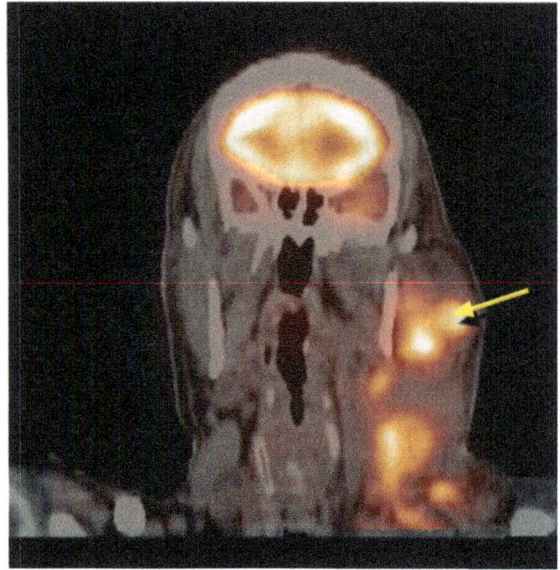

Image 1 (coronal)

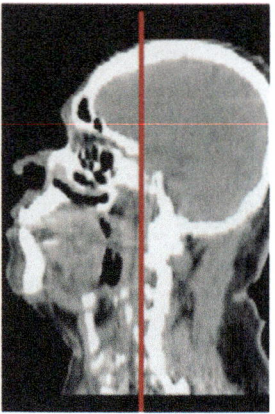

Localizer

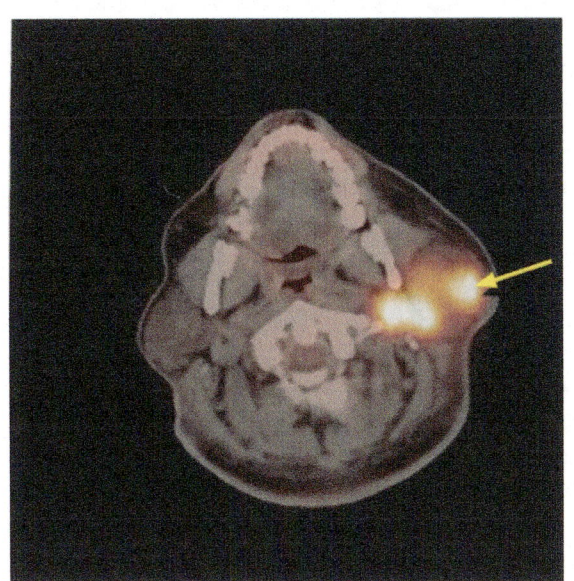

Image 2. Inspection of fused axial image revealed that the primary tumor was located in the left parotid (arrow).

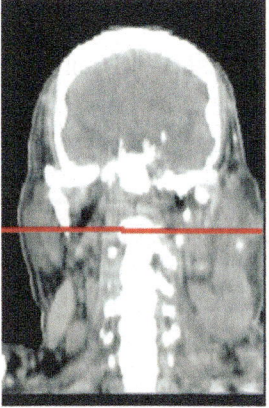

Image 2 (axial)   **Localizer**

Squamous Cell Carcinoma

Clinical History

Male patient with newly diagnosed squamous cell carcinoma of the neck.

PET/CT indication: Staging.

Findings

There are two foci of increased glycolytic activity in the right neck. The larger focus is located infero-medial to the right parotid gland and is consistent with a metastatic lymph node conglomerate; the second smaller focus, positioned more inferiorly at the level of C5, is also consistent with a metastatic lymph node.

Teaching Point

Randomized studies to determine the usefulness of intravenous contrast for PET/CT imaging have not been performed. However, it is our experience that intravenous contrast facilitates the interpretation of PET/CT of the head and neck region.

Image 1

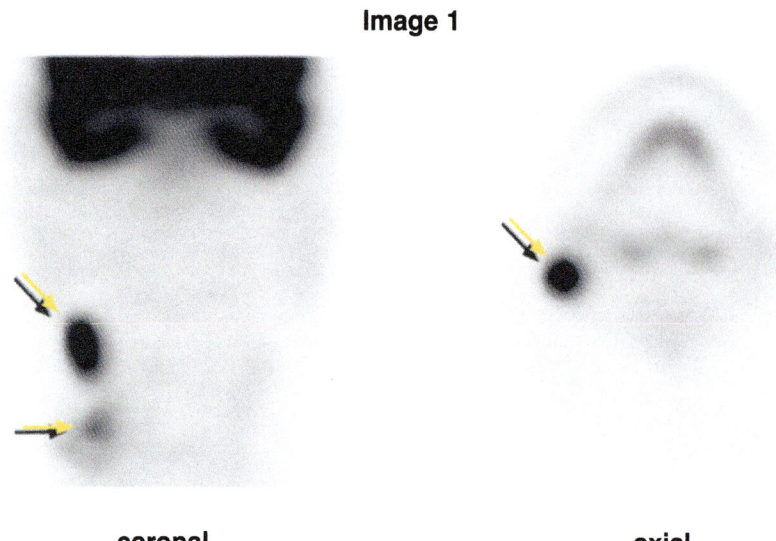

coronal   axial

Image 1. Coronal (left image) and axial PET (right image) depicting a large (arrows) and a small lymph node metastasis (lower arrow on coronal image).

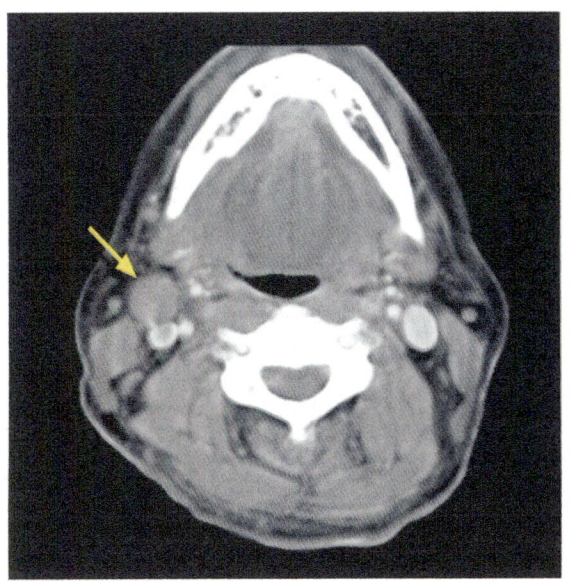

Image 2 (axial)

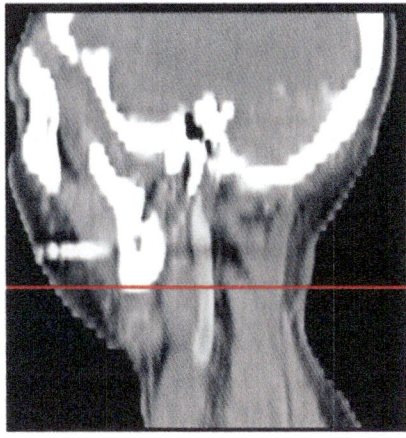

Localizer

Image 2. Axial contrast CT showing enlarged lymph node metastasis (arrow).

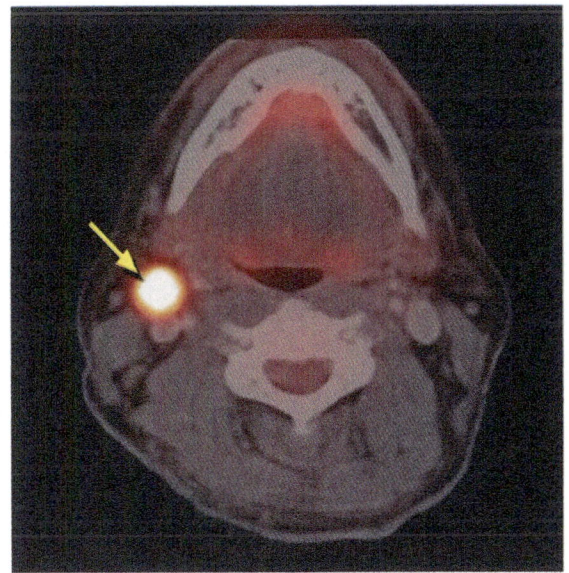

Image 3 (sagittal)

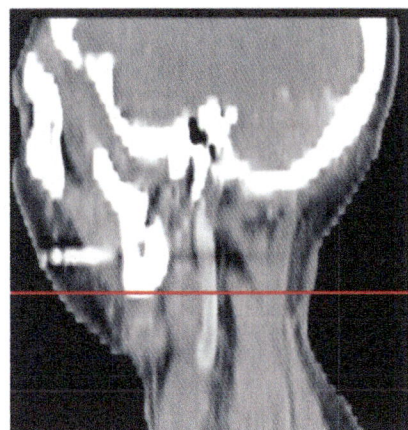

Localizer

Image 3. Fused axial image with hypermetabolic focus corresponding to enlarged lymph node (arrow).

Chapter 5

Solitary Pulmonary Nodules

Cases:

Chapter 5

SOLITARY PULMONARY NODULES

150,000 solitary pulmonary nodules (SPN), defined as single rounded lung lesions not associated with any other lung lesions or lymph-adenopathy, measuring ≤3 cm in maximal diameter, are diagnosed annually in the United States. PET imaging with FDG has largely focused on characterizing "indeterminate" SPNs as malignant or benign. The incidence of malignancy exceeds 40% in the large majority of reports. Benign SPNs might represent granuloma, infections, carcinoid, adenoma, hamartoma, fibrosis, and others. Bronchogenic carcinoma represents the majority of malignant solitary pulmonary nodules. The considerable number of benign solitary pulmonary nodules implies that a large number of biopsies performed are unnecessary. For example, 20% to 40% of lung biopsies produce benign tissue but result in significant morbidity. The diagnostic sensitivity and specificity of PET alone for characterizing solitary pulmonary nodules is high. PET is cost-effective for characterizing solitary pulmonary nodules. Because Medicare reimburses PET/CT at the same level as PET, these cost-effectiveness data also apply to PET/CT. PET/CT can be especially helpful for characterizing small lung nodules with only mildly increased glycolytic activity. The sensitivity of PET declines significantly, however, when solitary nodules are smaller than 8 mm.

Because the sensitivity of PET is less than 100% each solitary pulmonary nodule without glucose metabolic activity needs to be monitored in 3-month intervals by CT (or PET/CT). Despite a considerable number of false positive PET findings, PET positive solitary pulmonary nodules need to be considered malignant until proven otherwise. We consider a nodule suspicious for malignancy if it exhibits any glucose metabolic activity above background.

Key Indication for PET/CT: Tissue Characterization

Suggested Reading

Siegelman SS, Zerhouni EA, Leo FP, Khouri NF, Stitik FP. CT of the solitary pulmonary nodule. Am J Roentgenol. 1980;135(1):1-13.

Lowe VJ, Hoffman JM, DeLong DM, Patz EF, Coleman RE. Semiquantitative and visual analysis of FDG-PET images in pulmonary abnormalities. J Nucl Med. 1994;35(11): 1771-1776.

Dewan NA, Shehan CJ, Reeb SD, Gobar LS, Scott WJ, Ryschon K. Likelihood of malignancy in a solitary pulmonary nodule: comparison of Bayesian analysis and results of FDG-PET scan. Chest. 1997;112(2):416-422.

Lowe VJ, Fletcher JW, Gobar L, Lawson M, Kirchner P, Valk P, Karis J, Hubner K, Delbeke D, Heiberg EV, Patz EF,

Coleman RE. Prospective investigation of positron emission tomography in lung nodules. J Clin Oncol. 1998;16(3):1075-1084.

Gambhir SS, Shepherd JE, Shah BD, Hart E, Hoh CK, Valk PE, Emi T, Phelps ME. Analytical decision model for the cost-effective management of solitary pulmonary nodules. J Clin Oncol. 1998;16(6):2113-2125.

Gould MK, Maclean CC, Kuschner WG, Rydzak CE, Owens DK. Accuracy of positron emission tomography for diagnosis of pulmonary nodules and mass lesions: a meta-analysis. JAMA. 2001;285(7):914-924.

Solitary Pulmonary Nodule

Clinical History

70-year-old female patient with a solitary pulmonary nodule in the left upper lobe on CT.

PET/CT indication: Tissue Characterization.

Findings

A focus of moderately to severely increased glycolytic activity in the left upper lobe corresponds to a nodule measuring 1.5 cm on CT images. This is consistent with malignancy.

Histology: High grade spindle cell tumor.

Teaching Point

FDG-PET characterizes solitary pulmonary nodules with a high accuracy as benign or malignant. PET/CT might be especially helpful to characterize small nodules that can exhibit only mild FDG uptake. Every solitary pulmonary nodule with any degree of FDG uptake needs to be considered malignant until proven otherwise.

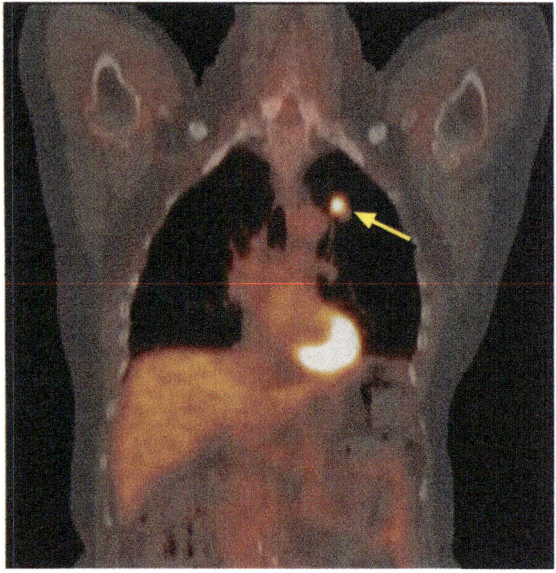

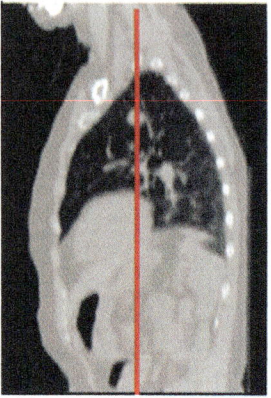

Image 1. Fused coronal image with hyper-glycolytic lung nodule in the left upper lobe (arrow).

Image 1 (coronal)

Localizer

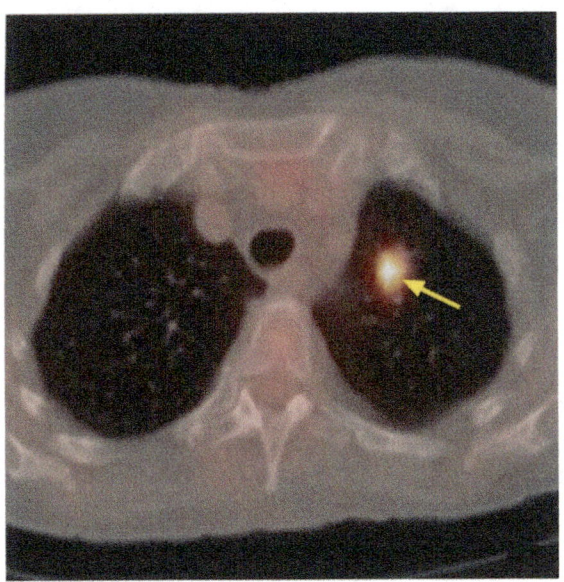

Image 2 (axial)

Image 2. Fused axial image demonstrating the hyper-glycolytic nodule (arrow).

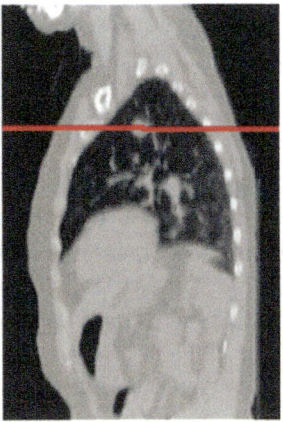

Localizer

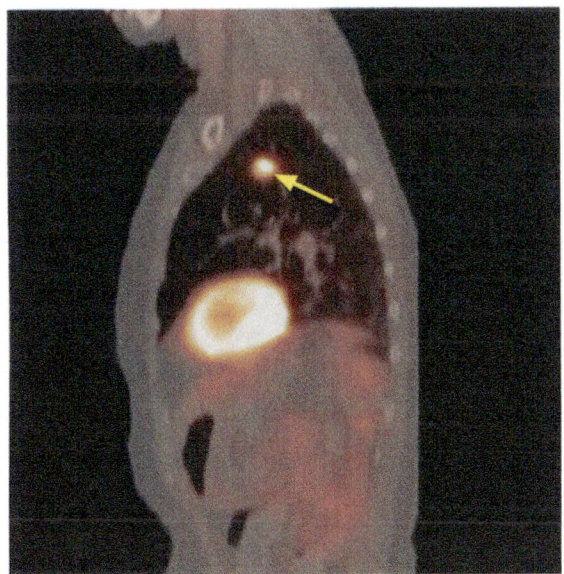

Image 3 (sagittal)

Image 3. Fused sagittal image depicting the hypermetabolic, malignant lung nodule (arrow).

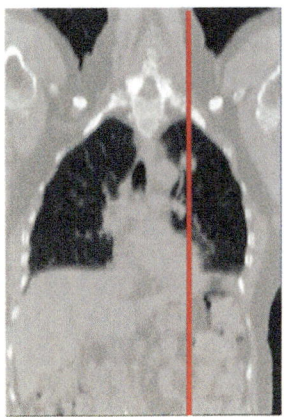

Localizer

Solitary Pulmonary Nodule

Clinical History

50-year-old female with history of Systemic Lupus and a left lower lobe solitary pulmonary nodule.

PET/CT indication: Lesion characterization.

Findings

Mildly increased paraspinal and para-aortic FDG uptake in the left lower lung. This might be consistent with malignancy. Because the uptake is very mild benign disease is more likely. However, biopsy is suggested to rule out malignancy.

Pathological Verification: Necrotizing granuloma secondary to coccidiomycosis infection.

Teaching Point

Even mildly increased FDG uptake in solitary pulmonary nodule does not rule out lung cancer. Thus, biopsy needs to be performed to rule out malignancy. Biopsy revealed granuloma in this patient.

Image 1. Fused coronal images showing left paraspinal focus of very mildly increased FDG uptake (arrow). Note the "mushroom artifact" due to respiratory motion.

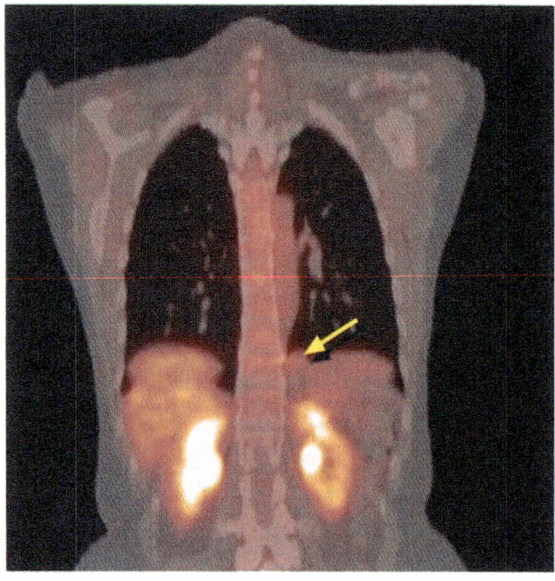

Image 1 (coronal)

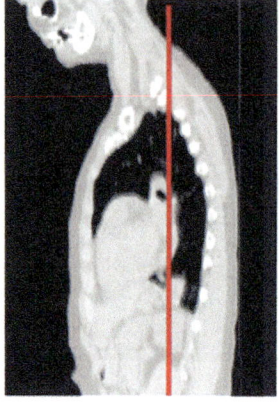

Localizer

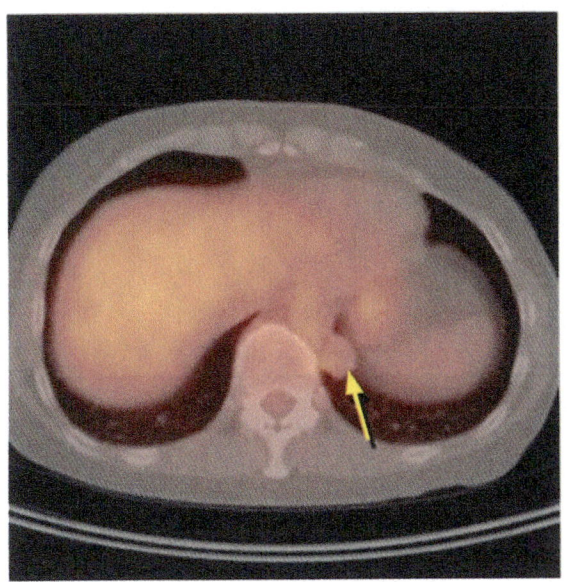

Image 2 (axial)

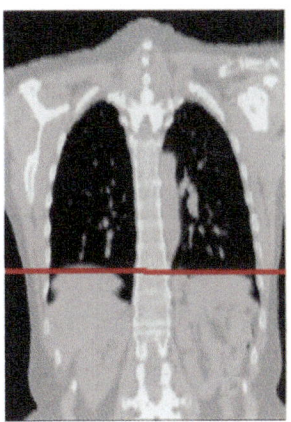

Localizer

Image 2. Fused axial image localizing the lung nodule with mildly increased FDG uptake to the left paraspinal region (arrow).

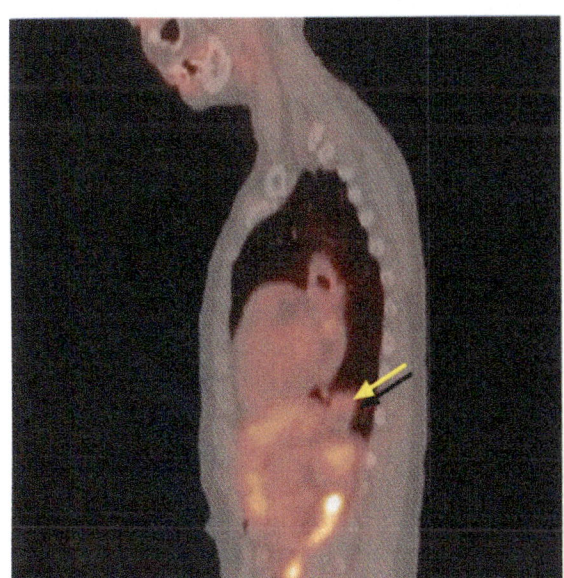

Image 3 (sagittal)

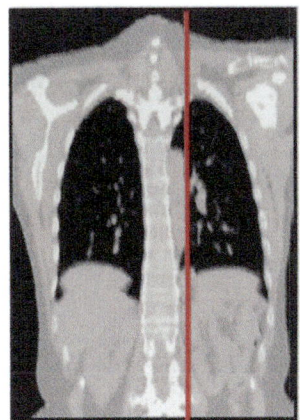

Localizer

Image 3. Sagittal image localizing the lung nodule to the base of the left lung with mildly increased FDG uptake (arrow).

Hamartoma

Clinical History

65-year-old male with incidental finding of solitary pulmonary nodule.

PET/CT indication: Lesion characterization.

Findings

A solitary left lung nodule demonstrates no significant FDG activity

Pathology Verification: Hamartoma.

Teaching Point

Solitary pulmonary nodules without glucose metabolic activity require CT follow up in 3-months intervals.

Image 1. Fused coronal image with FDG-negative solitary pulmonary nodule (yellow arrow). Note the prominent vascular structures on the right (red arrow).

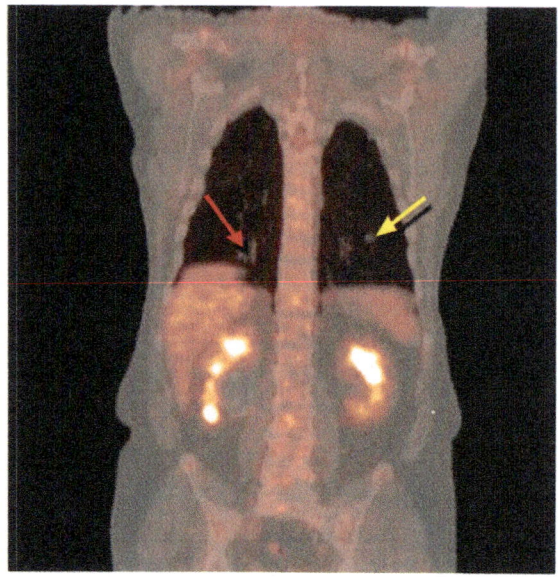

Image 1 (coronal)

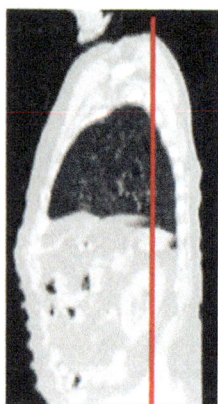

Localizer

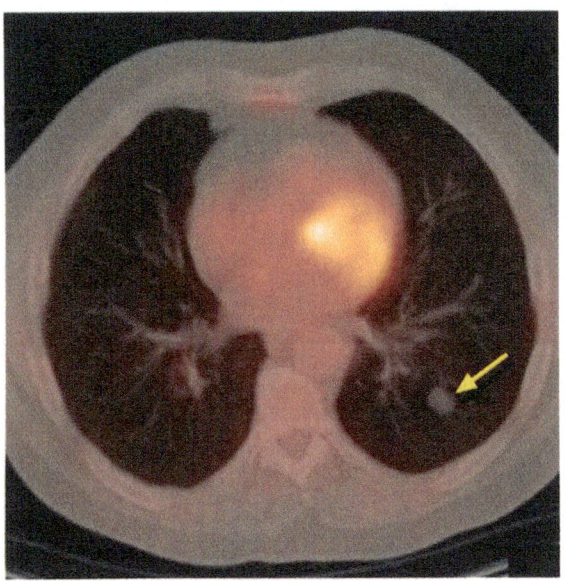

Image 2 (axial)

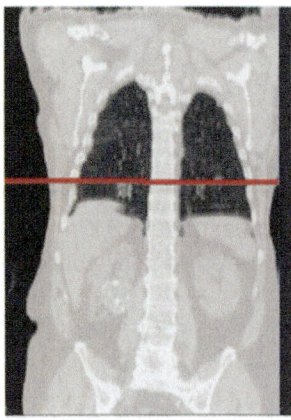

Localizer

Image 2. Fused axial image depicting the solitary pulmonary nodule without FDG uptake (arrow).

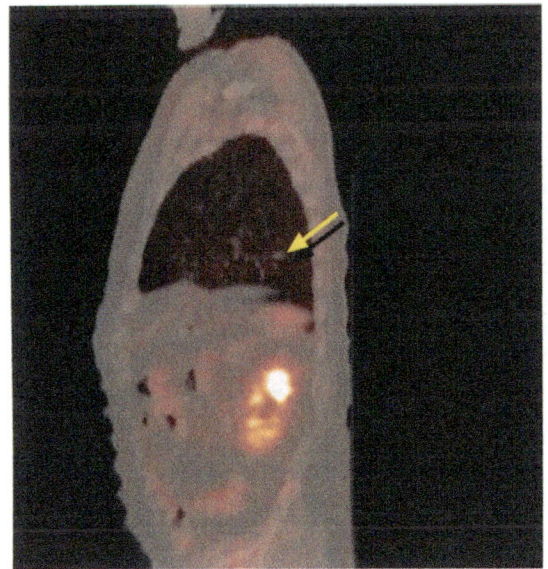

Image 3 (sagittal)

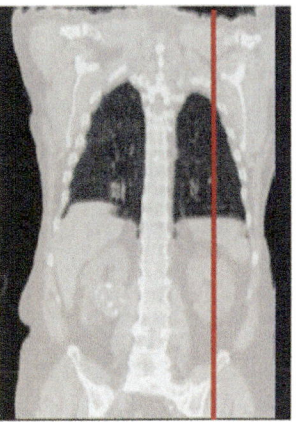

Localizer

Image 3. Fused sagittal image showing the solitary pulmonary nodule (arrow).

Coccidiomycosis

Clinical History

50-year-old male with left lower lobe pulmonary nodule.

PET/CT indication: Lesion characterization.

Findings

A nodule measuring 1.3 cm in greatest diameter is present in the left lower lobe on CT. There is no evidence of abnormal tracer activity on PET images to suggest malignancy.

Pathology Verification: Coccidiomycosis.

Teaching Point

Coccidiomycosis can be associated with intensely increased FDG uptake. In the current case, PET was true negative for malignancy. However, the specificity of FDG-PET for characterizing solitary lung nodules is below 85% in most studies. This is due to the fact that benign lesions can exhibit various degrees of increased FDG uptake.

Image 1. Fused coronal image depicting an ametabolic solitary pulmonary nodule of the left lower lobe (arrow).

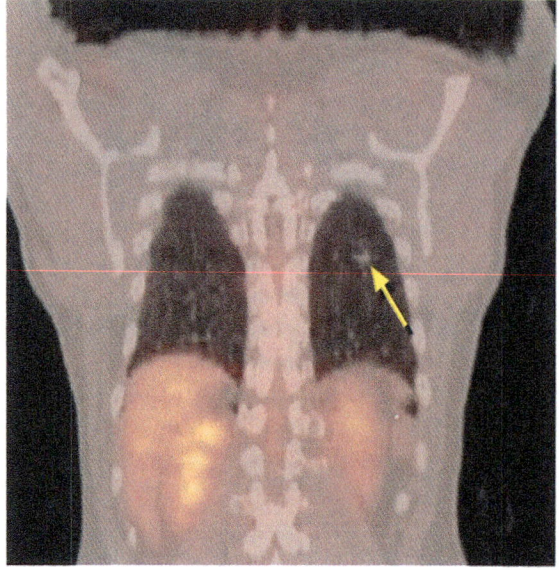

Image 1 (coronal)

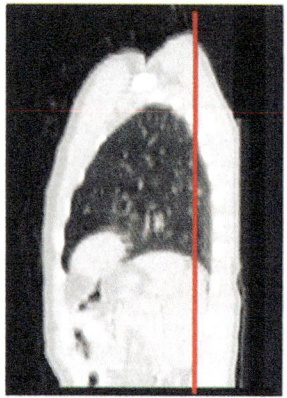

Localizer

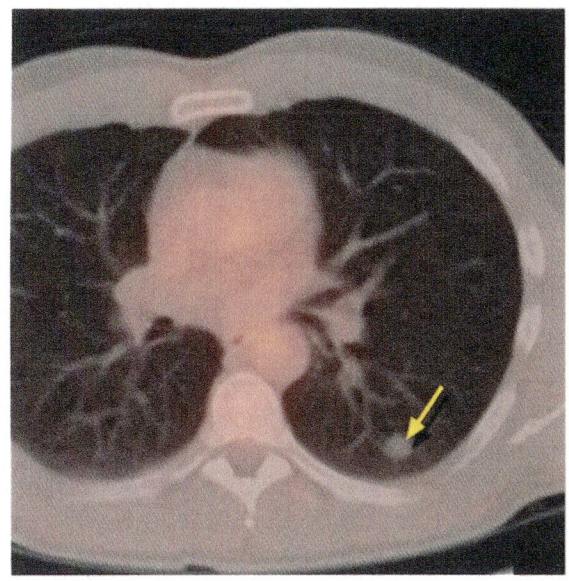

Image 2 (axial)

Image 2. The posterior left lung nodule without metabolic activity is shown on fused axial image (arrow).

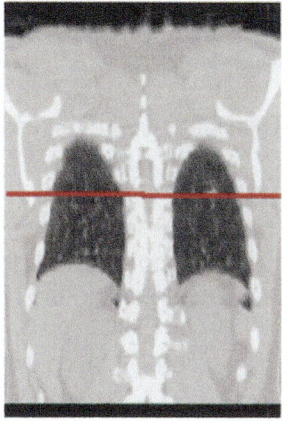

Localizer

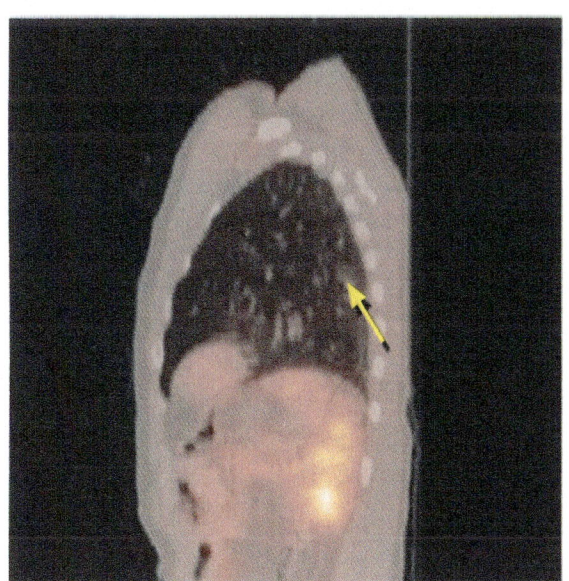

Image 3 (sagittal)

Image 3. Fused sagittal view of the ametabolic lung nodule (arrow).

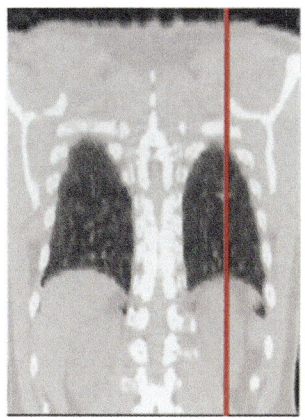

Localizer

Solitary Pulmonary Nodule

Clinical History

72-year-old male with history of smoking and asbestos exposure presents with left upper lobe lung nodule on CT.

PET/CT indication: Characterization of pulmonary nodule.

Findings

The lung nodule does not exhibit increased FDG uptake. The incidental finding of an area of increased FDG uptake in the right 7th rib laterally may be secondary to trauma.

Pathology verification: Benign disease

Teaching Point

Early detection and removal is the only way to cure lung cancer. Thus, PET/CT studies should be interpreted at high sensitivity levels. We consider even the mildest degree of FDG uptake in a solitary pulmonary nodule as suspicious for malignancy until proven otherwise. In the case of a negative PET scan, patients need to be followed by CT to avoid the consequences of false negative PET studies.

Image 1

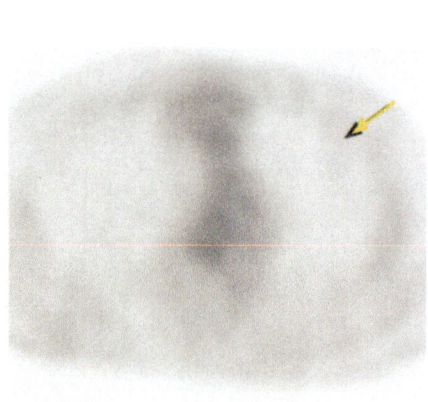 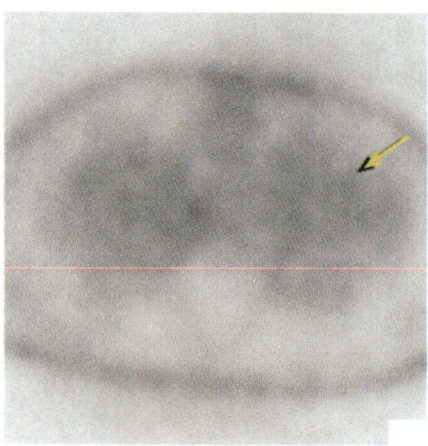

axial   axial

Image 1. Axial attenuation corrected (left image) and uncorrected (right image) PET without increased FDG uptake.

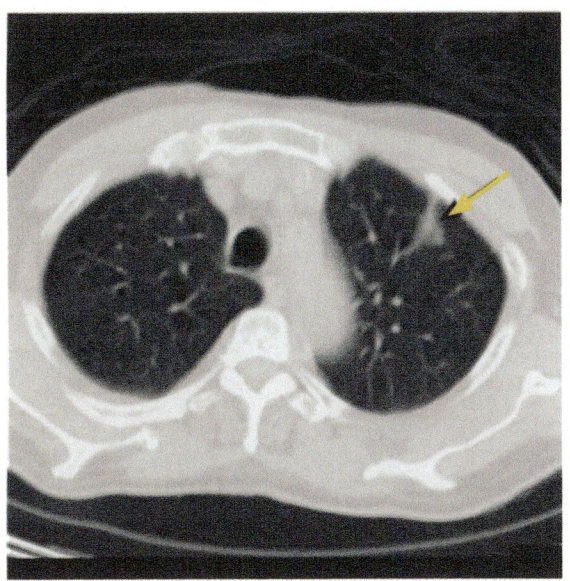

Image 2 (axial)

Image 2. Axial CT demonstrating the solitary pulmonary nodule in the left upper lobe (arrow).

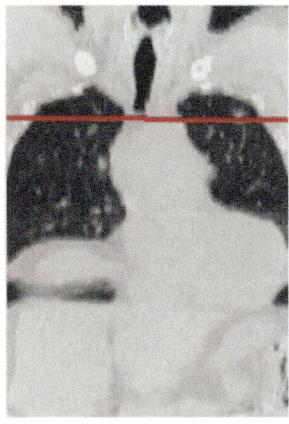

Localizer

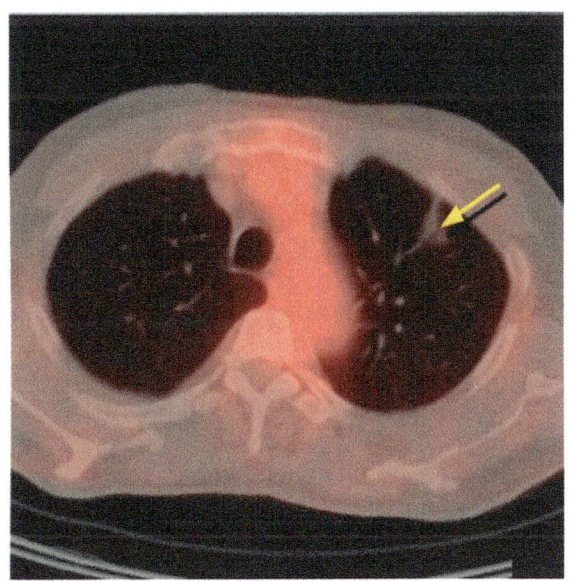

Image 3 (axial)

Image 3. Fused axial corrected image demonstrating the lung nodule without increased glucose metabolic activity (arrow).

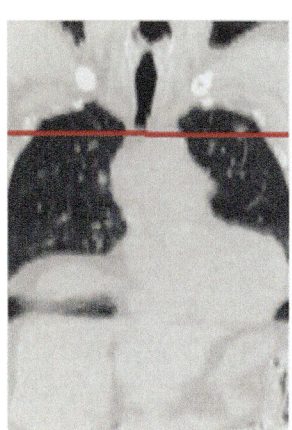

Localizer

Chapter 6

Lung Cancer

Cases:

Chapter 6

Lung Cancer

The incidence of lung cancer is increasing largely due to a continuing rise of smoking in women. The 5-year survival rate of lung cancer patients is 13%. FDG-PET diagnoses, stages and re-stages lung cancer with a high diagnostic accuracy that is superior to that of CT. PET has therefore been established as the standard of care for these indications.

There are, however, some limitations of PET that can be overcome with PET/CT. For instance, PET can determine presence but not the precise location of lymph node involvement. Exact localization is however important for establishing the correct patient stage and thus the appropriate treatment.

Early PET/CT studies suggest that PET/CT stages lung cancer with a higher accuracy than PET or CT alone or than PET and CT read side by side.

Key Indications for PET/CT: Diagnosis, Staging and Restaging

Suggested Reading

Dillemans B, Deneffe G, Verschakelen J, Decramer M. Value of computed tomography and mediastinoscopy in preoperative evaluation of mediastinal nodes in non-small cell lung cancer. A study of 569 patients. Eur J Cardiothorac Surg. 1994;8(1):37-42.

Valk PE, Pounds TR, Hopkins DM, Haseman MK, Hofer GA, Greiss HB, Myers RW, Lutrin CL. Staging non-small cell lung cancer by whole-body positron emission tomographic imaging. Ann Thorac Surg. 1995;60(6):1573-1582.

Scott WJ, Gobar LS, Terry JD, Dewan NA, Sunderland JJ. Mediastinal lymph node staging of non-small-cell lung cancer: a prospective comparison of computed tomography and positron emission tomography. J Thorac Cardiovasc Surg. 1996;111(3):642-648.

Gambhir SS, Hoh CK, Phelps ME, Madar I, Maddahi J. Decision tree sensitivity analysis for cost-effectiveness of FDG-PET in the staging and management of non-small-cell lung carcinoma. J Nucl Med. 1996;37(9):1428-1436.

Steinert HC, Hauser M, Allemann F, Engel H, Berthold T, von Schulthess GK, Weder W. Non-small cell lung cancer: nodal staging with FDG PET versus CT with correlative lymph node mapping and sampling. Radiology. 1997;202(2):441-446.

Vansteenkiste JF, Stroobants SG, De Leyn PR, Dupont PJ, Bogaert J, Maes A, Deneffe GJ, Nackaerts KL, Verschakelen JA, Lerut TE, Mortelmans LA, Demedts MG. Lymph node staging in non-small-cell lung cancer with FDG-PET scan: a prospective study on 690 lymph node stations from 68 patients. J Clin Oncol. 1998;16(6):2142-2149.

Weder W, Schmid RA, Bruchhaus H, Hillinger S, von Schulthess GK, Steinert HC. Detection of extrathoracic metastases by positron emission tomography in lung cancer. Ann Thorac Surg. 1998;66(3):886-892.

Dwamena BA, Sonnad SS, Angobaldo JO, Wahl RL. Metastases from non-small cell lung cancer: mediastinal staging in the 1990s—meta-analytic comparison of PET and CT. Radiology. 1999;213(2):530-536.

Pieterman RM, van Putten JW, Meuzelaar JJ, Mooyaart EL, Vaalburg W, Koeter GH, Fidler V, Pruim J, Groen HJ. Preoperative staging of non-small-cell lung cancer with positron-emission tomography. N Engl J Med. 2000;343(4):254-261.

Seltzer MA, Yap CS, Silverman DH, Meta J, Schiepers C, Phelps ME, Gambhir SS, Rao J, Valk PE, Czernin J. The impact of PET on the management of lung cancer: the referring physician's perspective. J Nucl Med. 2002;43(6):752-756.

Lardinois D, Weder W, Hany TF, Kamel EM, Korom S, Seifert B, von Schulthess GK, Steinert HC. Staging of non-small-cell lung cancer with integrated positron-emission tomography and computed tomography. N Engl J Med. 2003;348(25):2500-2507.

Antoch G, Stattaus J, Nemat AT, Marnitz S, Beyer T, Kuehl H, Bockisch A, Debatin JF, Freudenberg LS. Non-small cell lung cancer: dual-modality PET/CT in preoperative staging. Radiology. 2003;229(2):526-533.

Lung Cancer

Clinical History

This 82-year-old patient with non-small-cell carcinoma underwent a left upper lobectomy with lymph node dissection in 1997. A recent CT revealed a right lung mass.

PET/CT indication: Restaging.

Findings

A large focus of intense hypermetabolism in the posterior aspect of the right upper lobe is consistent with recurrent disease. Right hilar lymph node involvement and a left adrenal gland metastasis are present.

Teaching Point

Adrenal metastases can be difficult to diagnose with PET. Co-registered PET/CT images correctly assigned the left abdominal hypermetabolic focus to the left adrenal gland.

Image 1. Fused coronal image demonstrating right hilar and left adrenal involvement (arrows).

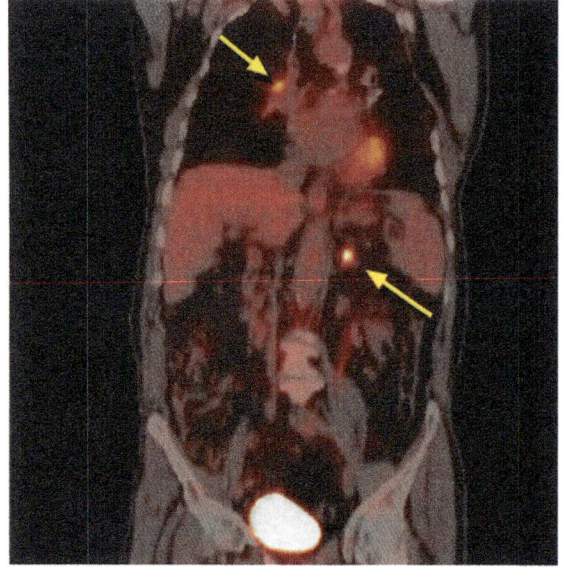

Image 1 (coronal)

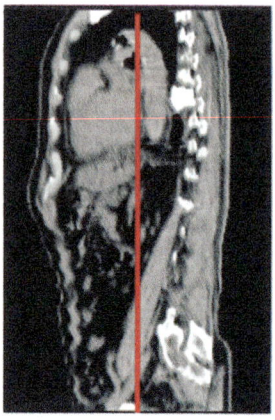

Localizer

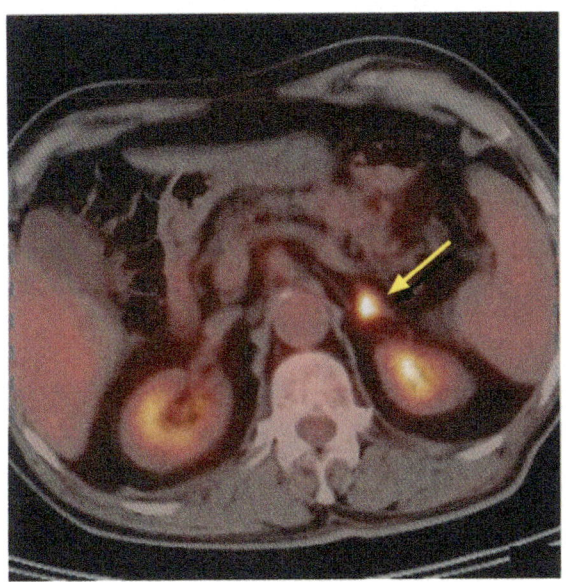

Image 2. Fused axial image with hypermetabolic focus in the left adrenal gland (arrow).

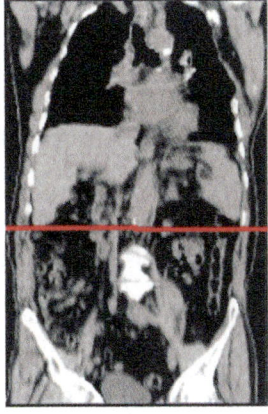

Image 2 (axial)

Localizer

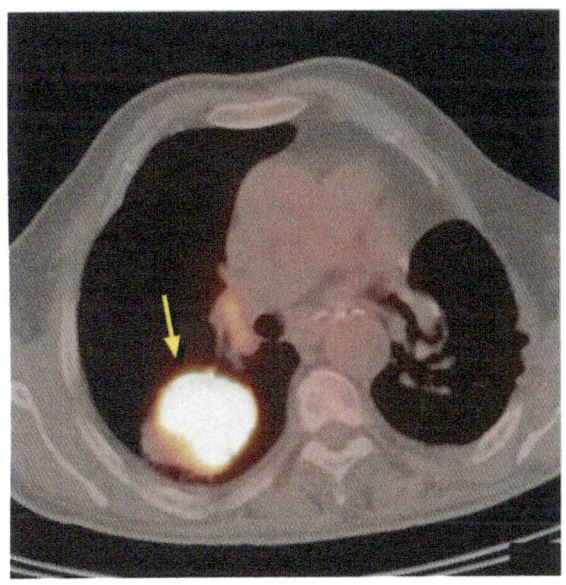

Image 3. Fused axial image with intensely hypermetabolic site of lung cancer recurrence (arrow).

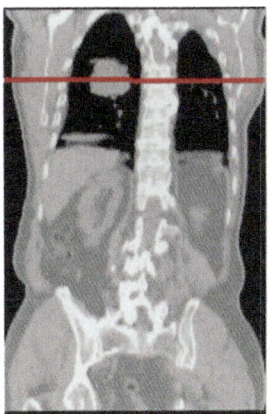

Image 3 (axial)

Localizer

Lung Cancer

Clinical History

51-year-old female patient with history of lung cancer and known bone metastases to the spine and the ribs.

PET/CT indication: Restaging.

Findings

Whole body PET/CT reveals multiple hypermetabolic bone lesions consistent with metastatic disease.

Teaching Point

Bone metastases can be assessed with PET/CT whereby FDG-PET provides more specific information than standard bone scanning. CT provides the exact anatomic localization of increased glycolysis. Note that PET alone could not reliably assign the large lesion shown below to bone.

Image 1. Large hypermetabolic lytic bone lesion involving vertebral body, transverse process and adjacent rib (arrows).

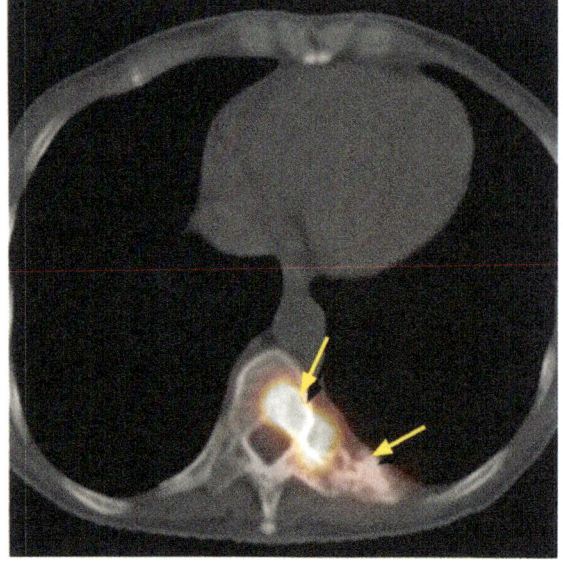

Image 1 (axial)

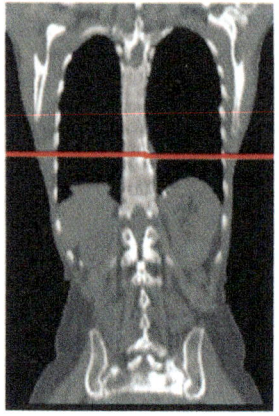

Localizer

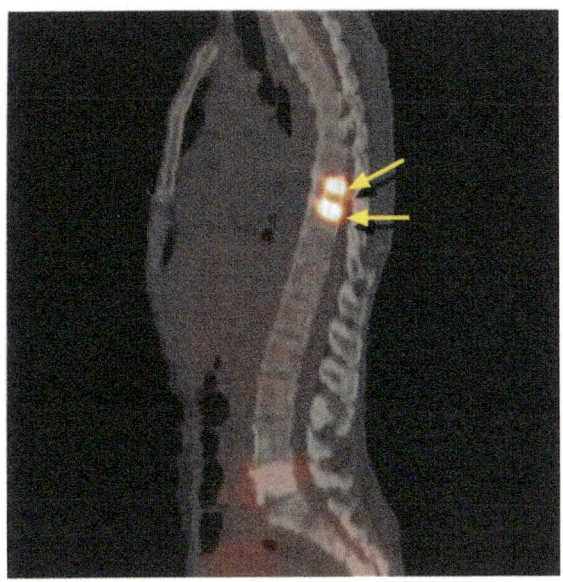

Image 2. Fused sagittal image demonstrates two hypermetabolic lesions in the distal thoracic spine (arrows).

Image 2 (sagittal)

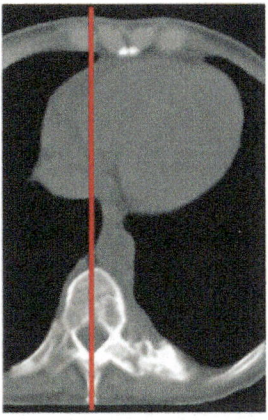

Localizer

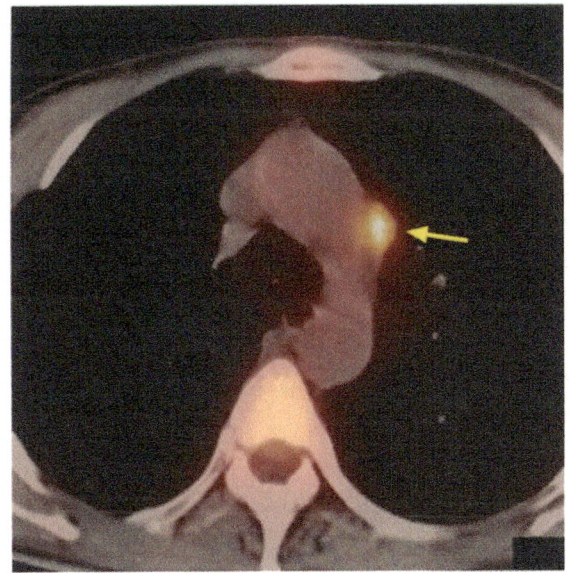

Image 3. In addition to bone lesions, the whole body scan revealed left-sided hilar lymph node involvement (arrow) as shown on fused axial image.

Image 3 (axial)

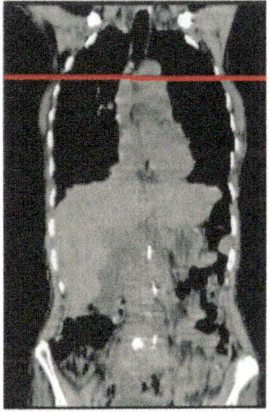

Localizer

Mucin-Producing Adenocarcinoma of the Lung

Clinical History

70-year-old patient with lung cancer who is status post radiation treatment and chemotherapy. The study was performed two months after the end of chemotherapy and radiation treatment.

PET/CT indication: Restaging.

Findings

Minimal, diffuse uptake is identified within the left upper lobe. This corresponds to an area of reticular nodular opacities on the CT that are suggestive of radiation change. A 2- to 3-cm soft tissue density in the left upper lung does not exhibit increased FDG uptake. Minimal, diffuse uptake in the upper lobe of the left lung is likely related to the patient's radiation therapy. No evidence to suggest recurrent or residual malignancy.

Teaching Point

CT revealed radiation changes and a residual mass in the left upper lobe. This was suspicious for residual malignancy. There was no FDG uptake in this area. PET findings were consistent with radiation changes but not with residual tumor. Thus, PET/CT was false negative for residual/recurrent lung cancer. Mucin-producing tumors are frequently false-negative by FDG-PET. This has been reported for mucin-producing broncho-alveolar carcinomas, pancreatic cancers and colorectal carcinomas.

Image 1. Fused coronal image demonstrating left upper lobe mass without FDG uptake. This was considered negative for malignancy (arrow). Biopsy performed one week later revealed mucin-producing adenocarcinoma. Note the bilateral "mushroom" artifacts.

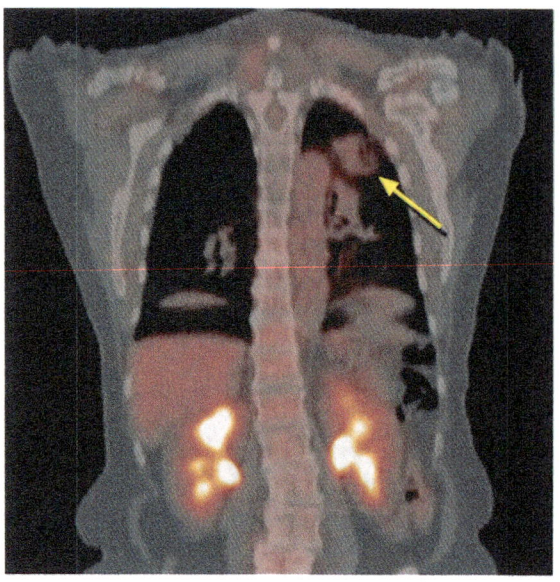

Image 1 (coronal)

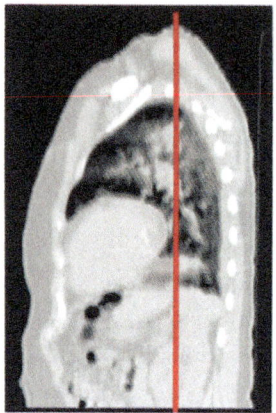

Localizer

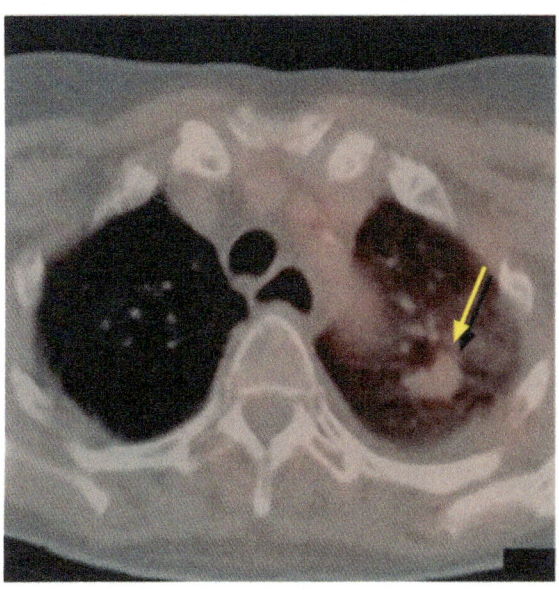

Image 2 (axial)

Image 2. Axial image demonstrating radiation-induced changes and a distinct left upper lobe mass on CT (arrow).

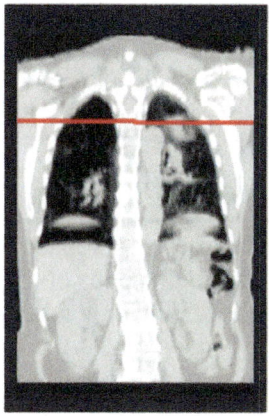

Localizer

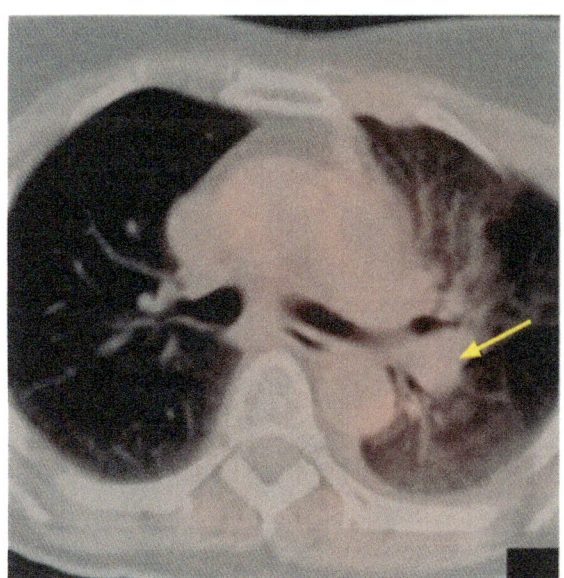

Image 3 (axial)

Image 3. Fused axial image demonstrating radiation-induced changes in lung parenchyma (arrow).

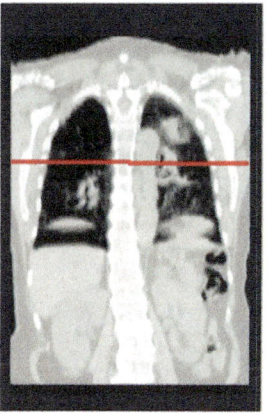

Localizer

Lung Cancer and Granuloma

Clinical History

64-year-old female patient with lung nodules detected on chest x-ray. PET performed at an outside institution two months before the PET/CT revealed foci of increased tracer activity in the left upper lobe and superior mediastinum, which were suggestive of metastatic disease.

PET/CT indication: Staging.

Findings

Two foci of mildly increased tracer activity in the superior mediastinum correspond to two pretracheal lymph nodes on CT. Foci of moderately increased tracer activity in the left suprahilar region and the left upper lobe also correspond to nodules on CT. Two nodules in the right lower lobe on CT measuring 1.8 cm and 0.6 cm do not exhibit increased activity on PET. These are therefore likely benign.

Teaching Point

Based on PET this patient was stage IIIA (ipsilateral lymph node involvement) and therefore a potential surgical candidate. CT revealed a contralateral right lower lobe nodule suggesting that the patient was stage IV. FDG uptake was not increased in this lesion. Subsequent biopsy revealed a granuloma in the right lower lobe. The case underscores the limitations of CT for characterizing lung masses as malignant or benign.

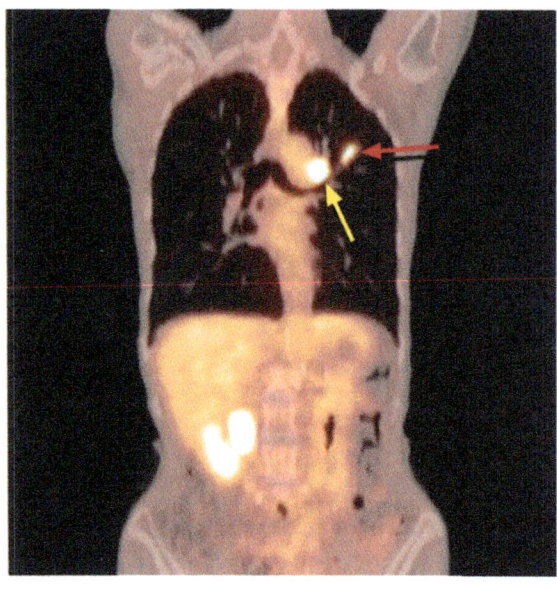

Image 1. Fused coronal image showing left hilar (yellow arrow) and left upper lobe (red arrow) hypermetabolic lesions consistent with non-small cell lung cancer with lymph node metastasis.

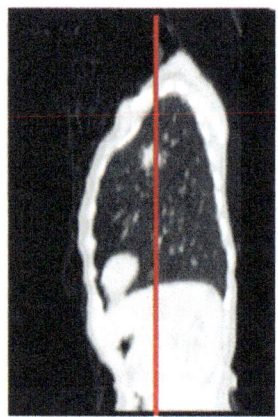

Image 1 (coronal)

Localizer

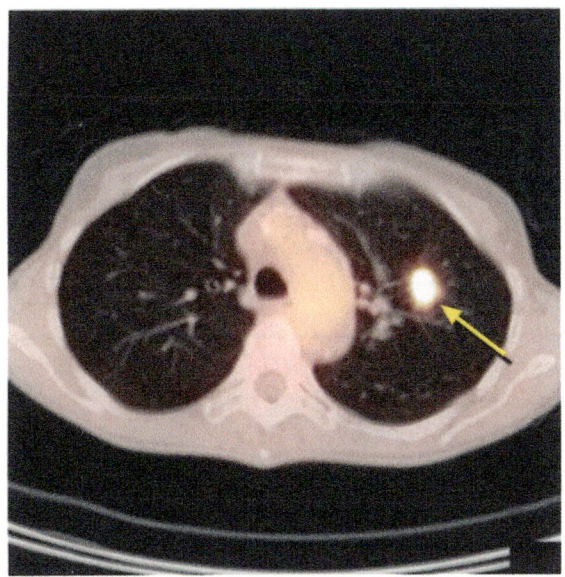

Image 2 (axial)

Image 2. Fused axial image of the primary tumor located in the left upper lobe (arrow).
Increased FDG uptake is consistent with malignancy. This was subsequently proven by biopsy.

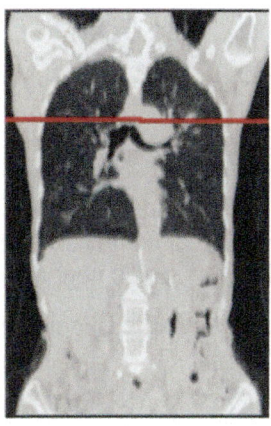

Localizer

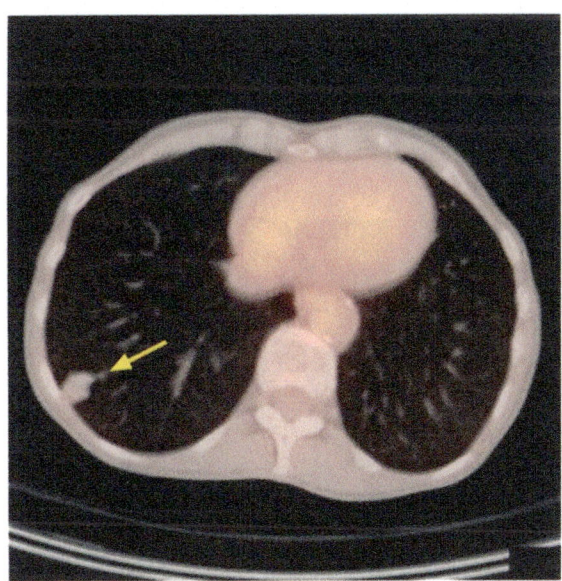

Image 3 (axial)

Image 3. An additional contralateral lung nodule without glycolytic activity (arrow) was identified on PET/CT. Biopsy of this lesion revealed granuloma.

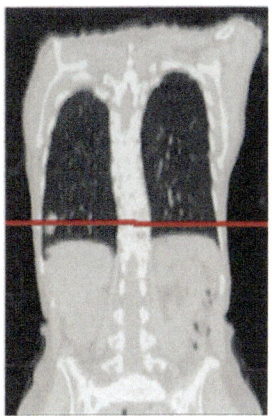

Localizer

Malignant and Benign Diseases

Clinical History

37-year-old female patient with multiple lung nodules and pulmonary fibrosis. Bronchoscopy was suspicious for lung malignancy.

PET/CT indication: Characterization of lung nodules.

Findings

1. Multiple bilateral diffuse foci of increased tracer activity are identified in the lungs. In the given clinical context, these foci are likely consistent with both fibrotic changes and malignancy which cannot be distinguished by PET/CT alone.

2. An intense focus is identified in the right iliac bone suspicious for a distant osseous metastasis.

Teaching Points

1. Benign (fibrosis and inflammation) and malignant diseases can co-exist and the intensity of FDG uptake can be very similar in inflammation and malignancy.

2. Mucin-producing adenocarcinoma frequently exhibits only mildly increased FDG uptake.

3. Whole body PET (and thus PET/CT) detects unexpected distant disease in about 10% of all lung cancer patients.

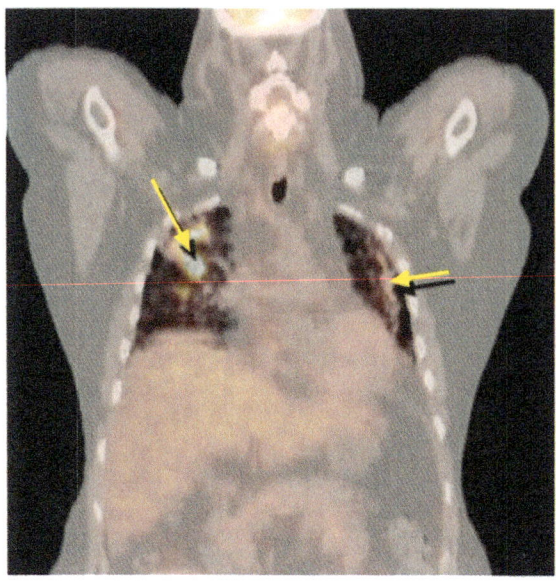

Image 1 (coronal)

Image 1. Fused coronal image with bilateral hypermetabolic lung lesions. FDG uptake in the right upper lobe appears to be more intense than in the left despite subsequent benign findings on biopsy.

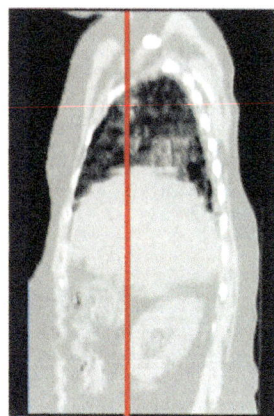

Localizer

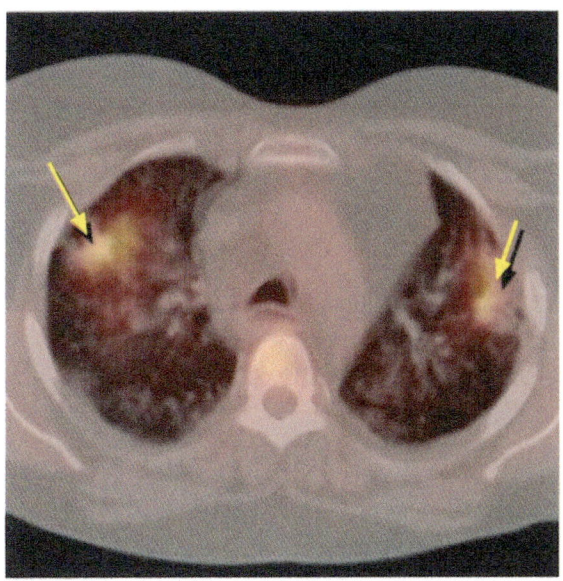

Image 2 (axial)

Image 2. Fused axial image showing bilateral lung lesions of similar intensity (arrows). Biopsy revealed mucin-producing adenocarcinoma on the left and benign inflammatory changes on the right.

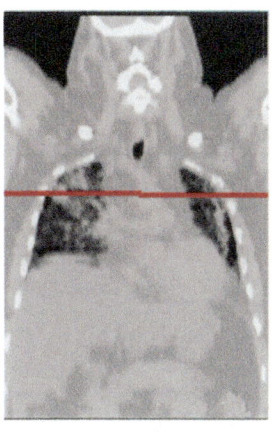

Localizer

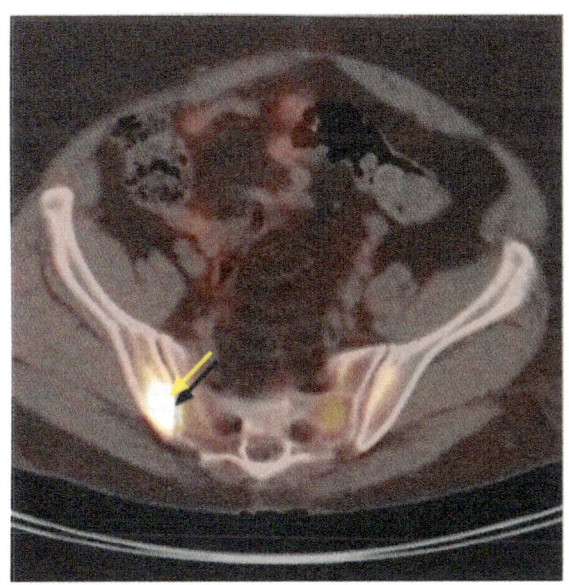

Image 3 (axial)

Image 3. Fused axial image with focally increased FGD uptake in the right posterior iliac wing consistent with metastatic disease (arrow).

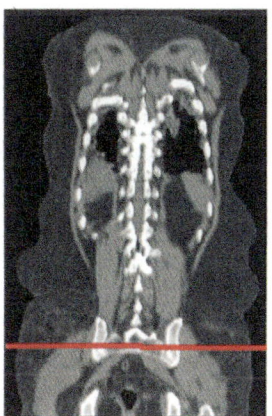

Localizer

Carcinoid

Clinical History

49-year-old female with hemoptysis and left upper lobe mass.

PET/CT indication: Characterization of pulmonary mass.

Findings

Diffusely increased tracer uptake in the left upper lung field is due to left upper lobe atelectasis. The left central hilar mass does not exhibit increased FDG uptake.

Verification: Well-differentiated Carcinoid.

Teaching Points

Neuroendocrine tumors do not consistently exhibit increased FDG uptake. Absent glycolytic activity in a suspicious mass does not obviate the need for biopsy.

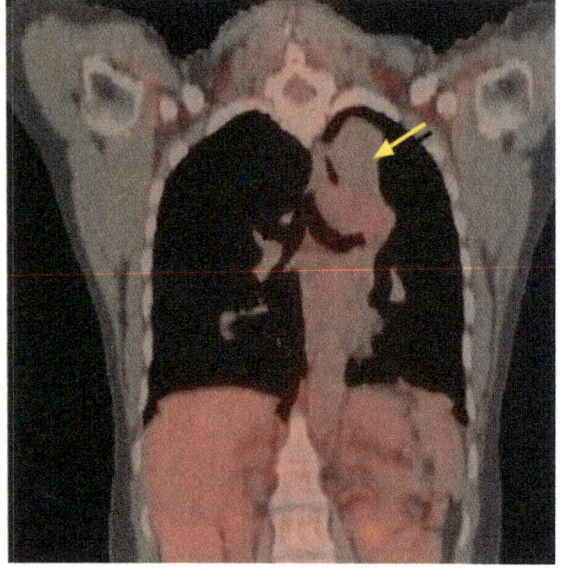

Image 1 (coronal)

Image 1. Fused coronal image depicting the large left upper lobe mass without significant FDG uptake (arrow).

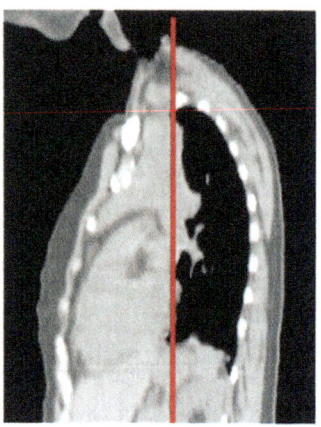

Localizer

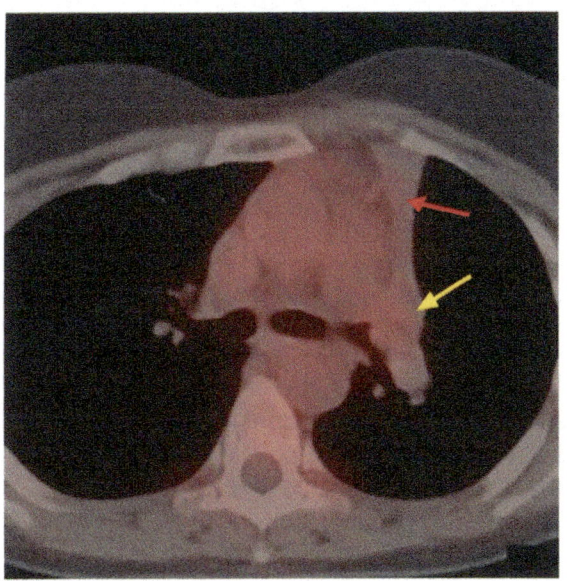

Image 2 (axial)

Image 2. Fused axial image demonstrating the left posterior hilar component of the mass (yellow arrow) extending to the anterior chest wall (red arrow). FDG uptake is not increased.

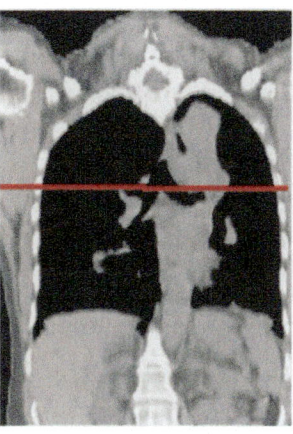

Localizer

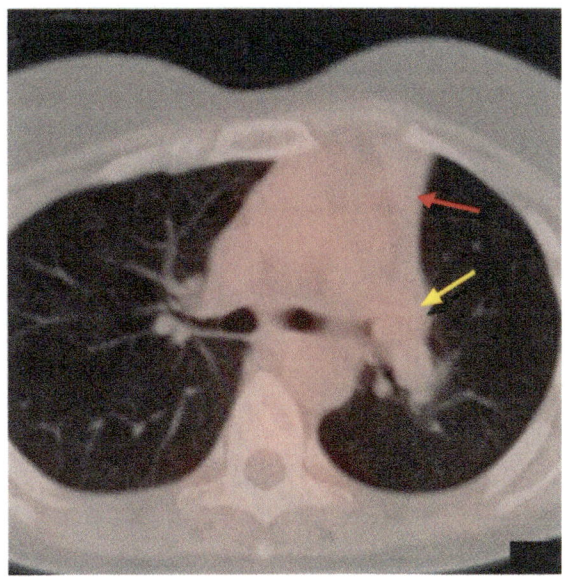

Image 3 (axial)

Image 3. Axial CT image set to lung window demonstrating the mass extending from the posterior left hilar region (yellow arrow) to the chest wall (red arrow).

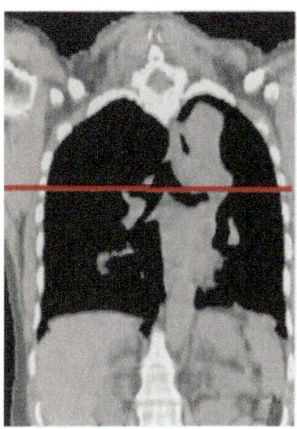

Localizer

Status post Pneumonectomy

Clinical History

78-year-old female with history of adeno-squamous lung carcinoma, status post left pneumonectomy.

PET/CT indication: Restaging.

Findings

A shift of the mediastinum to the left is noted. A focus of increased uptake is identified in the postero-medial left lower thorax posterior to the displaced right main bronchus. This is suspicious for right mediastinal/hilar lymph node metastasis. A small focus of mildly increased uptake in the right lower lobe is suspicious for a right lower lobe metastasis.

Teaching Points

The post-surgical anatomical distortion precludes accurate assessment of the PET study. Side by side visual analysis of PET and CT is also difficult and error prone. Image fusion provided more accurate topological information.

Image 1. Focus of increased FDG uptake in the mediastinum that has been shifted to the left (arrow). Note the mushroom artifact due to respiratory motion.

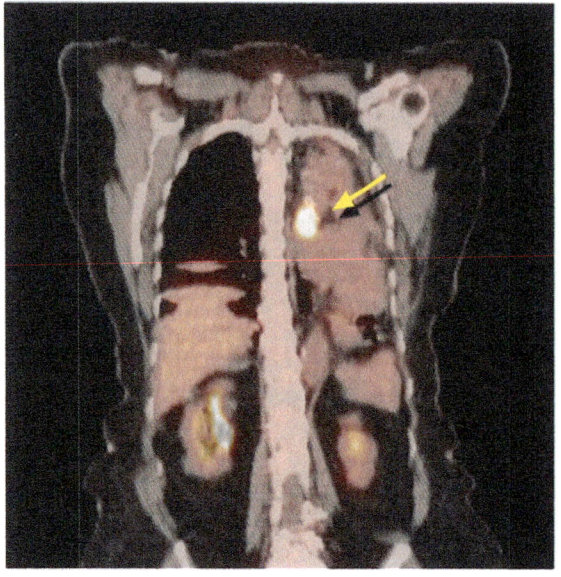

Image 1 (coronal)

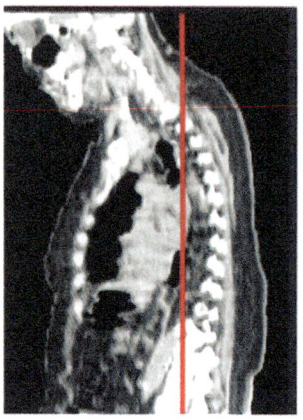

Localizer

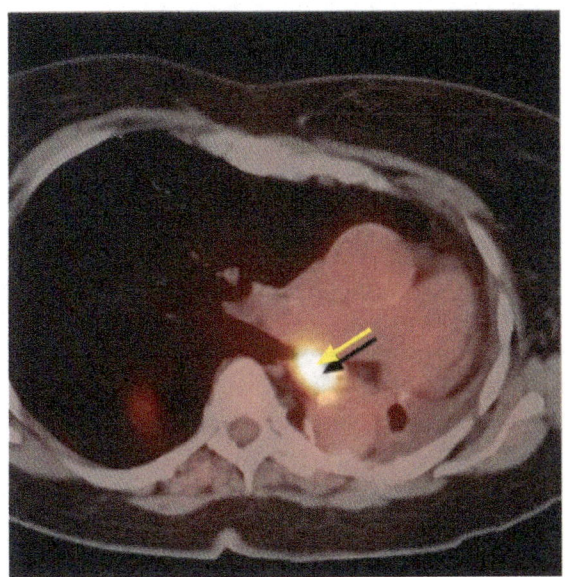

Image 2 (axial)

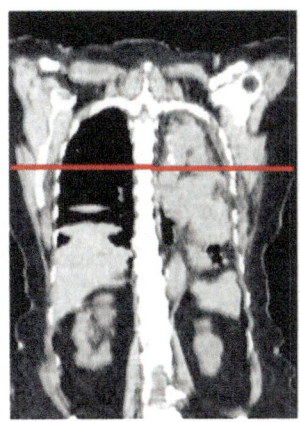

Localizer

Image 2. Fused axial image depicting suspicious hypermetabolic focus localized to left para-spinal region (arrow) behind the shifted right pulmonary artery.

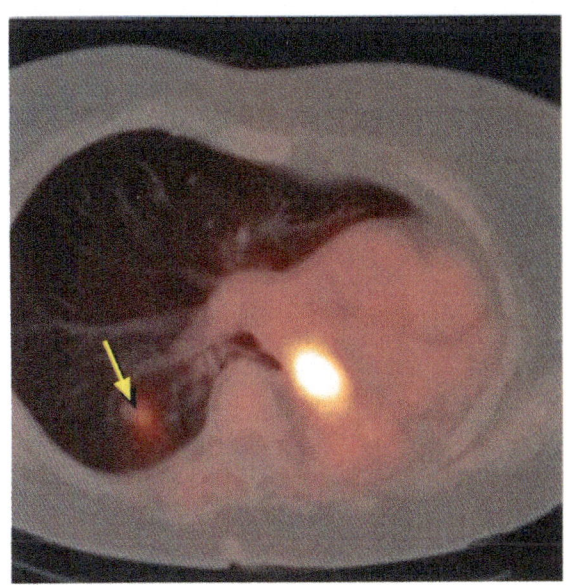

Image 3 (axial)

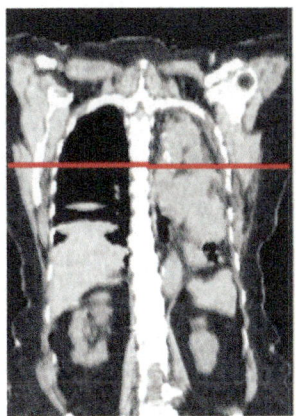

Localizer

Image 3. Fused axial image also revealed a second suspicious lesion with mildly increased FDG uptake corresponding to a small lung nodule seen on CT (arrow).

Pleural Carcinomatosis

Clinical History

66-year-old female with Non-Small Cell lung cancer who is status post chemotherapy.

PET/CT indication: Restaging.

Findings

Linear-nodular hypermetabolic activity surrounding the right lung together with hypermetabolic areas in the dependent portions of the right lower lobe suggest malignant pleural effusion and carcinomatosis of the pleura.

Teaching Points

Carcinomatosis of the pleura presents as a typical glucose metabolic pattern. Increased activity is linear and nodular and follows the surface of the lung . Differently, malignant or inflammatory effusions can present as moderately or severely increased FDG uptake in a diffuse fashion.

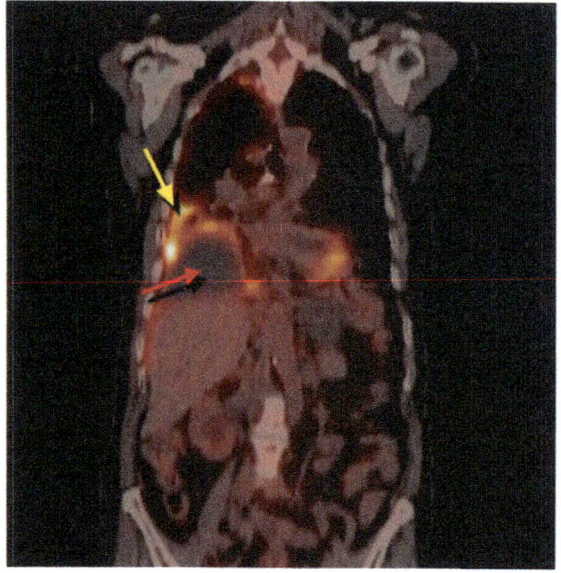

Image 1 (coronal)

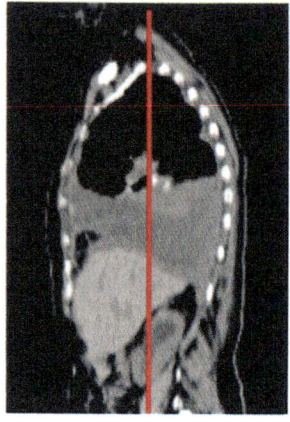

Localizer

Image 1. Linearly increased tracer activity is consistent with pleural involvement (yellow arrow). Note the hypodense fluid accumulation in the right lung base that does not exhibit increased FDG uptake (red arrow).

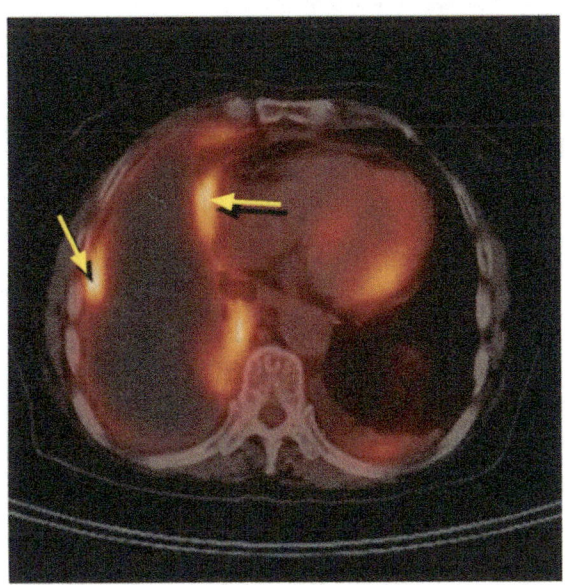

Image 2 (axial)

Image 2. Fused axial images with linear-to-nodular uptake pattern consistent with carcinomatosis of the pleura (arrows).

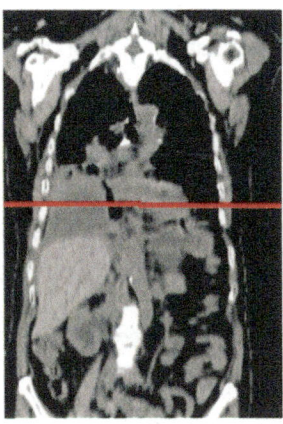

Localizer

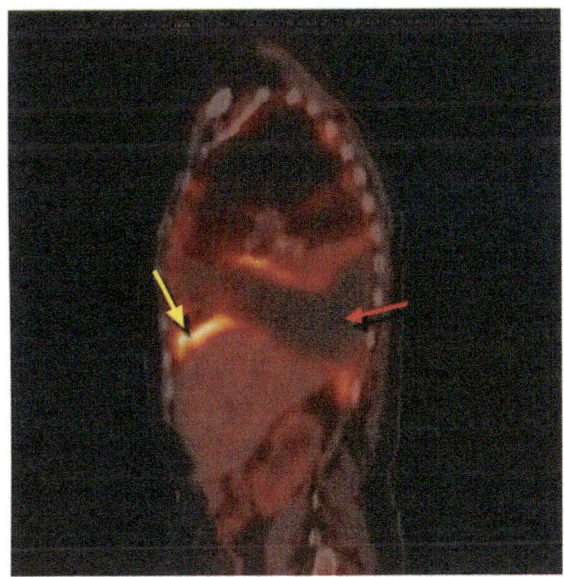

Image 3 (sagittal)

Image 3. Fused sagittal image with linear uptake pattern following the diaphragm (yellow arrow). The red arrow points to a pleural effusion.

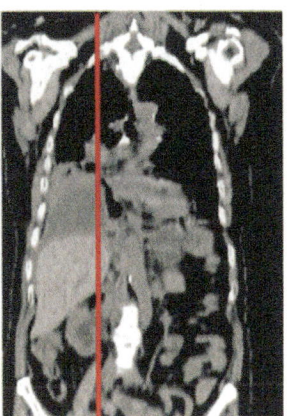

Localizer

Mesothelioma

Clinical History

76-year-old male with left-sided mesothelioma and pleural effusion.

PET/CT indication: Staging.

Findings

There are multiple foci of intensely increased FDG uptake throughout the entire pleural surface of the left lung and along the major fissure. The pattern of metabolic abnormalities is typical for mesothelioma but also for carcinomatosis of the pleura.

Pathology verification: Mesothelioma invading the lung.

Teaching Points

Mesothelioma and carcinomatosis of the pleura have very similar metabolic appearances. They are characterized by a pattern of intense metabolic activity that is both nodular and linear. The addition of CT permits to determining invasion of adjacent tissues. Malignant and inflammatory pleural effusions can exhibit normal or increased glucose metabolic activity.

Image 1

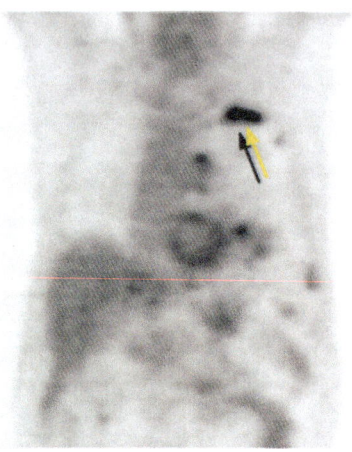
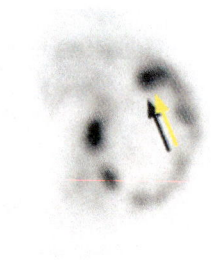

coronal   **axial**

Image 1. Coronal (left) and axial (right) FDG PET images displaying the typical nodular/linear pattern of mesothelioma (arrows).

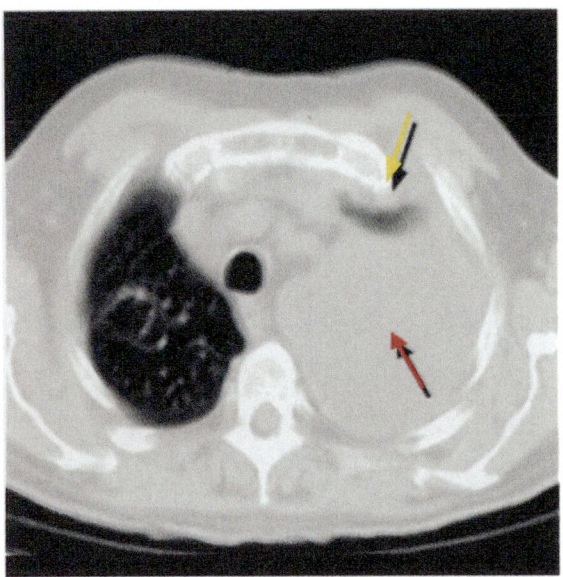

Image 2 (axial)

Image 2. Axial CT demonstrating anterior pleural mass (anterior arrow) corresponding to anterior focus of increased FDG uptake on axial PET (shown above). The posterior arrow denotes a pleural effusion.

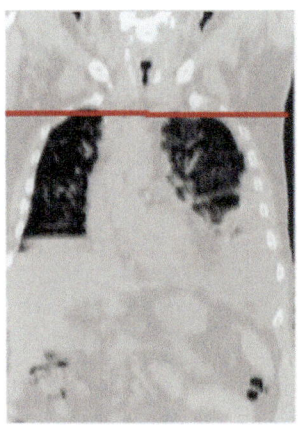

Localizer

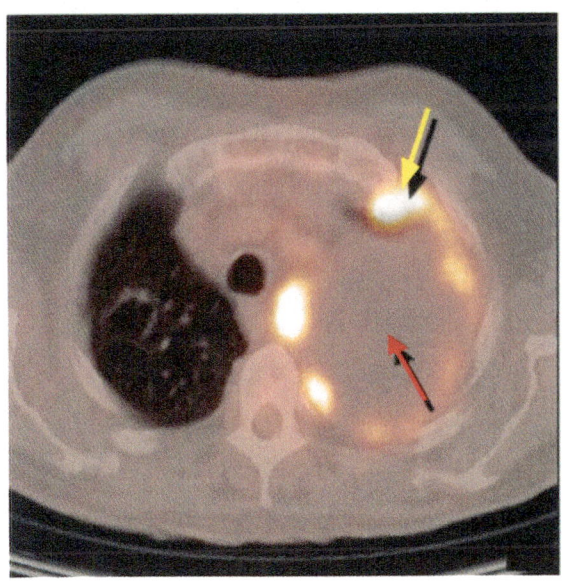

Image 3 (axial)

Image 3. Fused axial image demonstrating a pleural mass invading the left upper lobe (arrow). The pleural effusion (arrow) does not exhibit increased glycolysis.

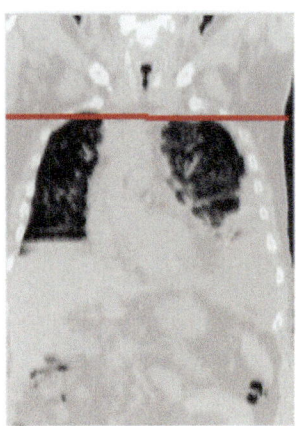

Localizer

Chapter 7

Cancers of the Gastrointestinal Tract

Cases:

Chapter 7

Cancers of the Gastrointestinal Tract

Colorectal Cancer

Colorectal cancer accounts for about 15% of all cancers in the United States. FDG-PET is used most frequently for restaging in patients who present with rising tumor markers or some equivocal finding on anatomical imaging or who are symptomatic after primary treatment has been completed. The ability of FDG-PET to determine extra-hepatic disease involvement can be limited by physiologically increased mucosal FDG uptake. PET/CT is especially useful for these cases. Further, PET/CT facilitates the characterization of small, mildly hyper-glycolytic liver lesions. This can be difficult with PET alone because of the relatively high physiological hepatic glycolytic activity.

Key Indications: Staging and Restaging

Esophageal Cancer

In the United States, esophageal cancer accounts for approximately 1% of all newly diagnosed cancers per year. FDG-PET is used to determine presence and extent of local tumor invasion, tumor size, lymph node involvement and the presence of metastases at the time of diagnosis. Preliminary data suggest that PET/CT can improve the staging accuracy achieved by PET alone.

Key Indications: Staging and Restaging

Pancreatic Cancer

Pancreatic cancer causes approximately 27,000 cancer deaths per year and was the fifth leading cause of cancer death in the United Sates in 1995. The 5-year survival rate is abysmal at 1-4%.
The ability of FDG-PET to differentiate benign from malignant pancreatic masses has been controversial. It appears that especially mucinous pancreatic cancers exhibit low glucose metabolic activities. The added value of PET/CT over PET has not yet been determined.

Key Indications: Tissue Characterization and Staging

Suggested Reading

Colorectal Cancer

Schiepers C, Penninckx F, De Vadder N, Merckx E, Mortelmans L, Bormans G, Marchal G, Filez L, Aerts R. Contribution of PET in the diagnosis of recurrent colorectal cancer: comparison with conventional imaging. Eur J Surg Oncol. 1995; 21(5):517-522.

Huebner RH, Park KC, Shepherd JE, Schwimmer J, Czernin J, Phelps ME, Gambhir SS. A meta-analysis of the literature for whole-body FDG PET detection of recurrent colorectal cancer. J Nucl Med. 2000;41(7):1177-1189.

Meta J, Seltzer M, Schiepers C, Silverman DH, Ariannejad M, Gambhir SS, Phelps ME, Valk P, Czernin J. Impact of 18F-FDG PET on managing patients with colorectal cancer: the referring physician's perspective. J Nucl Med. 2001;42(4):586-590.

Esophageal Cancer

Luketich JD, Friedman DM, Weigel TL, Meehan MA, Keenan RJ, Townsend DW, Meltzer CC. Evaluation of distant metastases in esophageal cancer: 100 consecutive positron emission tomography scans. Ann Thorac Surg. 1999;68(4):1133-1136.

Flamen P, Lerut A, Van Cutsem E, Cambier JP, Maes A, De Wever W, Peeters M, De Leyn P, Van Raemdonck D, Mortelmans L. The utility of positron emission tomography for the diagnosis and staging of recurrent esophageal cancer. J Thorac Cardiovasc Surg. 2000;120(6):1085-1092.

Pancreatic Cancer

Reske SN, Grillenberger KG, Glatting G, Port M, Hildebrandt M, Gansauge F, Beger HG. Overexpression of glucose transporter 1 and increased FDG uptake in pancreatic cancer. J Nucl Med. 1997;38(9):1344-1348.

Imdahl A, Nitzsche E, Krautmann F, Hogerle S, Boos S, Einert A, Sontheimer J, Farthmann EH. Evaluation of positron emission tomography with 2-[18F]fluoro-2-deoxy-D-glucose for the differentiation of chronic pancreatitis and pancreatic cancer. Br J Surg. 1999;86(2):194-199.

Fröhlich A, Diederichs CG, Staib L, Vogel J, Berger HG, Reske SN. Detection of liver metastases from pancreatic cancer using FDG PET. J Nucl Med. 1999;40(2):250-255.

Rose D, Delbeke D, Beauchamp R, Chapman WC, Sandler MP, et al. 18Fluorodeoxyglucose-positron emission tomography in the management of patients with suspected pancreatic cancer. Ann Surg. 1999; 229:729-737.

Cholangiocarcinoma

Clinical History

56-year-old male with unresectable cholangiocarcinoma. The patient underwent chemotherapy and radiation treatment.

PET/CT indication: Restaging.

Findings

Multiple focal areas of increased metabolic activity are located in the right hepatic lobe corresponding to low density CT lesions. These are consistent with metastatic disease. The remainder of the body shows no evidence for metastatic disease.

Teaching Point

Because of the high normal hepatic glycolytic activity liver metastases can be difficult to detect with PET alone. PET/CT facilitated identification and localization of lesions with mildly to moderately increased FDG uptake.

Image 1. Fused axial image reveals mildly increased FDG activity in the medial portion of the right liver lobe (arrow).

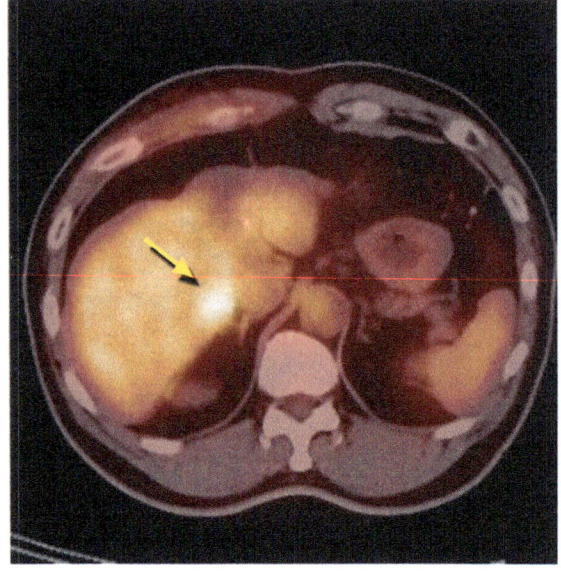

Image 1 (axial)

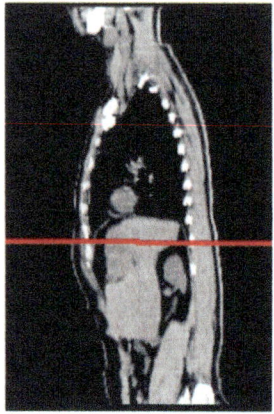

Localizer

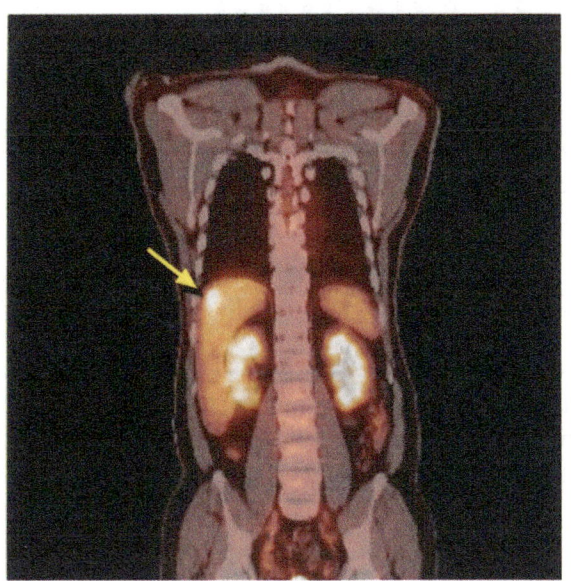

Image 2 (coronal)

Image 2. Fused coronal image depicting metastatic liver lesion in the lateral aspect of the right liver lobe (arrow).

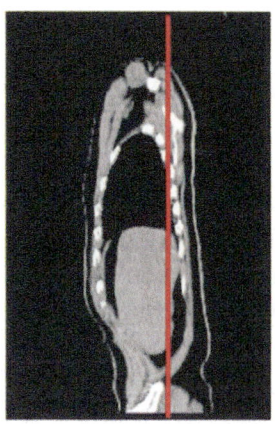

Localizer

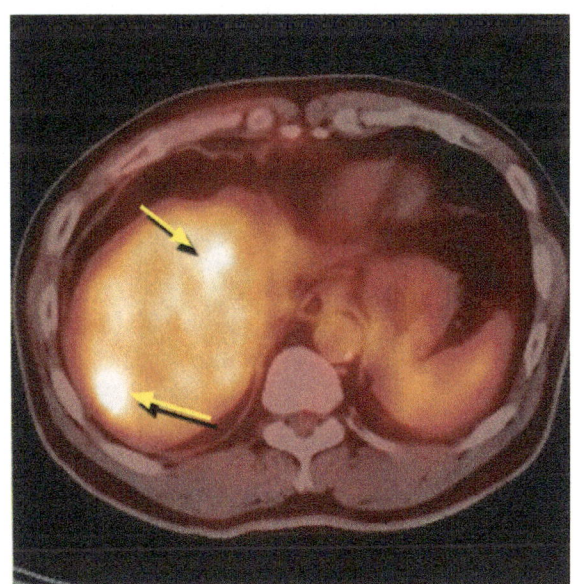

Image 3 (axial)

Image 3. Fused axial image with two metastatic liver lesions (arrows).

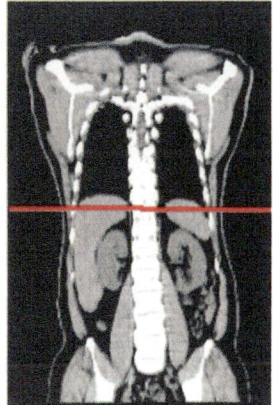

Localizer

Esophageal Cancer

Clinical History

A 66-year-old male who recently underwent chemotherapy for esophageal carcinoma.

PET/CT indication: Restaging.

Findings

Mild glucose metabolic activity throughout the lower esophagus is an unspecfifc finding. Focal hypermetabolism in the posterior right iliac wing lateral to the sacroiliac joint that is associated with a lytic lesion on CT is suspicious for metastatic disease.

Teaching Point

This case underscores the importance of a whole body survey for hypermetabolic distant lesions. The bone metastasis was unexpected and would not have been detected by standard limited CT alone. PET and PET/CT detect unexpected distant disease in a considerable number of cancer patients.

Image 1. Fused axial image of the pelvis with intensely hypermetabolic focus in the right iliac wing (focus).

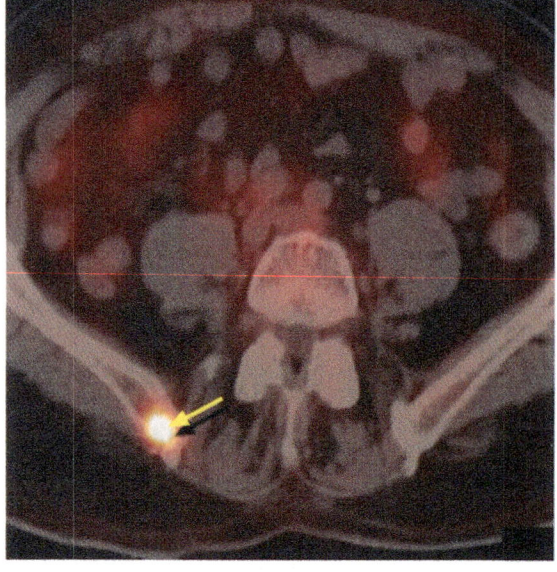

Image 1 (axial)

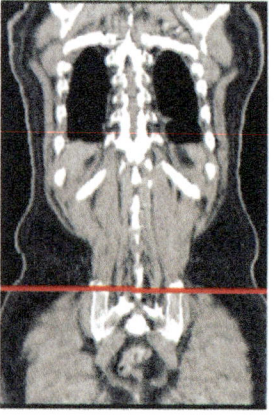

Localizer

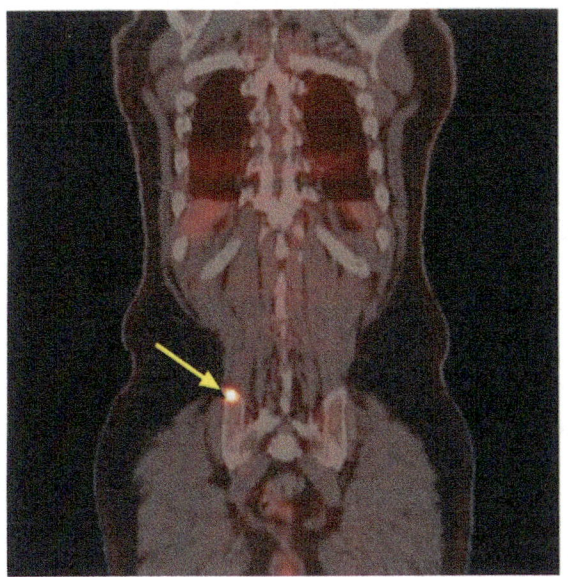

Image 2 (coronal)

Image 2. Fused coronal image demonstrating the hypermetabolic focus in the right iliac wing (arrow).

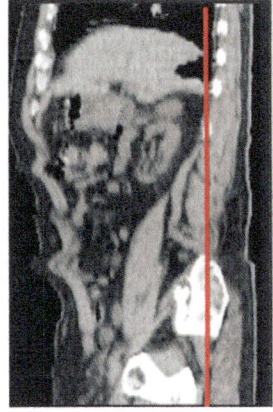

Localizer

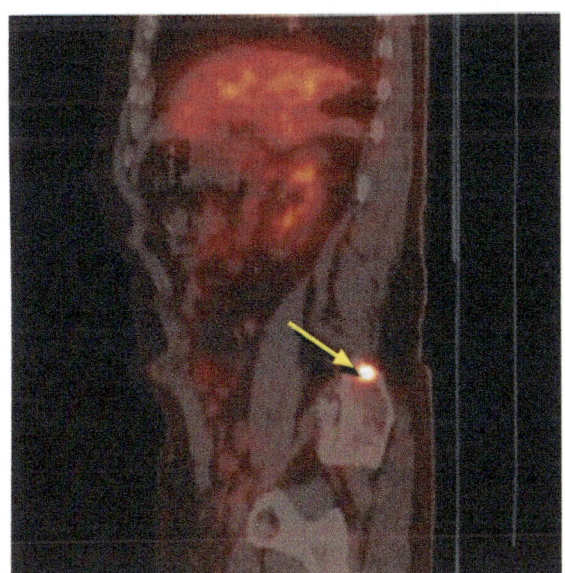

Image 3 (sagittal)

Image 3. Fused sagittal image with hypermetabolic iliac wing lesion (arrow).

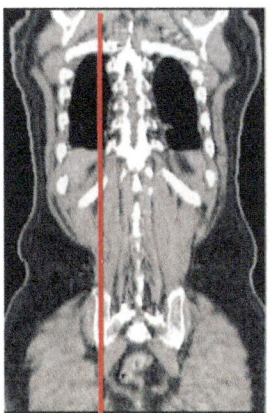

Localizer

Esophageal Carcinoma

Clinical History

69-year-old female with moderately differentiated adenocarcinoma of the esophagus.

PET/CT indication: Initial Staging

Findings

Focal hypermetabolism and wall thickening by CT at the gastro-esophageal junction is consistent with the primary carcinoma. No evidence for local adenopathy or metastatic disease.

Teaching Point

PET/CT is useful for staging of esophageal cancer. In this case, lymph node involvement and distant disease were ruled out.

Image 1. Intense hypermetabolism in the region of the gastro-esophageal junction subsequeuntly confirmed to be adenocarcinoma (arrow).

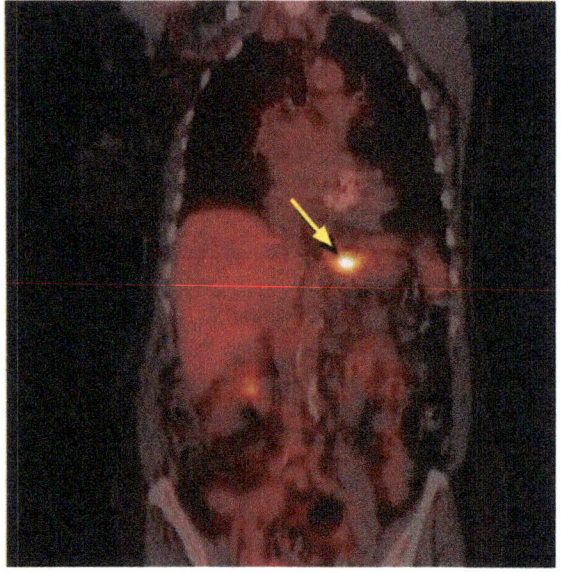

Image 1 (coronal)

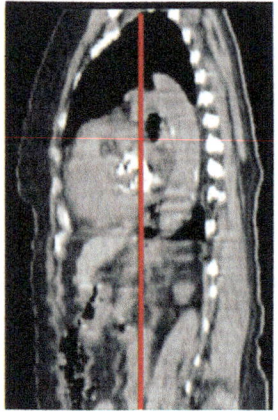

Localizer

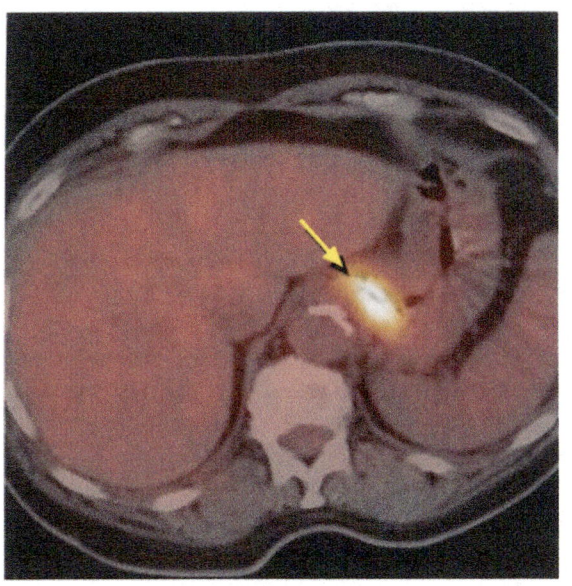

Image 2 (axial)

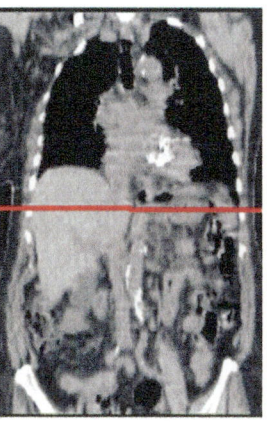

Localizer

Image 2. Axial image with localization of the hypermetabolic focus in the gastro-esophageal junction (arrow).

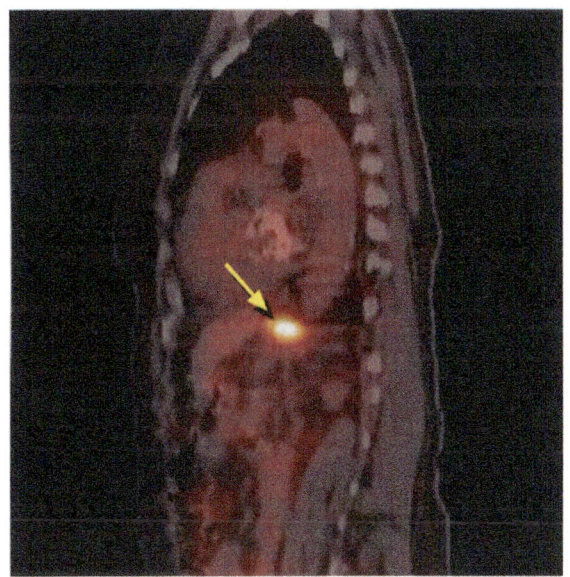

Image 3 (sagittal)

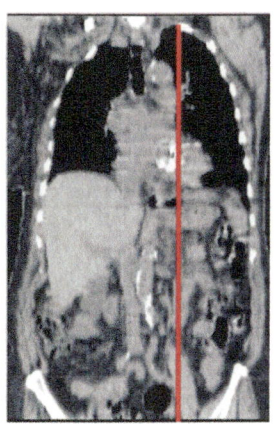

Localizer

Image 3. Sagittal image demonstrating the hypermetabolic focus in the gastro-esophageal junction (arrow).

Rectal Cancer

Clinical History

Patient with recently diagnosed rectal carcinoma.

PET/CT indication: Staging.

Findings

Abnormal glycolytic activity involving the rectum, representing the site of primary malignancy. An abnormal focus of FDG uptake in the right side of the posterior pelvis below the coccyx likely represents metastatic lymph node involvement.

Teaching Point

An outside contrast CT was negative for lymph node involvement and the non-contrast CT of this study was also interpreted as negative for nodal involvement. PET demonstrated focally increased uptake in the pelvis but the focus could not be localized to a specific structure. Thus, PET provided the metabolic information and CT the anatomical localization for correctly identifying lymph node involvement.

Image 1. Fused coronal image demonstrating the primary cancer site in the region of the rectum (arrow).

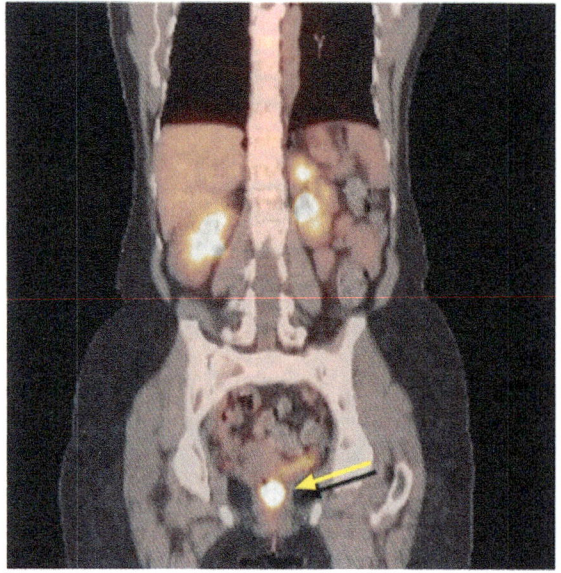

Image 1 (coronal)

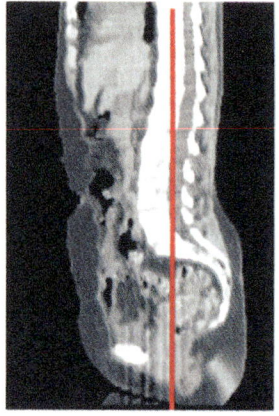

Localizer

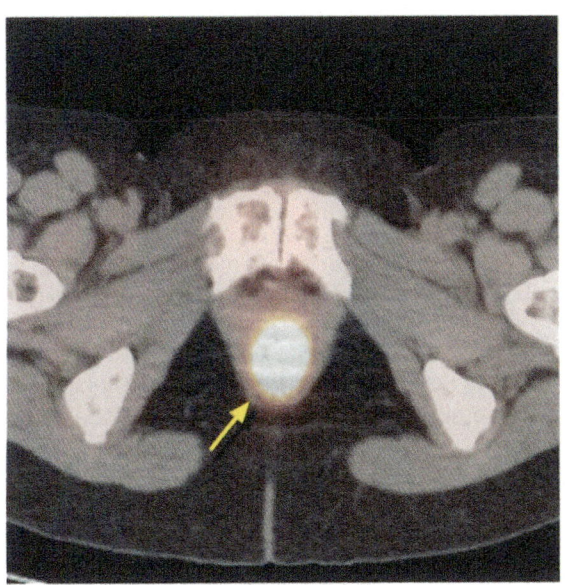

Image 2 (axial)

Image 2. Fused axial PET/CT image showing the large primary tumor (arrow).

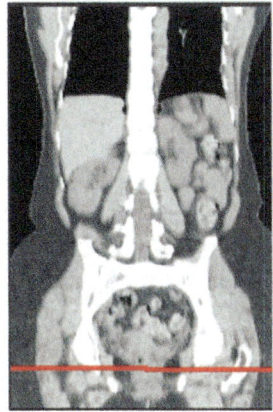

Localizer

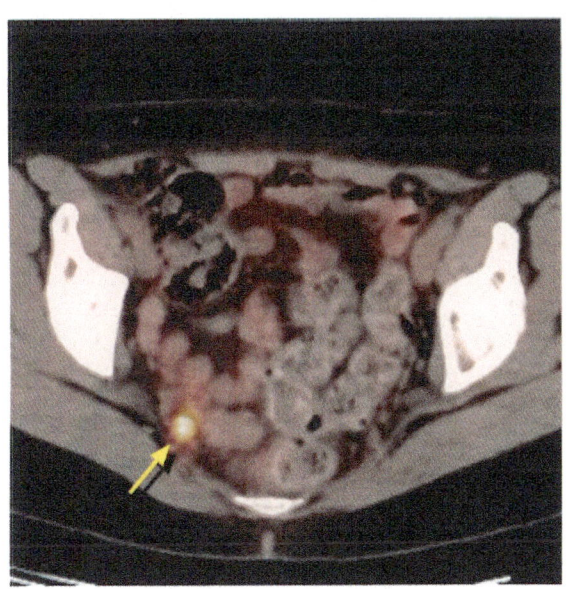

Image 3 (axial)

Image 3. Fused axial image depicting an abnormal focus of increased uptake in the right-sided posterior pelvis below the coccyx representingmetastatic lymph node involvement (arrow).

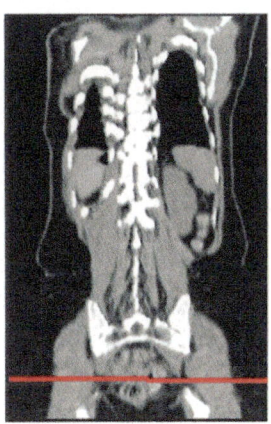

Localizer

Gallbladder and Pancreatic Cancer

Clinical History

62-year-old male with pancreatic and gallbladder cancer presents with rising tumor markers.

PET/CT indication: Restaging.

Findings

Mild hypermetabolic focus near the gallbladder fossa is suspicious for residual/recurrent tumor. Abnormal FDG uptake in the right posterior acetabulum corresponding to a lytic lesion on CT is consistent with bone metastasis.

Teaching Points

1. Physiologically increased glycolytic activity of the liver can render detection of small malignant lesions difficult. PET and CT alone might have been interpreted as equivocal for malignancy. Image fusion provided the correct answer.

2. Whole body evaluation is one of the key advantages of PET and PET/CT and revealed unexpected distant disease in this patient.

Image 1. This section of a fused coronal image reveals a small focus of mildly increased metabolic activity in the region of the gallbladder fossa (arrow).

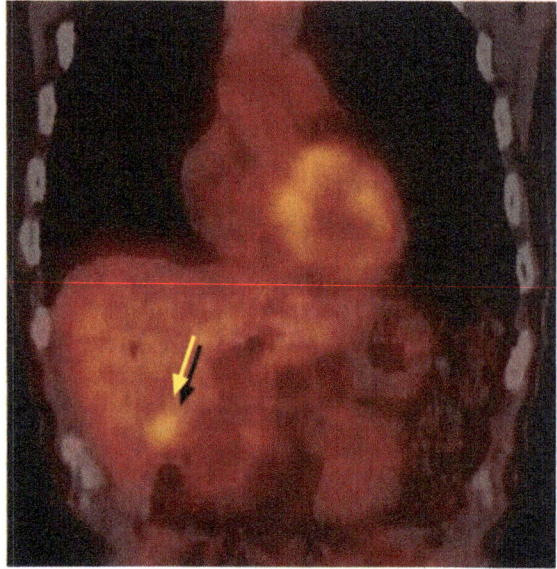

Image 1 (coronal)

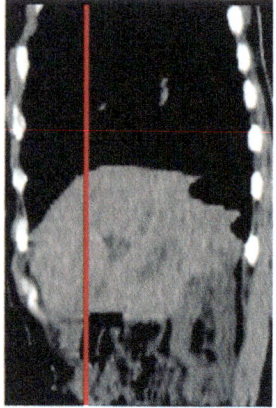

Localizer

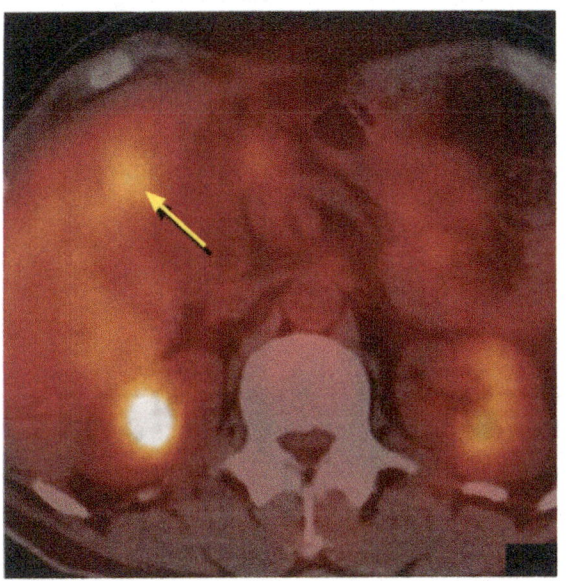

Image 2 (axial)

Image 2. Fused axial PET/CT and the CT images reveal that the hyper-glycolytic focus corresponded to a small low density CT lesion located in the region of the gall bladder fossa (arrows).

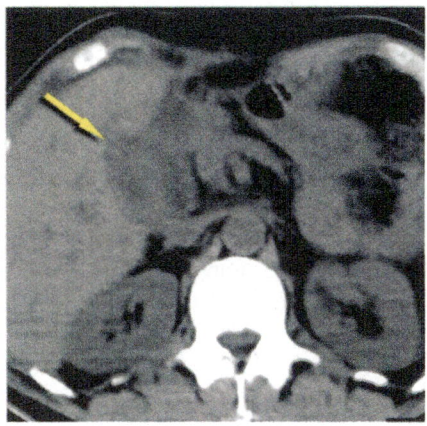

CT Image

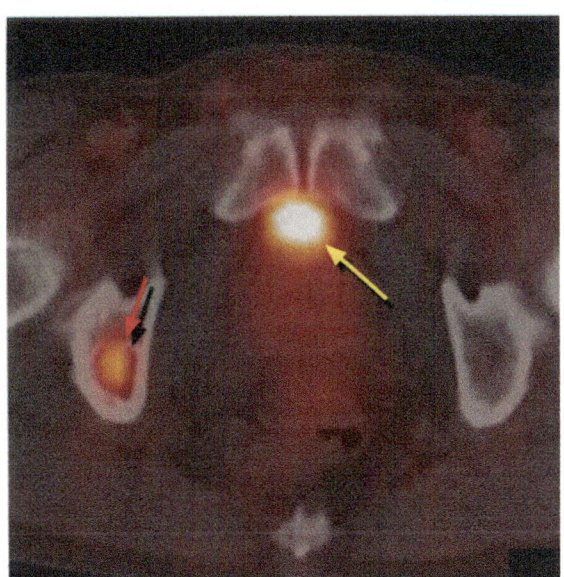

Image 3 (axial)

Image 3. Fused axial images depicting physiological activity in the urinary bladder (yellow arrow) but abnormal uptake in the acetabulum (red arrow). This is consistent with bone metastasis.

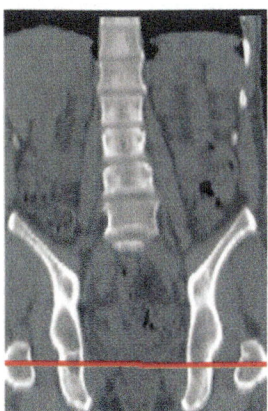

Localizer

Residual Tumor Viability

Clinical History

The patient is a 62-year-old male with colorectal carcinoma status post radio-ablation of multiple large hepatic lesions.

PET/CT indication: Restaging.

Findings

Increased FDG activity along the rim of a large hepatic mass noted on CT is consistent with metabolically active tumor cells in the periphery of the tumor.

Teaching Point

Note the dramatic discrepancy between the CT and PET findings. Only a small rim of mildly increased FDG uptake suggests small areas of viable tumor. Thus, the large CT mass is largely necrotic. The implications for biopsy and radiation planning are evident.

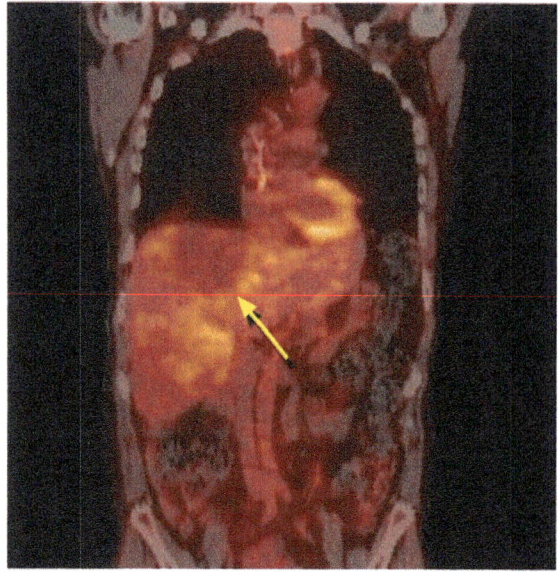

Image 1 (coronal)

Image 1. Fused coronal image demonstrating a mildly hypermetabolic rim (arrow) surrounding a large "mass" in the right liver lobe.

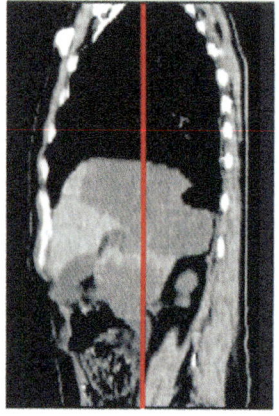

Localizer

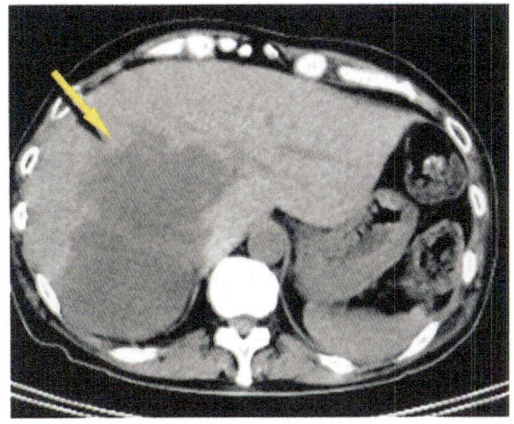

Image 2. Fused axial image demonstrating the hypermetabolic rim (arrows) surrounding the mass. The mass is best seen on the axial CT image (arrow).

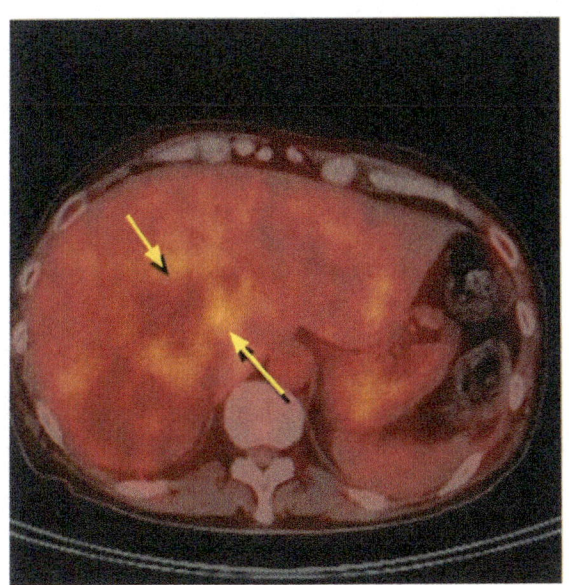

Image 2 (axial)

CT Image

Gastro-Esophageal Cancer With Unexpected Distant Disease

Clinical History

42-year-old male who was recently diagnosed with distal esophageal cancer.

PET/CT indication: Staging.

Findings

Multiple foci of hypermetabolic activity are located in thegastro-esophageal junction. In addition, multiple lesions are located in the left hepatic lobe, the celiac and paraaortic lymph node chains, the thoracic spine, the sacrum, the left and right rib cage, the lower thoracic prevertebral lymph nodes, and the left scapula. Overall findings are consistent with widespread metastatic disease.

Teaching Point

Whole body staging is important for determining resectability in many cancer patients. In this particular case PET/CT revealed unexpected extensive disease and conservative/palliative rather than surgical treatment was initiated.

Image 1. Extensive distal esophageal and gastric involvement is demonstrated on this fused axial image (arrows).

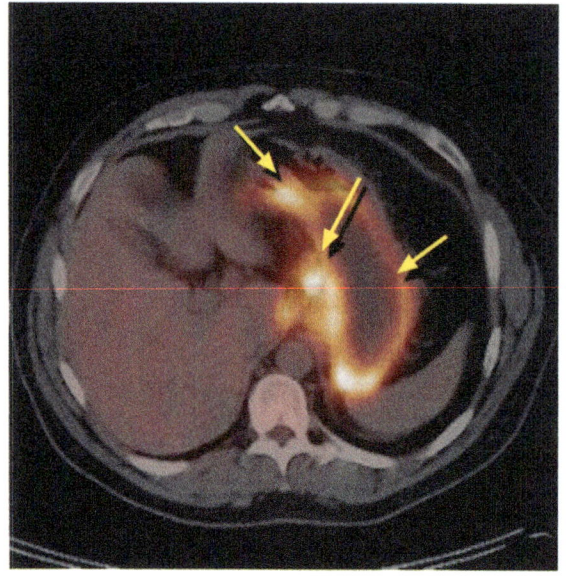

Image 1 (arial)

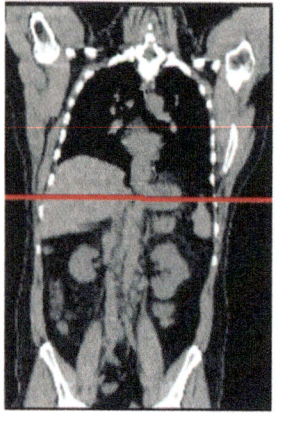

Localizer

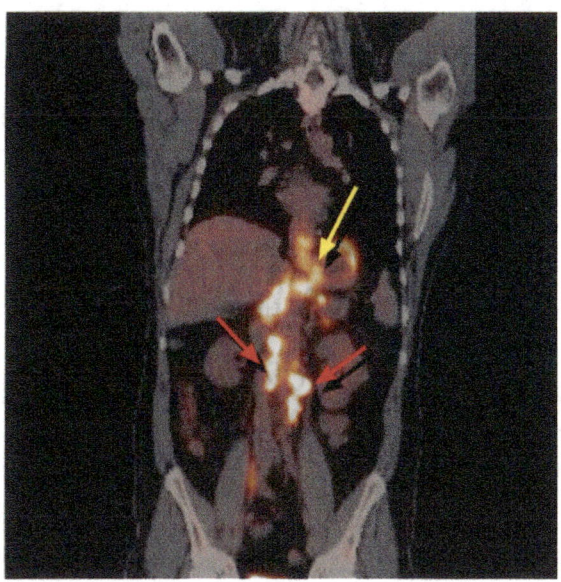

Image 2. Coronal view showing the distal esophageal and gastric tumor (yellow arrow) and the paraaortic lymph node involvement (red arrows).

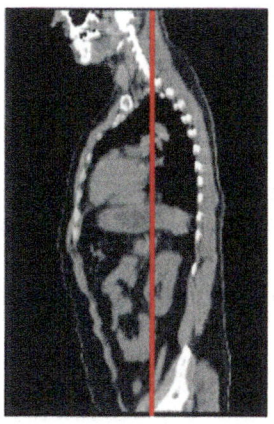

Image 2 (coronal)

Localizer

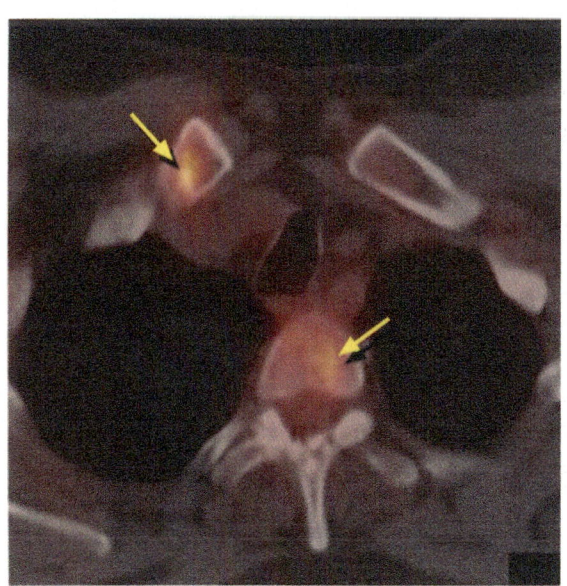

Image 3. Incidental finding of metastatic lesions of the right clavicle and the thoracic spine shown on the axial fused PET/CT (arrows). Coronal PET alone demonstrated a focused of increased uptake (arrow) in this region that could not be assigned to a specific anatomic structure. Note the abnormal activity in the stomach region on PET (arrrow).

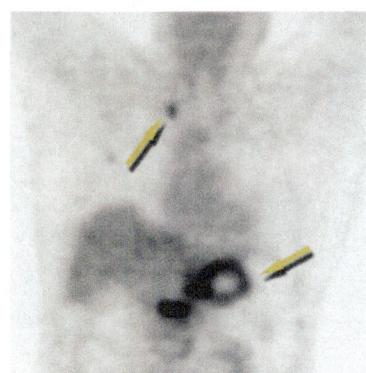

Image 3 (axial)

PET Image

Metastatic Rectal Carcinoma

Clinical History

60-year-old male with history of rectal carcinoma, status post resection, chemotherapy and radiation treatment.

PET/CT indication: Restaging.

Findings

A left adrenal mass is identified on CT that demonstrates peripheral hypermetabolic activity. This is consistent with a partially necrotic adrenal metastasis.

Teaching Point

Review of PET images alone would suggest prominent stomach or bowel activity. The adrenal mass with increased glucose metabolic activity was revealed only through image fusion.

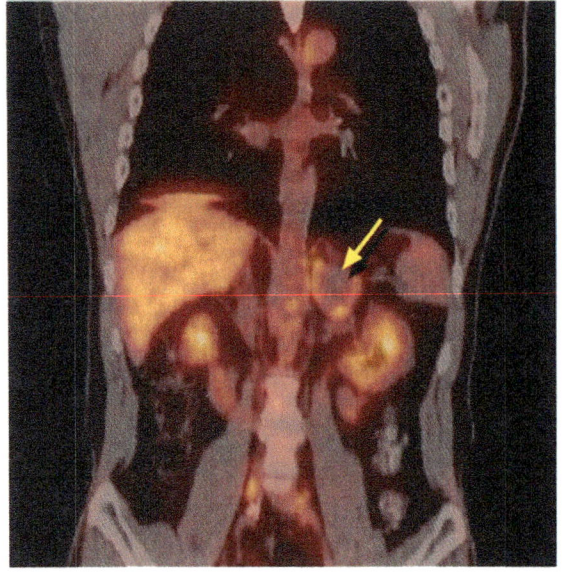

Image 1 (coronal)

Image 1. Fused coronal image demonstrating a rim of hypermetabolic activity surrounding a photopenic area located in the left adrenal gland (arrow).

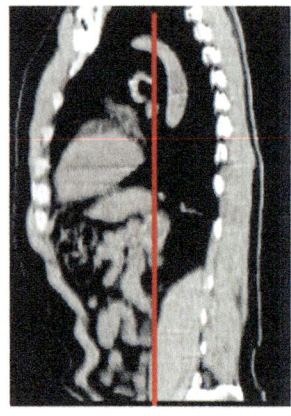

Localizer

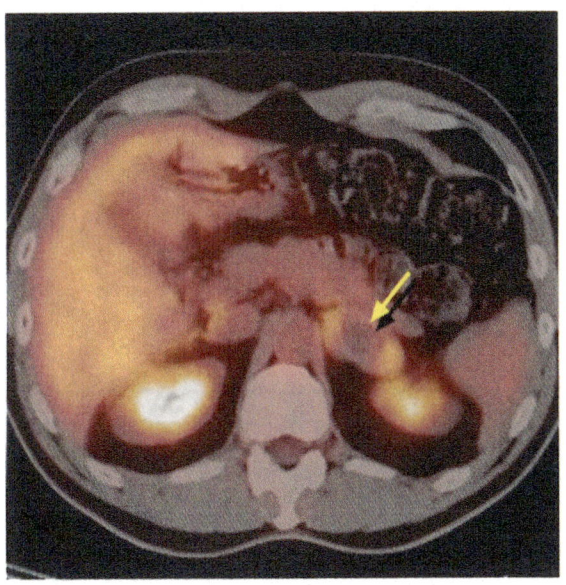

Image 2. Axial fused image depicting the left adrenal gland with its hypermetabolic rim (arrow).

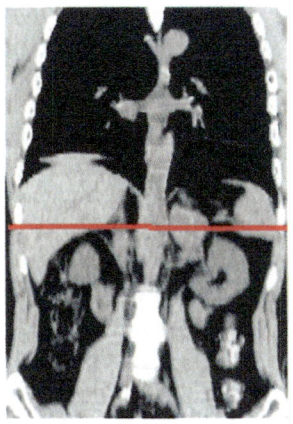

Image 2 (axial)

Localizer

Image 3. Sagittal view of adrenal metastasis.

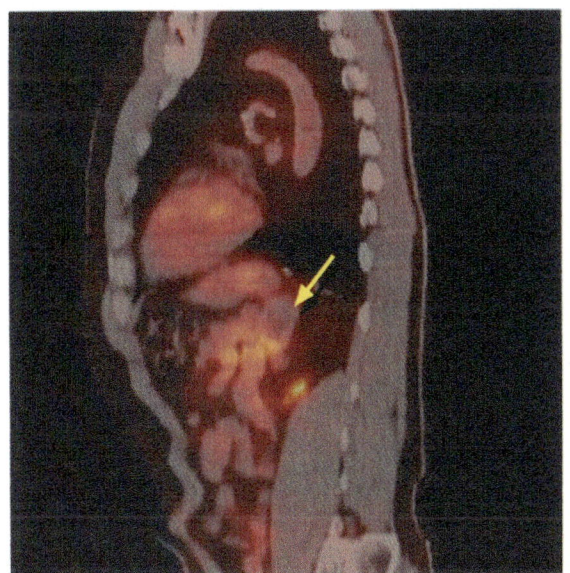

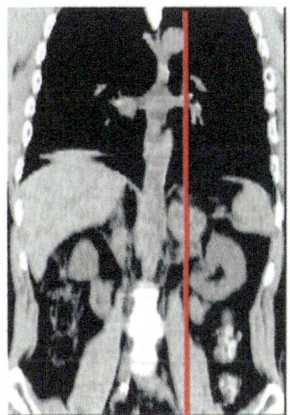

Image 3 (sagittal)

Localizer

Colon and Hepatocellular Cancer

Clinical History

67-year-old patient with colon carcinoma and a history of chronic hepatitis B. A recent MRI of the abdomen demonstrated cirrhotic liver with a 5 x 5cm lesion in the right liver lobe.

PET/CT indication: Staging.

Findings

A large, about 2-cm focus of intense tracer uptake in the descending colon is consistent with the primary tumor. There is no evidence of abnormal glucose metabolic activity in the liver. However, primary hepatic malignancy does not consistently exhibit hypermetabolic activity.

Teaching Point

Liver metastases from colon cancer exhibit intensely increased glucose metabolic activity. In contrast, hepatocellular carcinoma is frequently metabolically quiescent. Thus, the hypodense lesion is more likely explained by second primary rather than colon cancer metastasis.

Image 1. Fused coronal image demonstrating intensely increased glucose metabolic activity consistent with the known primary colon cancer (arrow).

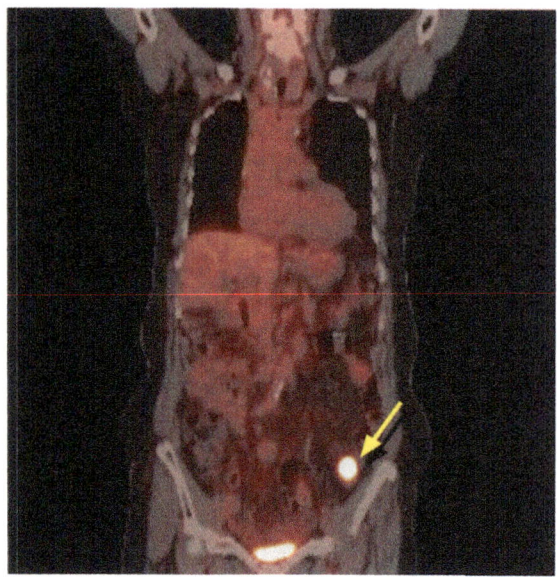

Image 1 (coronal)

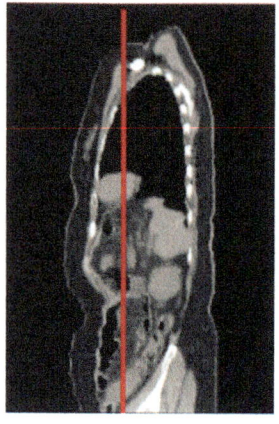

Localizer

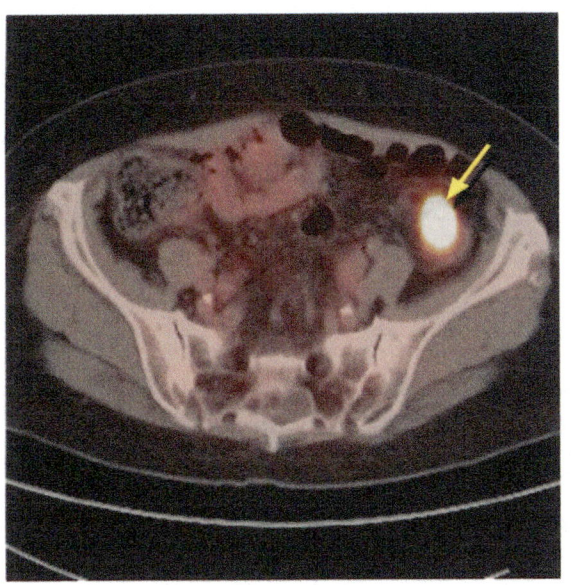

Image 2. Fused axial image showing the primary tumor (arrow).

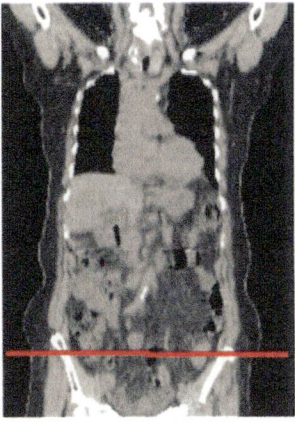

Image 2 (axial)

Localizer

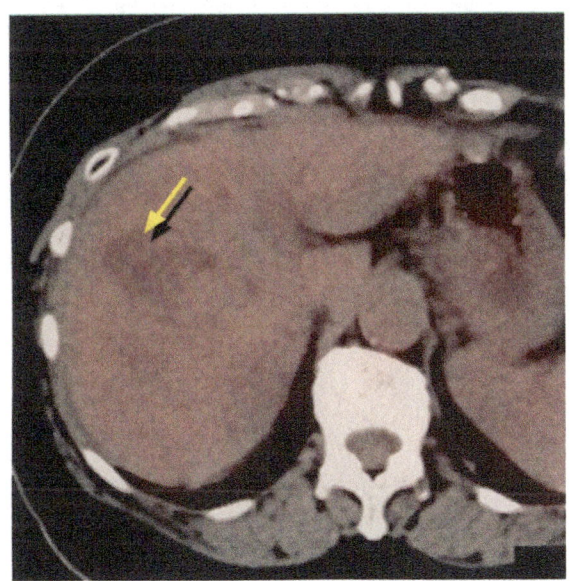

Image 3. Hypodense liver lesion without glucose metabolic activity (arrow) shown on axial fused image. The absent glucose metabolic activity suggests hepatocellular cancer rather than colon cancer metastasis.

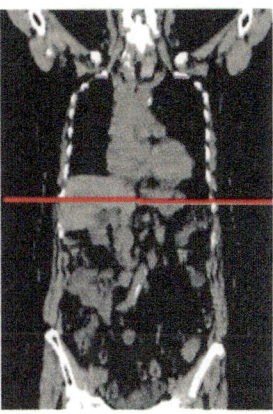

Image 3 (axial)

Localizer

Pancreatic Cancer

Clinical History

72-year-old female with incidental finding of pancreatic mass.

PET/CT indication: Characterization of pancreatic mass.

Findings

A focus of intense tracer uptake in the region of body of the pancreas which is not well-delineated on the non-contrast CT exam. This is suggestive of pancreatic malignancy.

Pathology Verification: Biopsy revealing pancreatic cancer.

Teaching Point

FDG-PET is useful to differentiate benign from malignant pancreatic masses.

Image 1. Fused coronal image showing an area of increased glucose metabolism in the pancreas indicating the presence of malignant tumor (arrow).

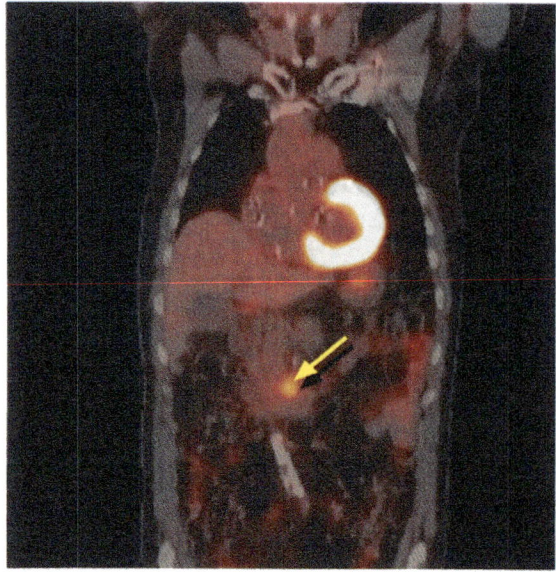

Image 1 (coronal)

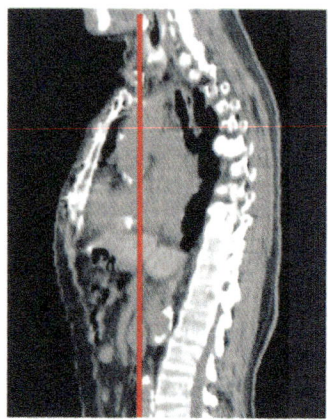

Localizer

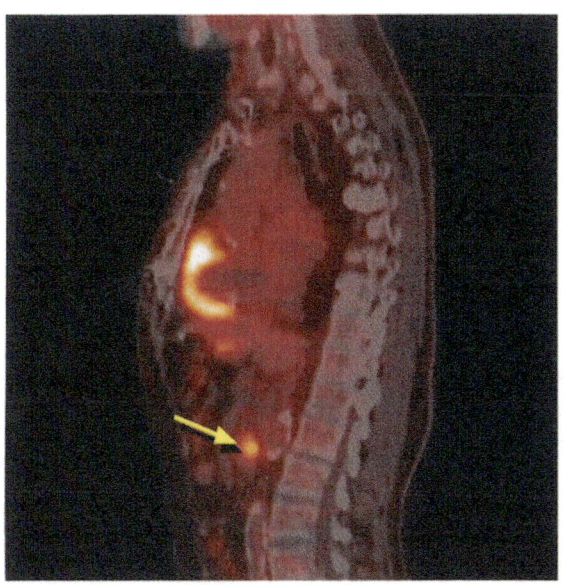

Image 2 (sagittal)

Image 2. Fused sagittal image showing an area of increased glucose metabolism in the pancreas indicating the presence of malignant tumor (arrow).

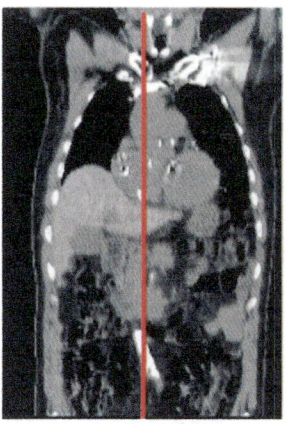

Localizer

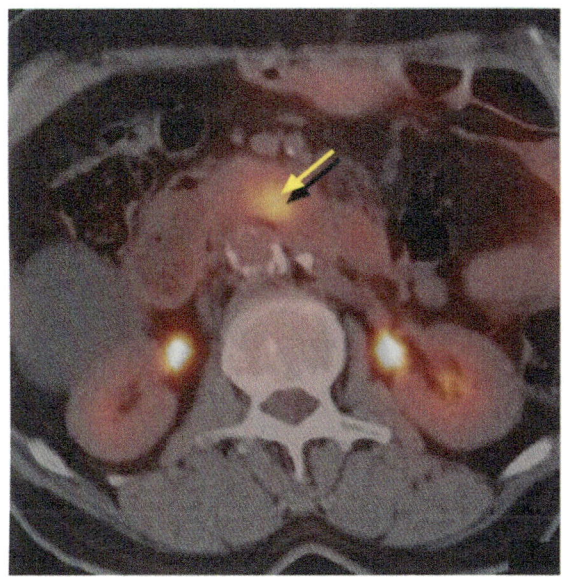

Image 3 (axial)

Image 3. Fused axial image demonstrating the primary pancreatic malignancy (arrow).

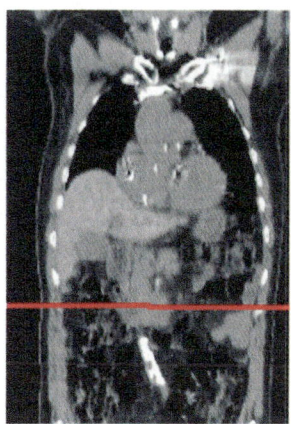

Localizer

Gastric Cancer

Clinical History

56-year-old female with history of unresectable gastric cancer and recent chemotherapy.

PET/CT indication: Restaging.

Findings

Focal area of increased metabolic activity is seen in the region of the lesser curvature corresponding to the patient's known gastric carcinoma.

Teaching Point

Stomach cancer exhibits markedly increased FDG uptake. In this case, the FDG uptake pattern allowed the differentiation between normal and abnormal segments of the stomach. This is critical for proper biopsy planning.

Image 1. Coronal PET image demonstrating focally increased FDG uptake in the stomach (arrow).

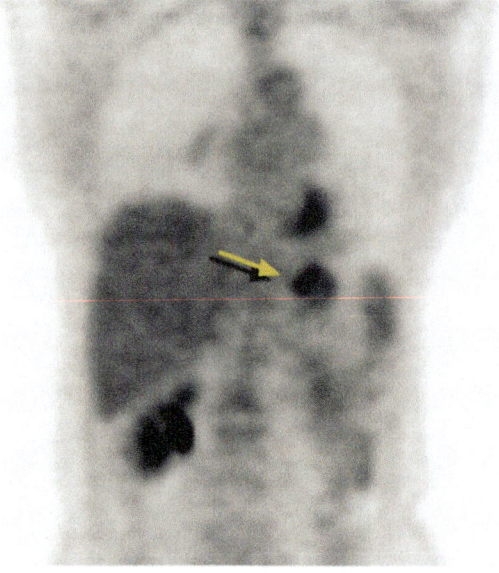

Image 1 (coronal)

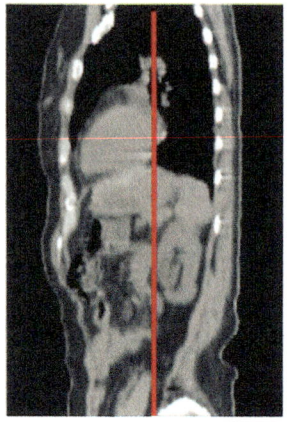

Localizer

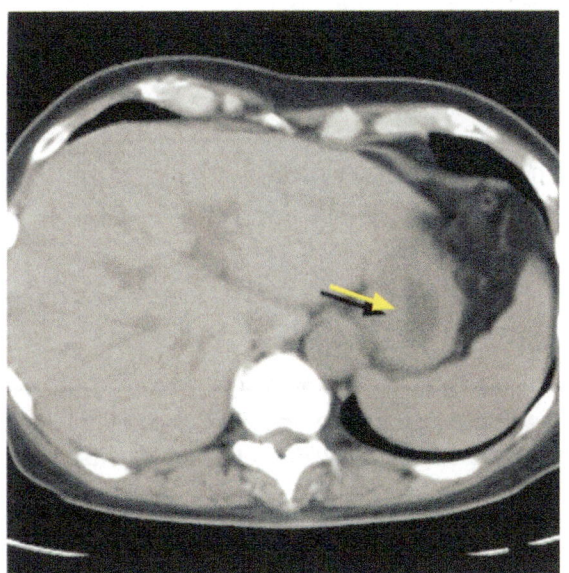

Image 2. Axial CT image depicting thickened stomach wall (arrow).

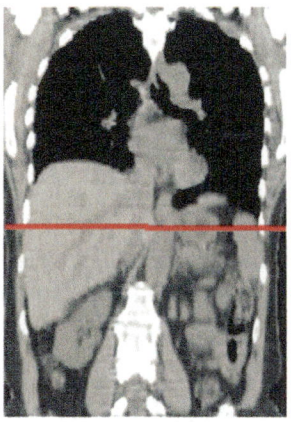

Image 2 (axial)

Localizer

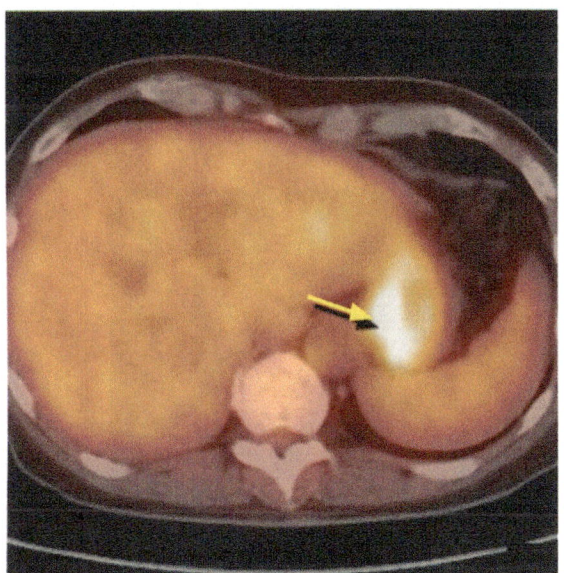

Image 3. Fused axial image identifying the tumor-involved portion of the stomach wall (arrow).

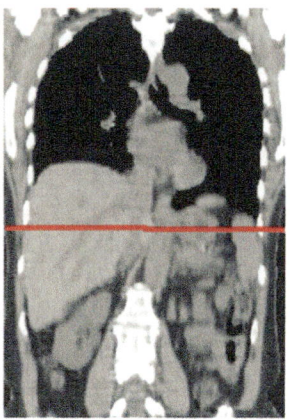

Image 3 (axial)

Localizer

Carcinoma of the Appendix

Clinical History

40-year-old female recently diagnosed with carcinoma of the appendix.

PET/CT indication: Staging.

Findings

Three moderately sized irregular-shaped hypermetabolic lesions are noted within the left lobe of the liver just superior to the porta hepatis. These are consistent with metastatic disease.

Teaching Point

Lesion localization was impossible with PET alone. Co-registered CT images helped identify the anatomical localization of metastatic lesions. Conversely PET helped identify hepatic metastasis that did not have a detectable anomaly on non-contrast CT images.

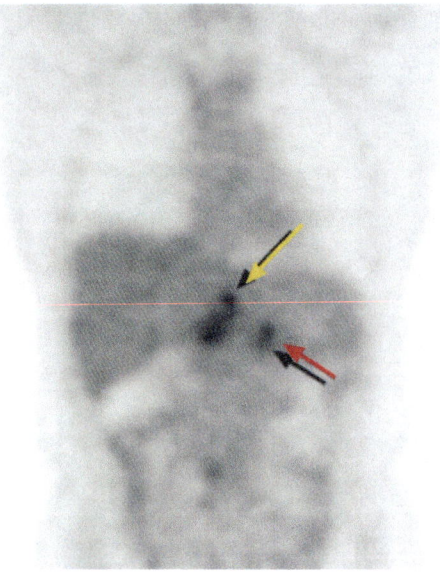

Image 1. Coronal PET images demonstrating several hypermetabolic foci in the left liver lobe (yellow arrow) and porta hepatis (red arrow).

Image 1 (coronal)

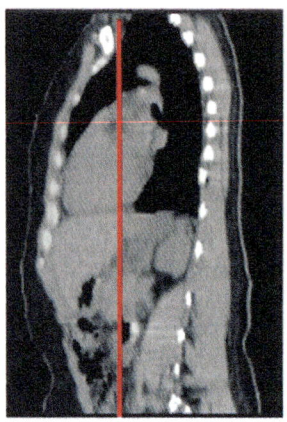

Localizer

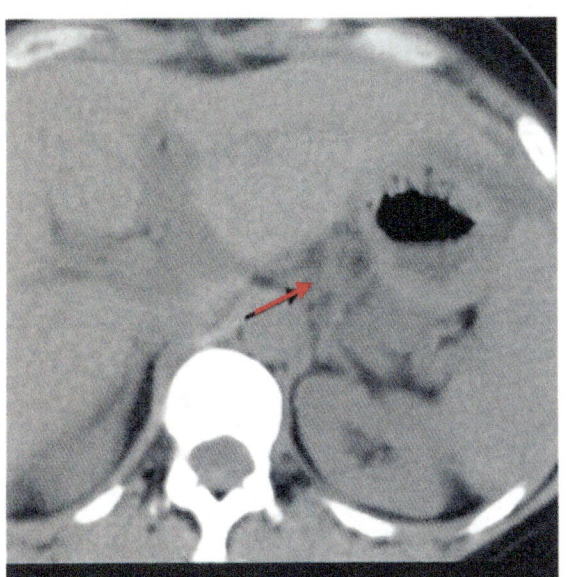

Image 2. Axial CT image with enlarged lymph node in the porta hepatis (arrow).

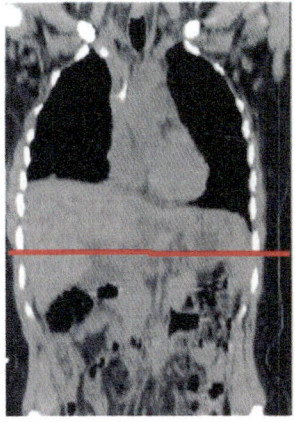

Image 2 (axial)

Localizer

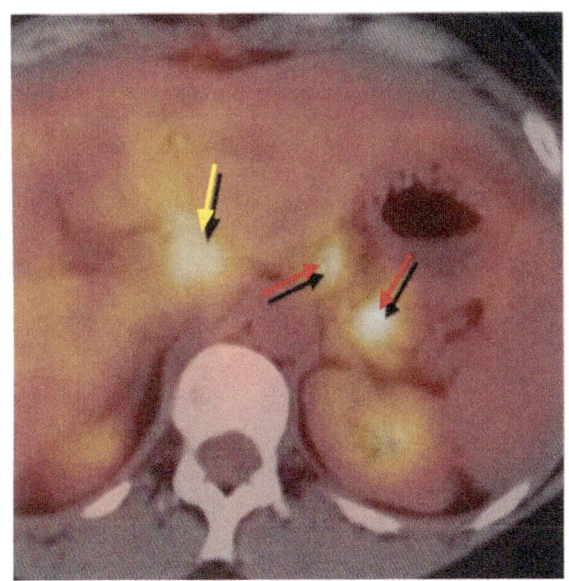

Image 3. Fused axial image demonstrating several hypermetabolic lesions (arrows).

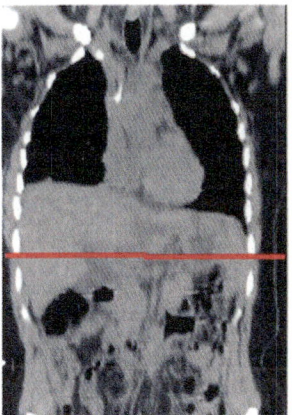

Image 3 (axial)

Localizer

Small Liver Metastasis from Colon Cancer

Clinical History

62-year-old male with colon cancer and suspected liver metastasis.

PET/CT indication: Restaging.

Findings

A round hypodense lesion with a maximum diameter of 0.9 cm is seen in the lateral edge of the right liver lobe, which exhibits mildly increased FDG uptake. This is suspicious for liver metastasis.

Teaching Point

Because of the considerable normal glucose metabolic activity of the liver, small lesions with mildly increased FDG uptake can be missed or misinterpreted. The small focus of increased uptake corresponded to a small hypodense liver lesion on CT. Thus, CT facilitated lesion detection and localization.

This patient had a barium swallow with subsequent barium accumulation in the stomach. This resulted in a photopenic area surrounded by a hypermetabolic rim.

Thus, depending on their density, contrast agents can induce "pseudo-FDG uptake" due to inappropriate attenuation correction.

Image 1. Coronal PET image demonstrate a small mildly hypermetabolic focus at the lateral edge of the right liver lobe (left arrow). A photopenic area in the region of the stomach is surrounded by a hypermetabolic rim ("pseudo-FDG uptake"; right arrow).

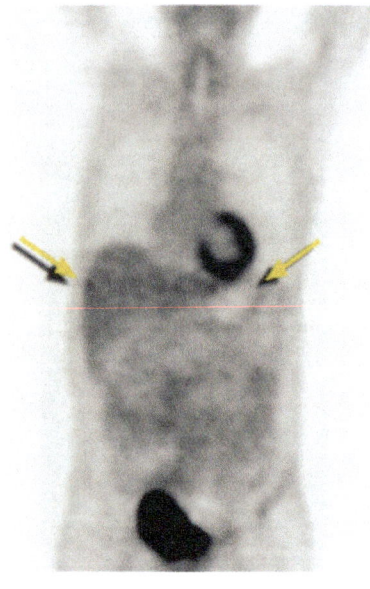

Image 1 (coronal)

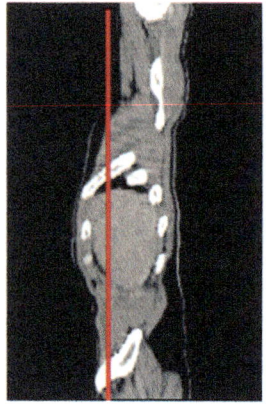

Localizer

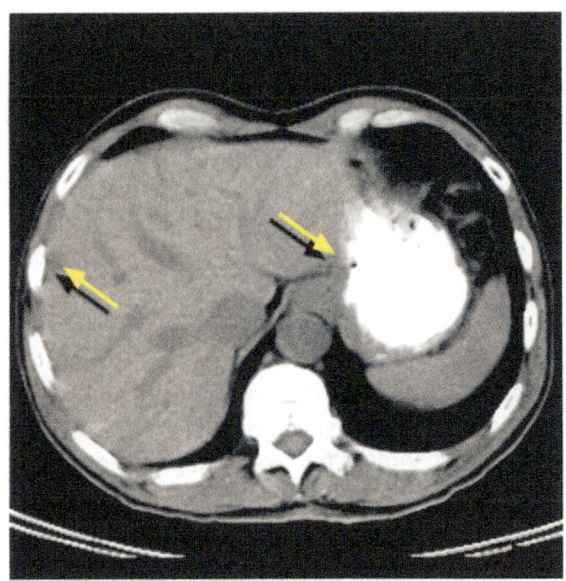

Image 2. Axial CT demonstrating a 9 mm hypodense liver lesion (left arrow) and the barium accumulation in the stomach (right arrow).

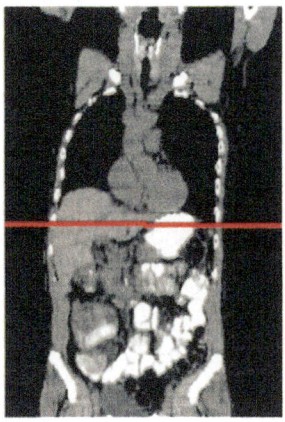

Image 2 (axial)

Localizer

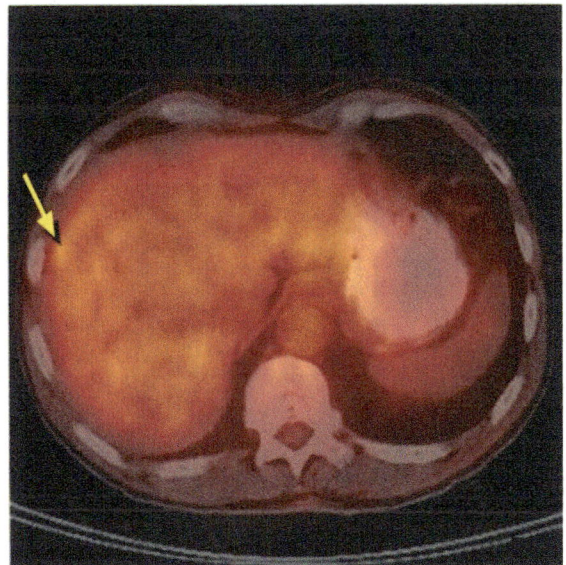

Image 3. Fused axial PET/CT image with the small hypermetabolic liver lesion (arrow).

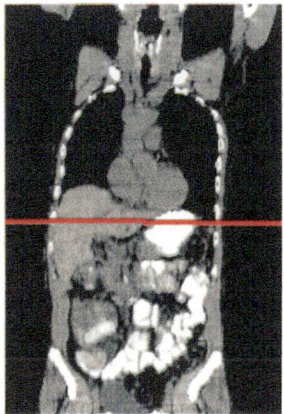

Image 3 (axial)

Localizer

Recurrent and Metastatic Colon Cancer

Clinical History

A 79-year-old male with colon cancer, status post colon resection, and chemotherapy.

PET/CT indication: Restaging.

Findings

A large, intense focus of increased metabolic activity is located between the pancreas and aorta. The CT shows a corresponding soft tissue mass. This is consistent with metastatic lymph nodes. Focally increased FDG uptake is also noted in the recto-sigmoid region. CT suggests thickening of the colon in this region. This is concerning for recurrent or residual malignancy.

Pathology verification: Positive for tumor recurrence and metastatic lymph nodes.

Teaching Point

Even large foci of increased FDG uptake can be difficult to localize with PET alone. CT provides better lesion localization.

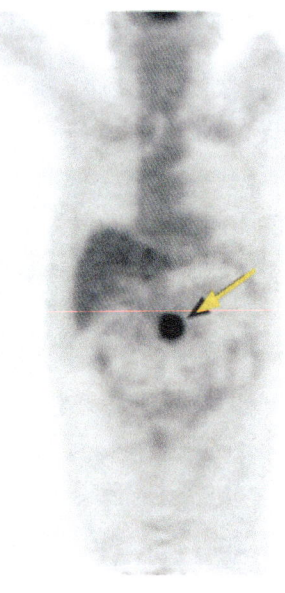

Image 1 (coronal)

Image 1. Coronal PET with large mid-abdominal focus of increased FDG uptake (arrow). The exact localization of this focus is not possible with FDG-PET.

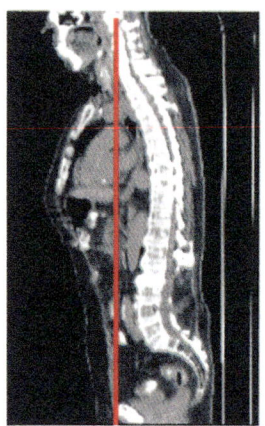

Localizer

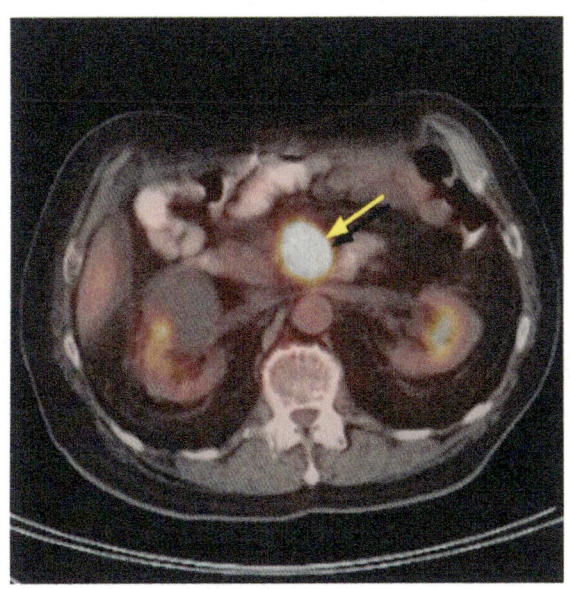

Image 2 (axial)

Image 2. Axial fused image showing intense FDG uptake in a large pre-aortic mass consistent with metastatic lymph node involvement (arrow).

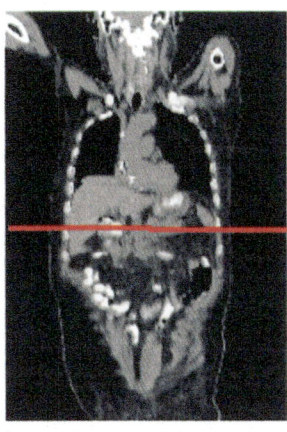

Localizer

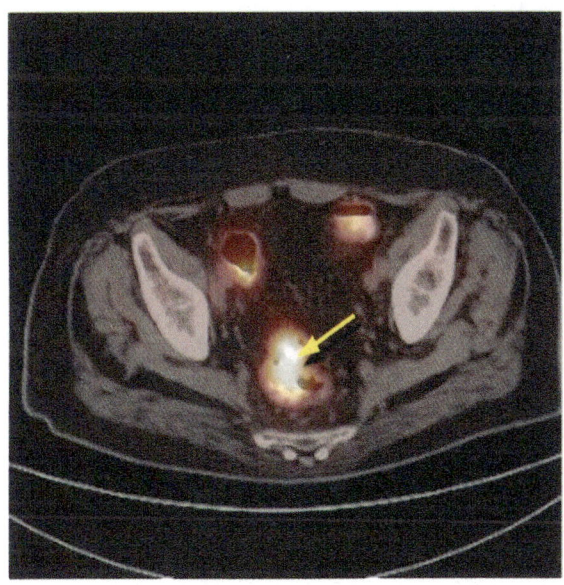

Image 3 (axial)

Image 3. Fused axial image with markedly increased FDG uptake corresponding to the thickened bowel wall (arrow). This is consistent with local disease recurrence.

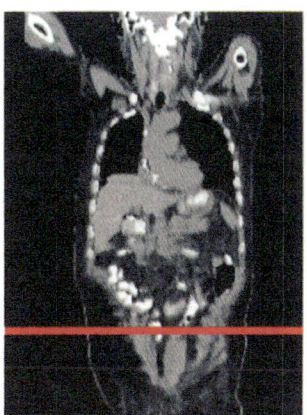

Localizer

Rectal Carcinoma

Clinical History

59-year-old female with recently diagnosed rectal adenocarcinoma. Two PET-CT studies were performed, one pre and one post chemotherapy.

PET/CT indication: Study I: Staging; Study II: Treatment monitoring.

Findings

PET/CT I: Moderately increased glucose metabolic activity is noted in the posterior lower pelvis. This correlates with a large rectal soft tissue mass, the site of the primary cancer.

PET/CT II: Interval resolution of the focally increased metabolic uptake in the rectum following chemotherapy.

Teaching Point

FDG-PET remains the most appropriate imaging modality to monitor treatment effects in many cancers.

Image 1

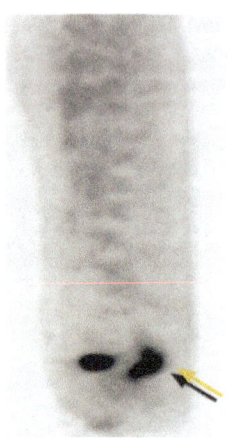 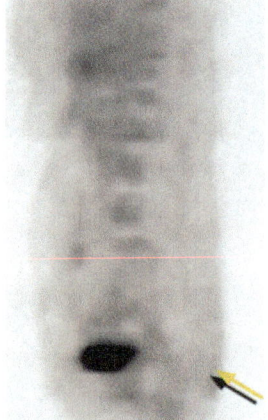

sagittal   sagittal

Image 1. Sagittal PET images obtained before (left) and after chemotherapy (right). Arrows point to the region of the primary tumor. Note the complete resolution of metabolic activity after treatment.

Image 1

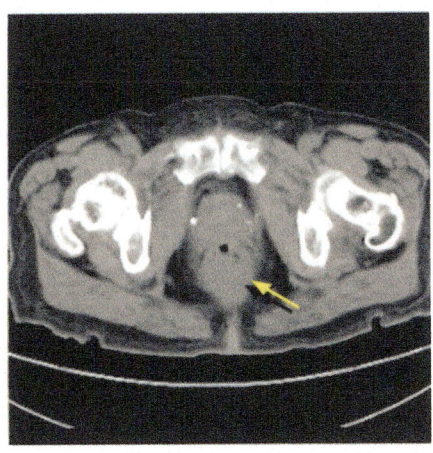 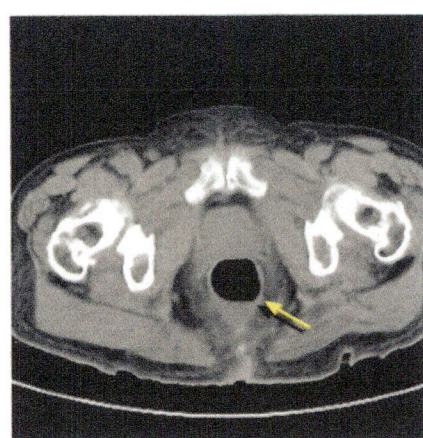

axial   axial

Image 2. Pre- (left) and post-treatment (right) axial CT images. The rectal wall is thickened and the lumen almost obstructed prior to chemotherapy (arrow on left image). Note the normal rectal wall and the patent lumen after chemotherapy (arrow in right image).

Image 1

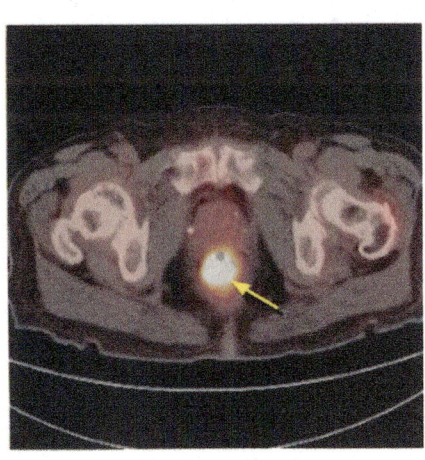 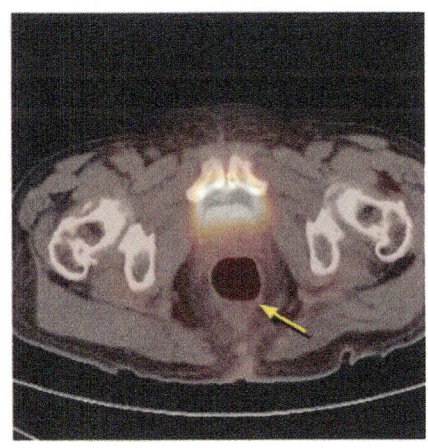

axial   axial

Image 3. Fused axial images with intense glucose metabolic activity prior to treatment (left arrow). The hypermetabolic activity is no longer seen after treatment (right arrow).

Sigmoid Colon Cancer

Clinical History

Patient with a history of sigmoid colon cancer presents with minimally elevated tumor markers.

PET/CT indication: Restaging.

Findings

A focus of moderately increased FDG uptake is located near the hepato-duodenal ligament and appears to correlate to a lymph node measuring approximately 2.8 x 2cm. This is suspicious for a malignant lymph node.

Teaching Point

FDG-PET is useful to identify unknown primary cancers and also to identify the source for rising tumor markers.

Image 1. Coronal PET with focally increased uptake (arrow) that cannot be localized to a specific anatomical structure.

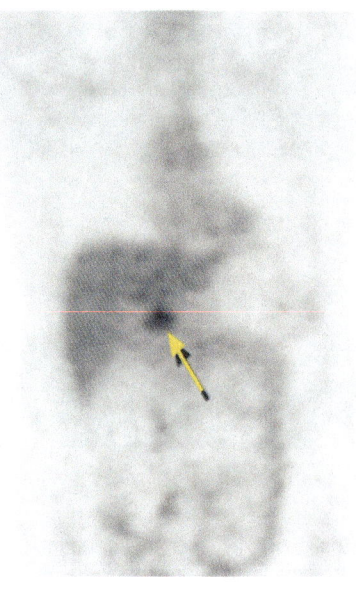

Image 1 (coronal)

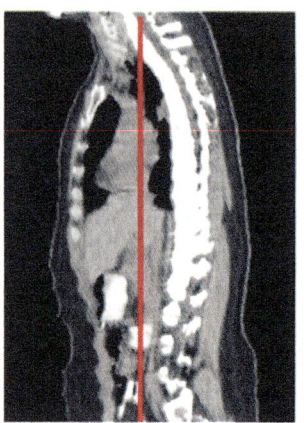

Localizer

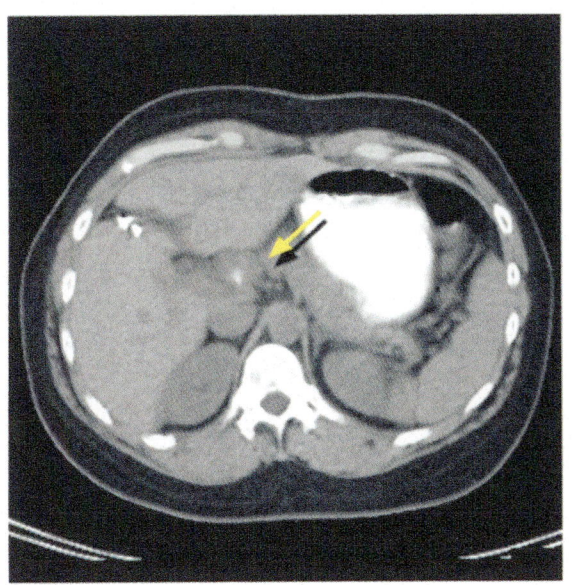

Image 2 (axial)

Image 2. Axial CT demonstrating extra-hepatic enlarged lymph node with small area of calcification (arrow).

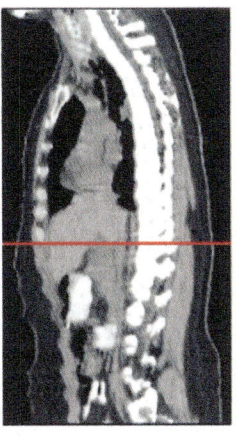

Localizer

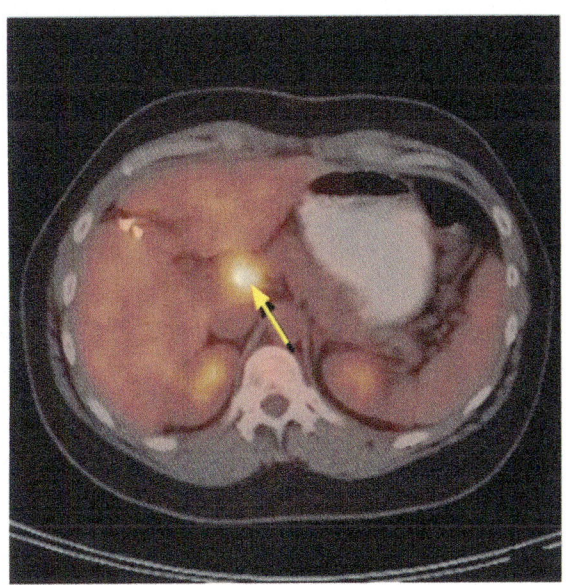

Image 3 (axial)

Image 3. Fused axial image localizing the hypermetabolic focus (arrow) to an enlarged lymph node.

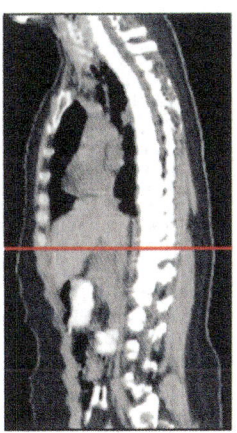

Localizer

Chapter 8

Lymphoma

Cases:

Chapter 8

Lymphoma

Lymphoma, i.e., Hodgkin's disease (HD), and Non-Hodgkin's lymphoma (NHL) are the fifth most common types of cancer diagnosed and the third most common form of cancer deaths in the United States. FDG-PET diagnoses and stages lymphoma with a higher diagnostic accuracy than any other non-invasive imaging modality. Restaging of the disease with PET after treatment is important because lymphoma is a curable disease even if first-line treatment fails. The question, whether PET/CT adds to the information provided by PET alone has not been examined. However, preliminary data from our institution suggest that PET/CT alters the clinical stage as determined by PET alone in about 20% of the patients.

Key Indications: Staging, Restaging, treatment Monitoring

Suggested Reading

Okada J, Yoshikawa K, Itami M, Imaseki K, Uno K, Itami J, Kuyama J, Mikata A, Arimizu N. Positron emission tomography using fluorine-18-fluorodeoxyglucose in malignant lymphoma: a comparison with proliferative activity. J Nucl Med. 1992;33(3):325-329.

Hoh CK, Glaspy J, Rosen P, Dahlbom M, Lee SJ, Kunkel L, Hawkin RA, Maddahi J, Phelps ME. Whole-body FDG-PET imaging for staging of Hodgkin's disease and lymphoma. J Nucl Med. 1997;38(3):343-348.

de Wit M, Bumann D, Beyer W, Herbst K, Clausen M, Hossfeld DK. Whole-body positron emission tomography (PET) for diagnosis of residual mass in patients with lymphoma. Ann Oncol. 1997;8(Suppl 1):S57-S60.

Carr R, Barrington SF, Madan B, O'Doherty MJ, Saunders CA, van der Walt J, Timothy AR. Detection of lymphoma in bone marrow by whole-body positron emission tomography. Blood. 1998;91(9):3340-3346.

Römer W, Hanauske AR, Ziegler S, Thödtmann R, Weber W, Fuchs C, Enne W, Herz M, Nerl C, Garbrecht M, Schwaiger M. Positron emission tomography in non-Hodgkin's lymphoma: assessment of chemotherapy with fluorodeoxyglucose. Blood. 1998;91(12):4464-4471.

Jerusalem G, Beguin Y, Fassotte MF, Najjar F, Paulus P, Rigo P, Fillet G. Whole-body positron emission tomography using 18F-fluorodeoxyglucose for posttreatment evaluation in Hodgkin's disease and non-Hodgkin's lymphoma has higher diagnostic and prognostic value than classical computed tomography scan imaging. Blood. 1999;94(2):429-433.

Zinzani PL, Magagnoli M, Chierichetti F, Zompatori M, Garraffa G, Bendandi M, Gherlinzoni F, Cellini C, Stefoni V, Ferlin G, Tura S. The role of positron emission tomography (PET) in the management of lymphoma patients. Ann Oncol. 1999;10(10): 1181-1184.

Spaepen K, Stroobants S, Dupont P, Van Steenweghen S, Thomas J, Vandenberghe P, Vanuytsel L, Bormans G, Balzarini J, De Wolf-Peeters C, Mortelmans L, Verhoef G. Prognostic value of positron emission tomography (PET) with fluorine-18 fluorodeoxyglucose ([18F]FDG) after first-line chemotherapy in non-Hodgkin's lymphoma: is [18F]FDG-PET a valid alternative to conventional diagnostic methods? J Clin Oncol. 2001;19(2):414-419.

Schöder H, Meta J, Yap C, Ariannejad M, Rao J, Phelps ME, Valk PE, Sayre J, Czernin J. Effect of whole-body 18F-FDG PET imaging on clinical staging and management of patients with malignant lymphoma. J Nucl Med. 2001;42(8):1139-1143.

Filmont JE, Czernin J, Yap C, Silverman DH, Quon A, Phelps ME, Emmanouilides C. Value of F-18 fluorodeoxyglucose positron emission tomography for predicting the clinical outcome of patients with aggressive lymphoma prior to and after autologous stem-cell transplantation. Chest. 2003;124(2):608-613.

Schiepers C, Filmont JE, Czernin J. PET for staging of Hodgkin's disease and non-Hodgkin's lymphoma. Eur J Nucl Med Mol Imaging. 2003;30(Suppl 1):S82-S88.

Freudenberg LS, Antoch G, Schutt P, Beyer T, Jentzen W, Muller SP, Gorges R, Nowrousian MR, Bockisch A, Debatin JF. FDG-PET/CT in re-staging of patients with lymphoma. Eur J Nucl Med Mol Imaging. 2003;In press.

Lymphoma

Clinical History

24-year-old woman with Hodgkin's lymphoma who recently underwent chemotherapy. CT performed at another institution suggested residual anterior mediastinal mass.

PET/CT indication: Treatment monitoring.

Findings

Intensely increased, partially symmetric FDG accumulation is noted in the head and neck regions correlating to areas of brown fat on CT. Areas of increased tracer activity do not correlate to any mass lesions on CT. They likely represent a normal physiological variant.

Teaching Point

CT revealed an anterior mediastinal mass and was interpreted as positive for residual disease. PET showed several areas of increased glucose metabolic activity, some of which were interpreted as residual disease by PET alone. Importantly, the PET "abnormalities" did not correlate to the location of the CT abnormalities. Upon further review of the fused images all areas of increased glycolysis corresponded to physiological structures such as fat, blood pool or muscle. Image co-registration resulted in a true negative interpretation of the study.

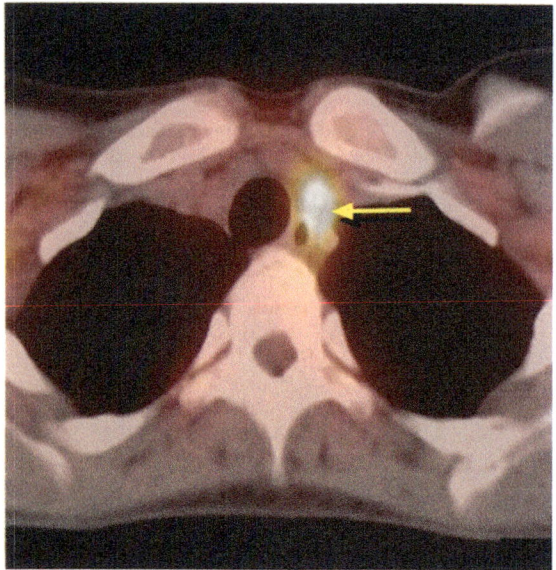

Image 1 (axial)

Image 1. Fused axial image demonstrating increased blood pool activity and FDG uptake in fat tissue (arrow).

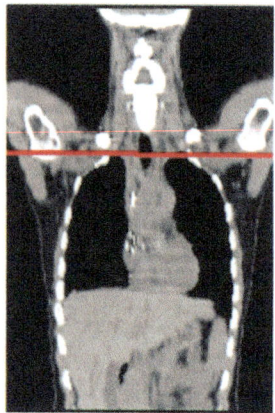

Localizer

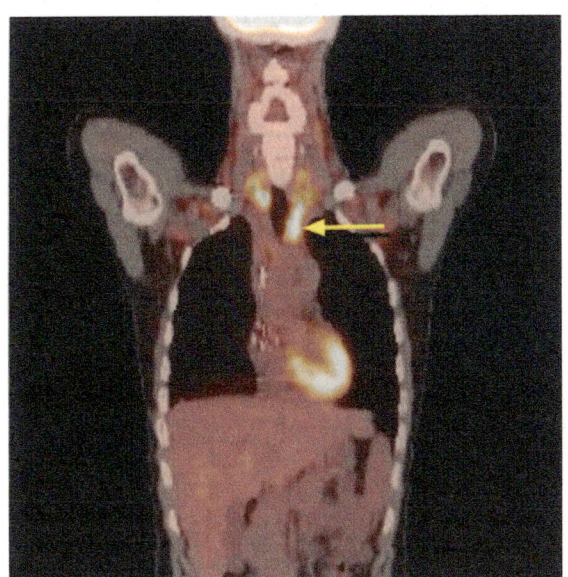

Image 2 (coronal)

Image 2. Fused coronal Image showing increased FDG uptake in the left para-treacheal region (arrow). This corresponded to perivascular fat on CT.

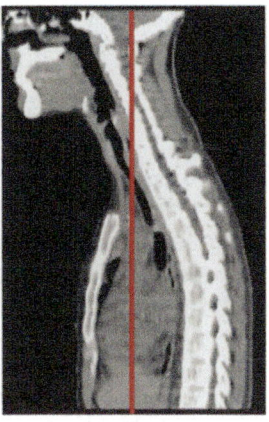

Localizer

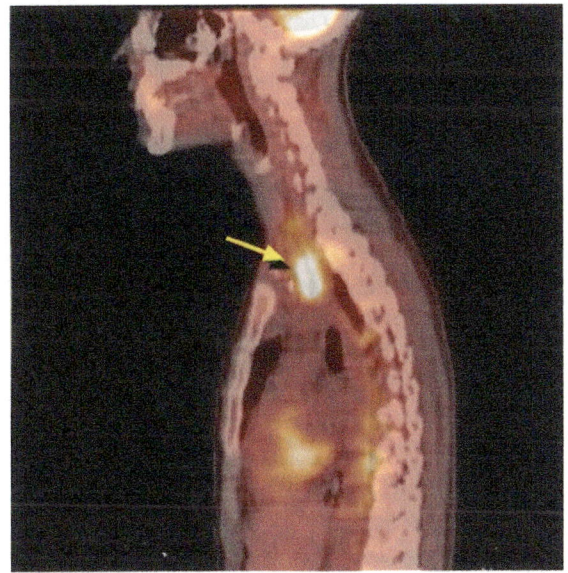

Image 3 (sagittal)

Image 3. Sagittal Image demonstrating increased FDG uptake in the left para-treacheal region (arrow) corresponding to fat on CT.

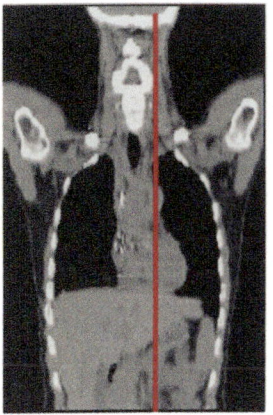

Localizer

Chronic Myelogenous Leukemia

Clinical History

74-year-old male with CML without history of chemotherapy. Red blood count is within normal limits.

PET/CT indication: Restaging.

Findings

Diffusely increased FDG uptake is present in the bone marrow of the bilateral humeral heads, the sternum, spine, pelvis, bilateral clavicles, rib cage and bilateral femur. Marked spleno-megaly is observed. Findings are consistent with myelo-proliferative disease.

Teaching Point

The pattern of diffusely increased bone marrow activity most frequently occurs in patients following chemotherapy due to regenerating bone marrow. Other reasons for diffusely increased marrow activity include anemia, treatment with granulocyte colony stimulating factor or erythropoetin, or in the case presented here, diffuse bone marrow infiltration due to a hematological malignancy. This patient had a normal red blood cell count and no previous chemotherapy.

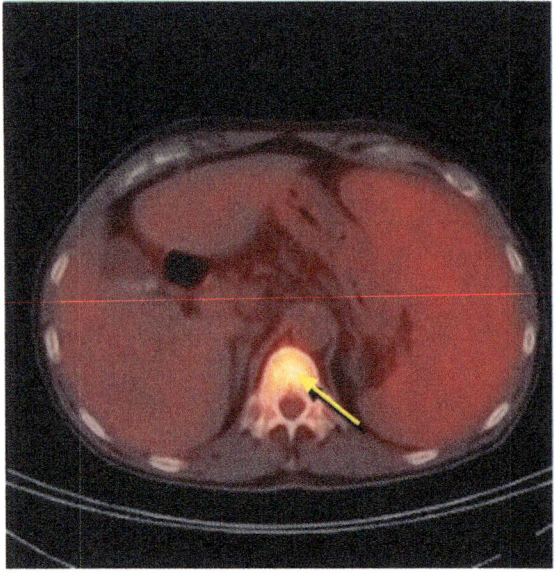

Image 1 (axial)

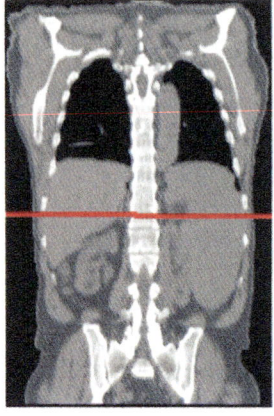

Localizer

Image 1. Fused axial image of a vertebral body demonstrating increased FDG accumulation in bone marrow due to diffuse bone marrow infiltration.

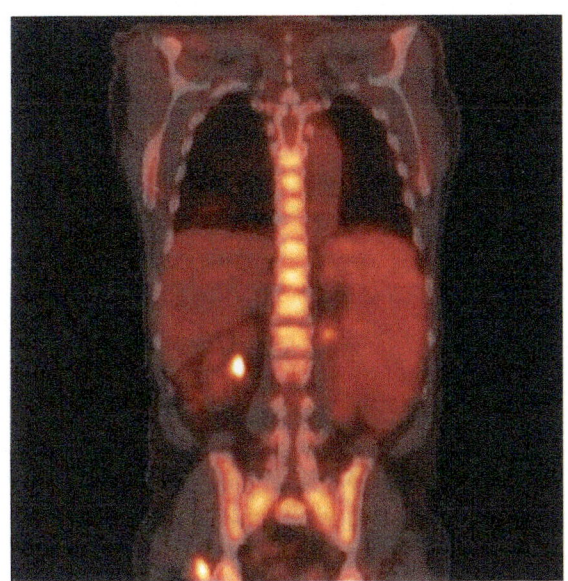

Image 2. Fused coronal image demonstrating increased FDG activity corresponding to diffuse bone marrow infiltration of the axial skeleton.

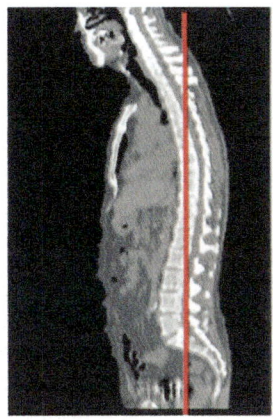

Image 2 (coronal)

Localizer

Image 3. Fused sagittal image with diffusely increased bone marrow activity.

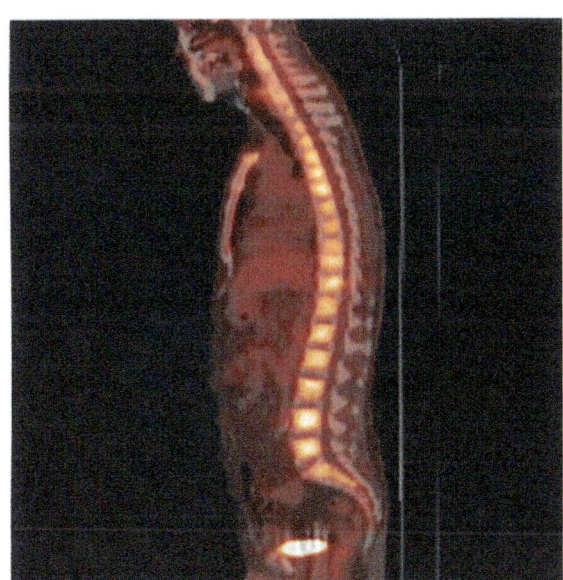

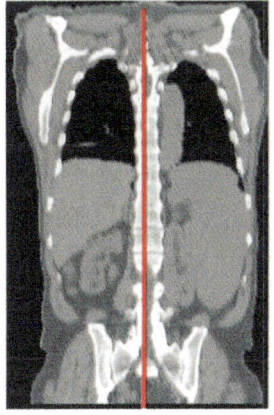

Image 3 (sagittal)

Localizer

Hodgkin's Lymphoma

Clinical History

This 39-year-old female patient was recently diagnosed with Hodgkin's lymphoma (biopsy of a right supraclavicular lymph node). An outside MRI reported right supraclavicular, bilateral axillary, anterior mediastinal, and right paratracheal masses as well as an enlarged lymph node in the AP window.

PET/CT indication: Staging.

Findings

Several foci of abnormally increased glycolytic activity consistent with lymphoma are identified. All correlate with lesions seen on the MRI and are located as follows: The posterior right neck, the right and left supraclavicular regions, left and right axillae, the right paratracheal region, the right lateral anterior mediastinum, and the AP window.

Teaching Point

PET is the gold standard for staging, restaging and monitoring treatment of lymphoma. Very few patients benefit from additional CT or even contrast CT studies.

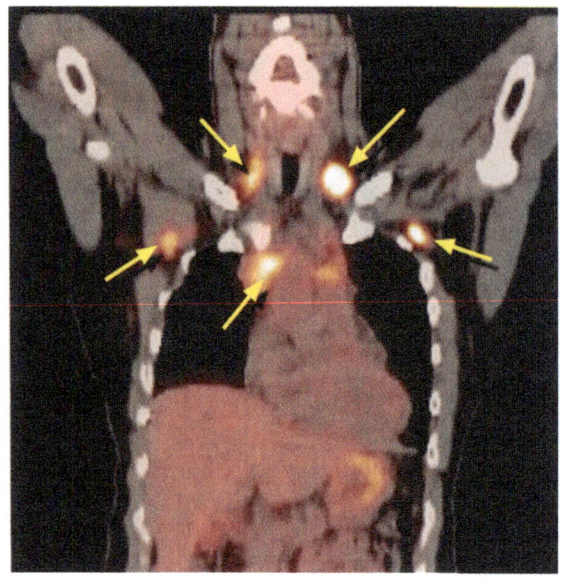

Image 1 (coronal)

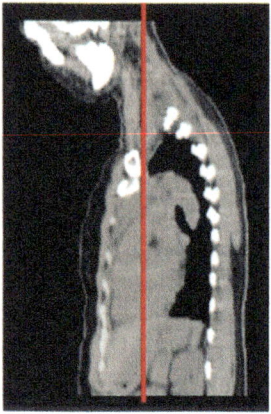

Localizer

Image 1. Fused coronal image with bilateral mediastinal, right paratracheal and left supraclavicular hypermetabolic lesions corresponding to enlarged lymph nodes on CT (arrows).

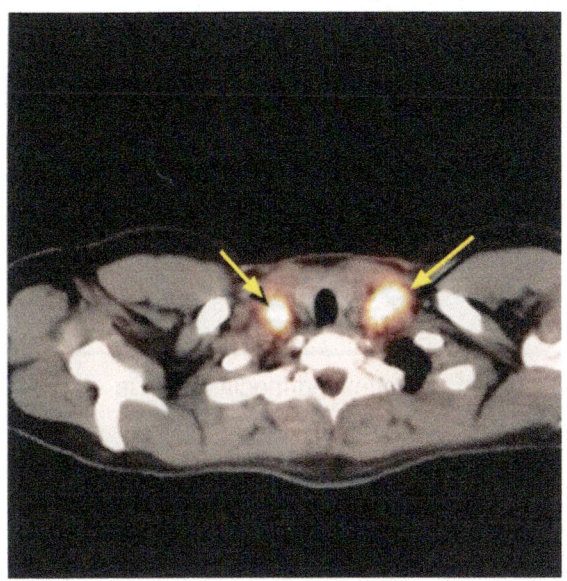

Image 2 (axial)

Image 2. Fused axial image demonstrating the bilateral supraclavicular lymphadenopathy (arrows).

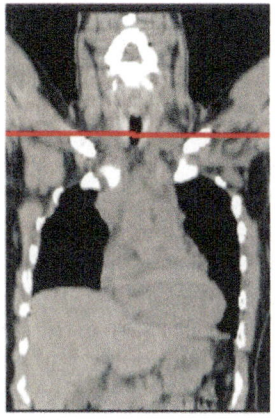

Localizer

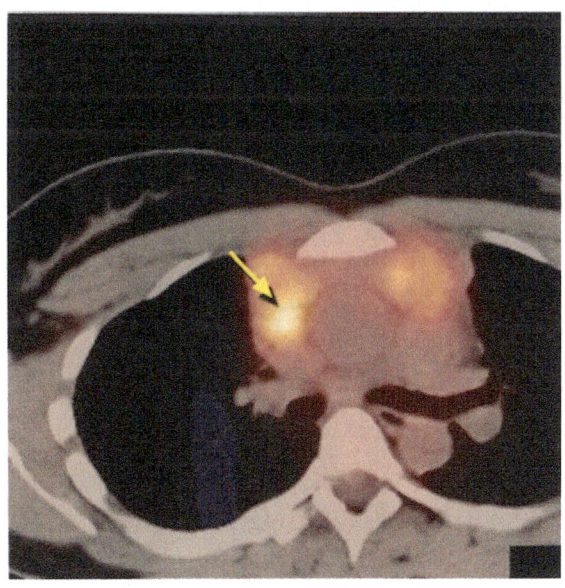

Image 3 (axial)

Image 3. Fused axial image with extensive hypermetabolic anterior mediastinal lymphadenopathy (arrow).

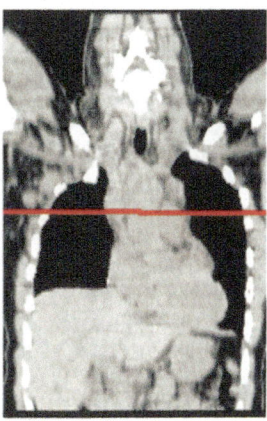

Localizer

Treatment Response

Clinical History

A 42-year-old female patient with recurrent large cell B-cell lymphoma is studied with PET/CT during chemotherapy. The pre-treatment and post-treatment scans are shown.

Findings

Pretreatment Study: Increased metabolic activity within the left-sided mediastinum is consistent with lymphadenopathy.

Post-treatment Study: Complete resolution of the abnormal metabolic activity in the mediastinum during chemotherapy. No metabolic evidence for residual lymphoma was present. Decrease in size of the mediastinal mass by CT was noted.

Teaching Point

FDG-PET predicts treatment response and patient outcome with a much higher accuracy than CT alone. Post-treatment tissue alterations such as scar or inflammation can present as residual masses on CT, which is frequently misinterpreted as residual disease.

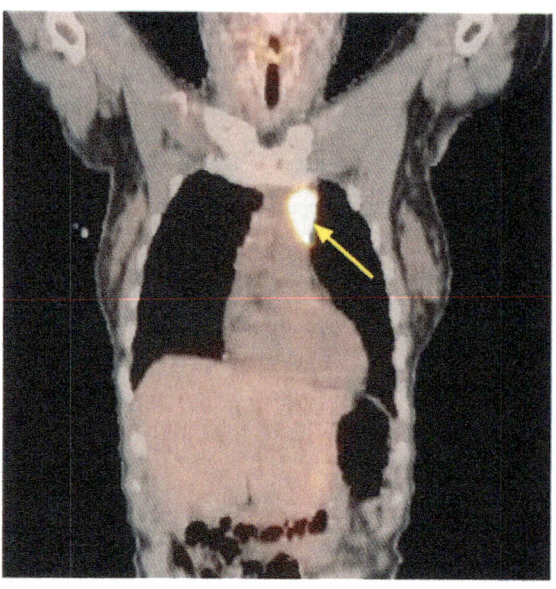

Image 1. A fused coronal view reveals a hypermetabolic left anterior mediastinal mass (arrow) prior to treatment.

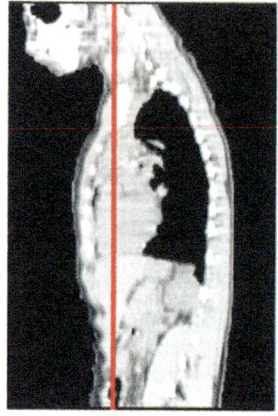

Image 1 (coronal)

Localizer

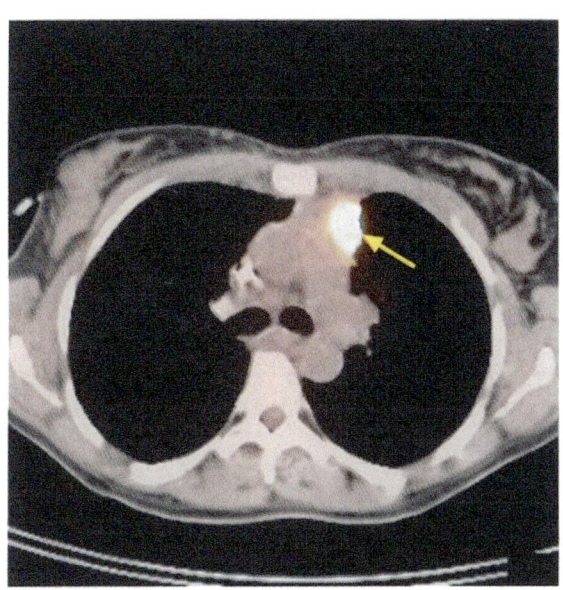

Image 2. Fused axial image demonstrating the hypermetabolic mediastinal mass.

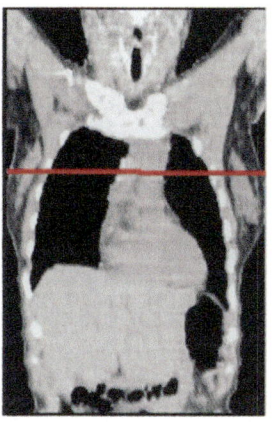

Image 2 (axial)

Localizer

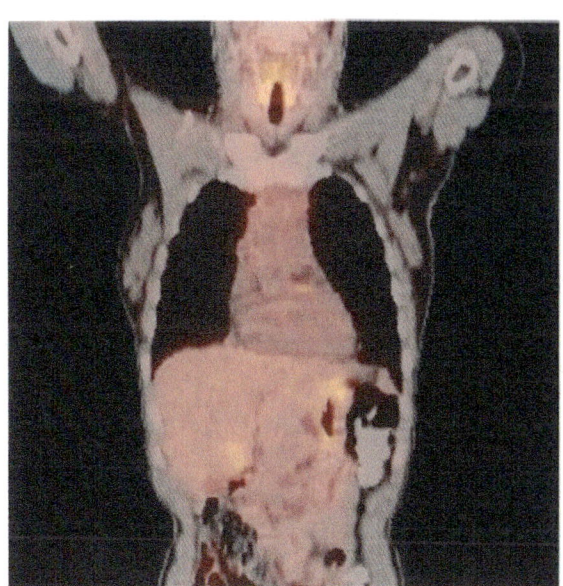

Image 3. Fused coronal image with complete resolution of the metabolic abnormality after treatment.

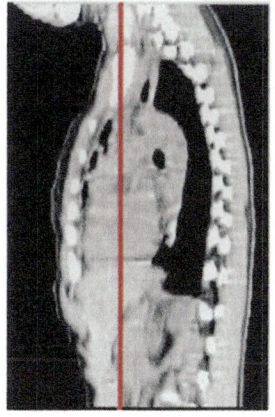

Image 3 (coronal)

Localizer

Localization of Malignant Lymph Node

Clinical History

13-year-old female patient with Hodgkin's Disease is studied after radiation- and chemo-therapy.

PET/CT indication: Restaging.

Findings

Increased glycolytic activity in a right axillary lymph node is suspicious for residual disease.

Teaching Point

PET/CT greatly facilitates the localization of hypermetabolic foci.

Image 1. Fused axial image demonstrating hypermetabolic right axillary lymph node (arrow).

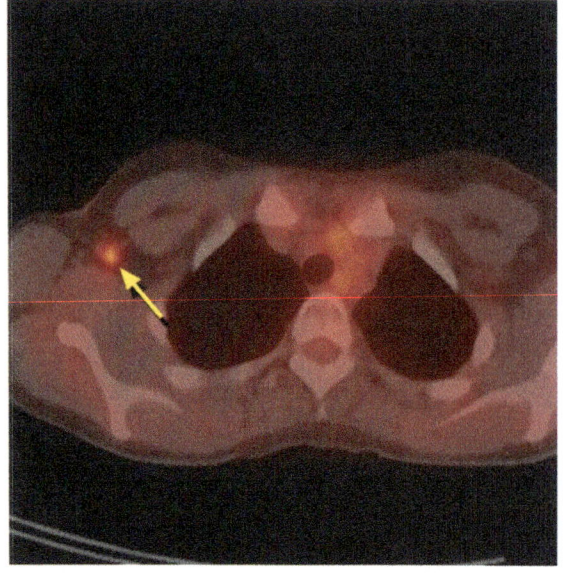

Image 1 (axial)

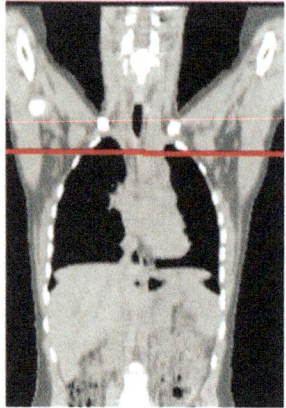

Localizer

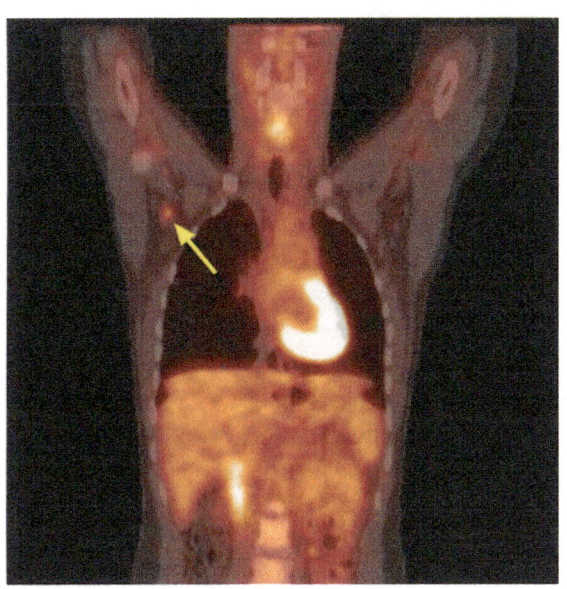

Image 2 (coronal)

Image 2. Fused coronal image with single hypermetabolic focus corresponding to an enlarged lymph node (arrow).

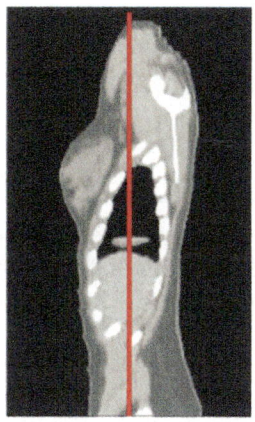

Localizer

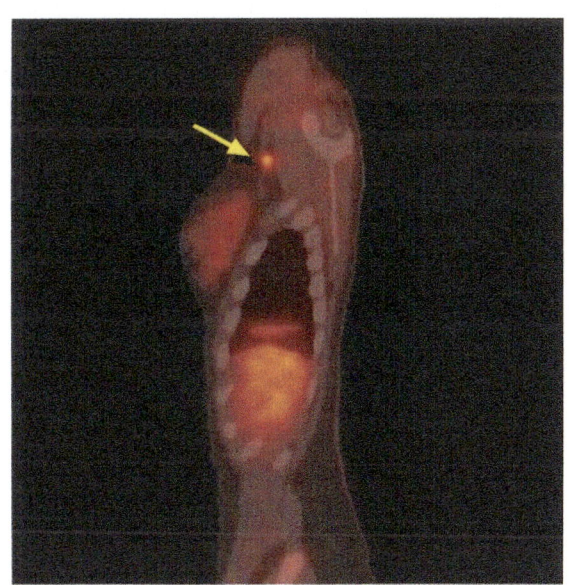

Image 3 (sagittal)

Image 3. Sagittal image in the same patient. Note the "mushroom" artifact due to respiratory diaphragmatic motion (arrow).

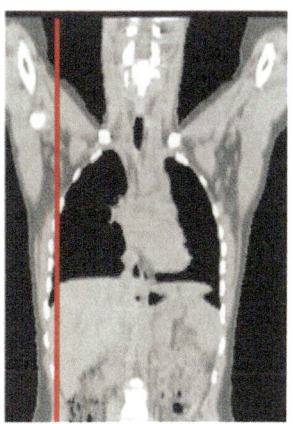

Localizer

Lymphoma

Clinical History

12-year-old male with Hodgkin's disease.

PET/CT indication: Restaging.

Findings

Multiple foci of increased FDG uptake corresponding to tumor lesions on CT. Of particular interest is a hypermetabolic lesion in the right lung base corresponding to a nodule just above the diaphragm on CT images

Teaching Point

Focally increased uptake in the liver-lung interface can frequently not be reliably assigned to liver or lung by PET alone. PET/CT provides accurate lesion localization.

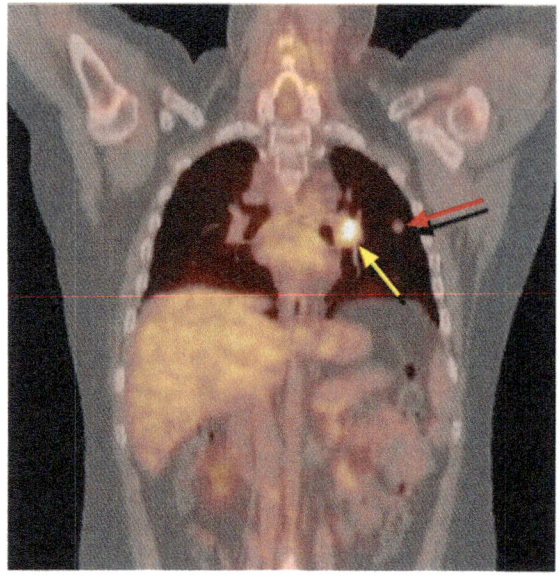

Image 1. Increased FDG uptake corresponding to a left mediastinal lesion (yellow arrow) and a smaller lesion in the left lung (red arrow) shown on fused coronal image.

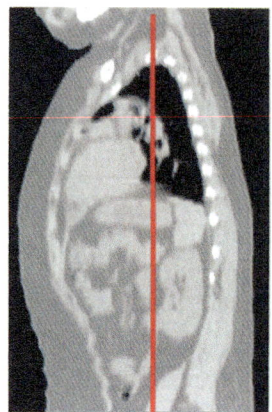

Image 1 (coronal)

Localizer

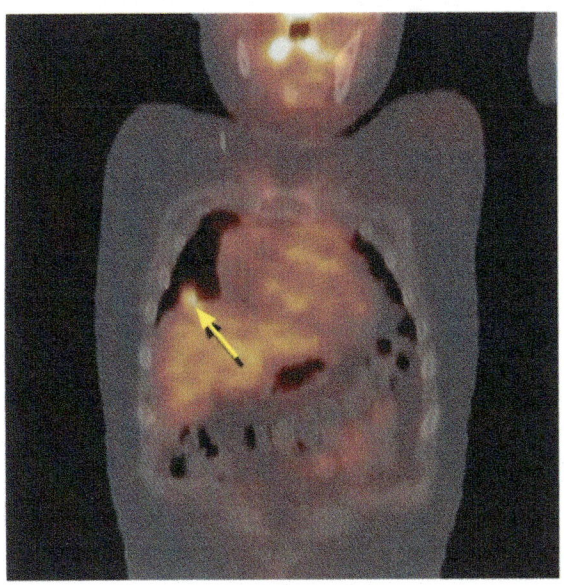

Image 2 (coronal)

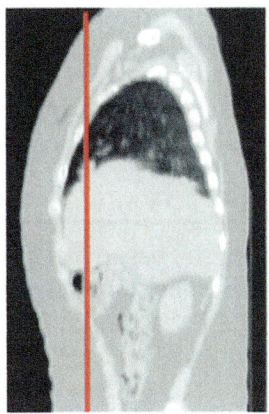

Localizer

Image 2. Fused coronal image depicting increased FDG uptake in a lesion located at the base of the right lung.

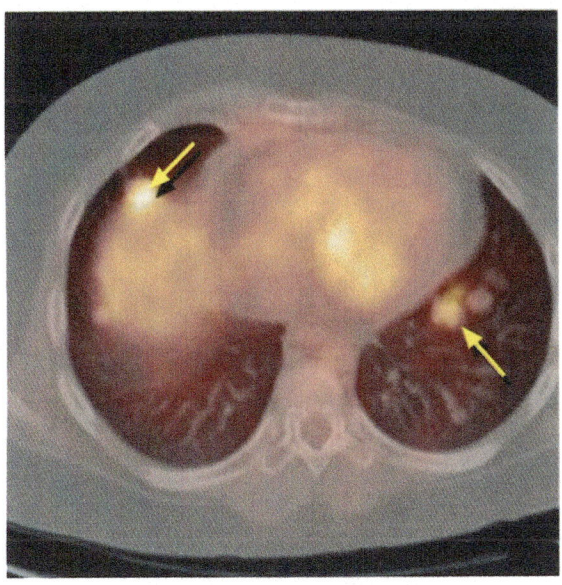

Image 3 (axial)

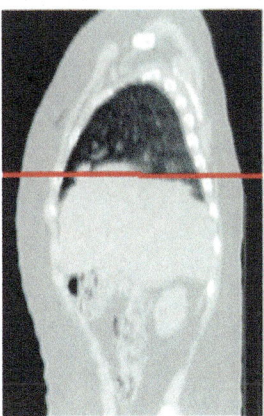

Localizer

Image 3. Fused axial view with increased FDG uptake in lesions located at the base of both lungs.

Non-Hodgkin's Lymphoma

Clinical History

35-year-old female with Non-Hodgkin's Lymphoma. The patient is currently undergoing her last cycle of chemotherapy.

PET/CT indication: Treatment monitoring.

Findings

A mediastinal soft tissue mass exhibits no glucose metabolic activity. Reactive bone marrow hyperplasia is consistent with marrow regeneration during chemotherapy.

Teaching Point

The positive predictive value of CT masses during or after treatment for lymphoma is low. Masses can consist of scar, necrosis or inflammation. In contrast, both the positive and negative predictive values of PET for treatment response are very high. Note the dramatic discrepancy between anatomical (CT) and molecular imaging findings.

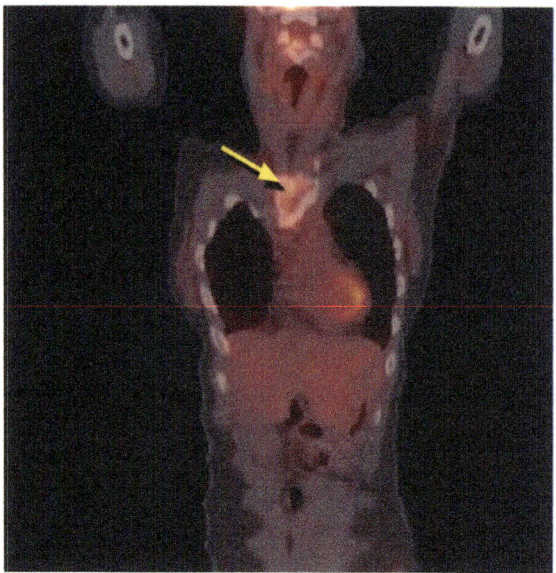

Image 1. Increased FDG uptake in the sternum consistent with regenerating marrow during chemotherapy (fused coronal image).

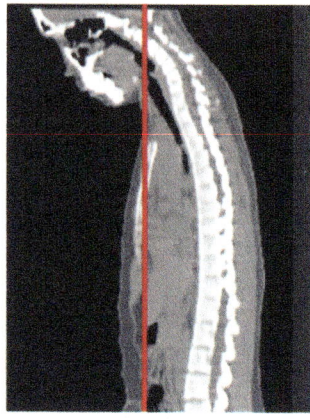

Image 1 (coronal)

Localizer

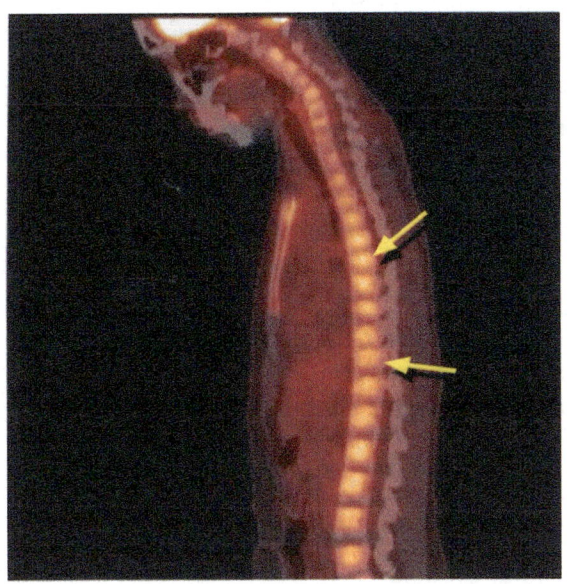

Image 2 (sagittal)

Image 2. Diffusely increased bone marrow activity (arrows) consistent with regenerating marrow during chemotherapy.

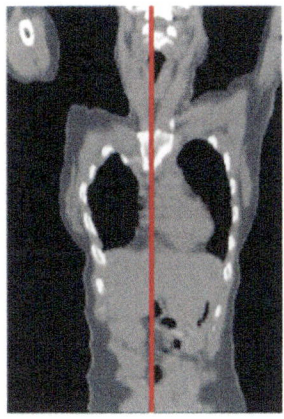

Localizer

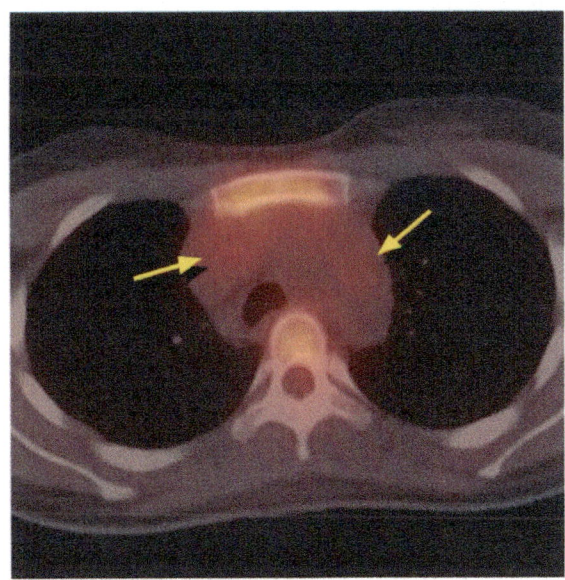

Image 3 (axial)

Image 3. Fused axial image depicting a large anterior mediastinal mass without increased glucose metabolic (arrows). This is consistent with scar tissue.

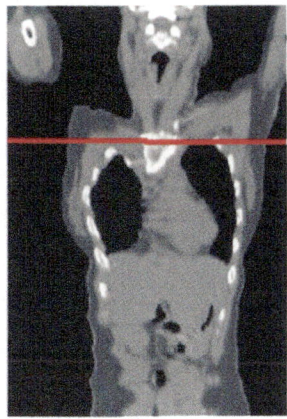

Localizer

Lymphoma Staging

Clinical History

62-year-old male with newly diagnosed left neck lymphoma.

PET/CT indication: Staging.

Findings

Intense hypermetabolic focus medial and posterior to the angle of the left mandible corresponds to a mass seen on CT. This is consistent with lymphoma.
A small-to-moderate sized focus of increased FDG uptake in the right neck posterior to the hyoid bone corresponds to a small lymph node seen on CT. This is also consistent with malignancy.

Histological Verification:
Left cervical lymph node biopsy: Follicular lymphoma, Grade 3.

Teaching Point

PET alone was equivocal for malignancy in the right neck. CT alone was negative for lymph node involvement by size criteria (less than 1 cm). PET/CT correctly diagnosed contralateral lymph node involvement.

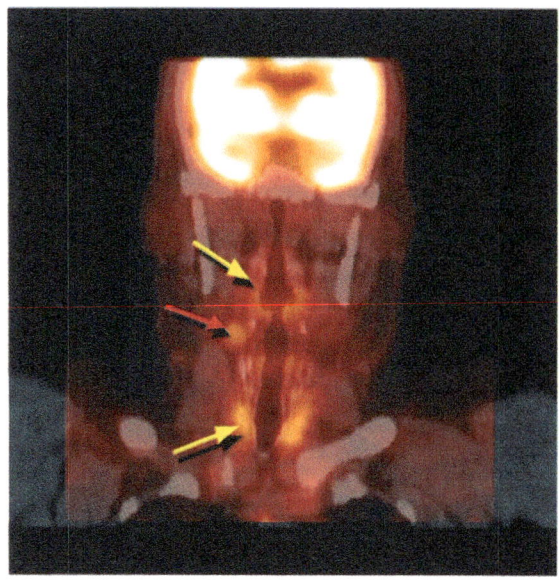

Image 1 (coronal)

Image 1. Fused coronal image identifying small hypermetabolic lymph node (red arrow). Upper arrow denotes physiologically increased vocal cord activity. The lower arrow points to normal thyroid activity.

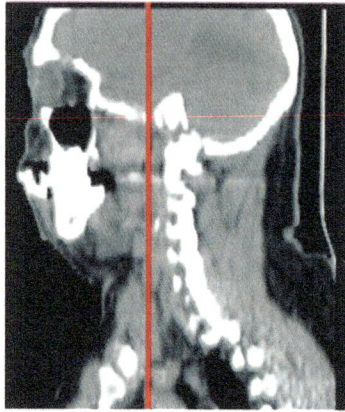

Localizer

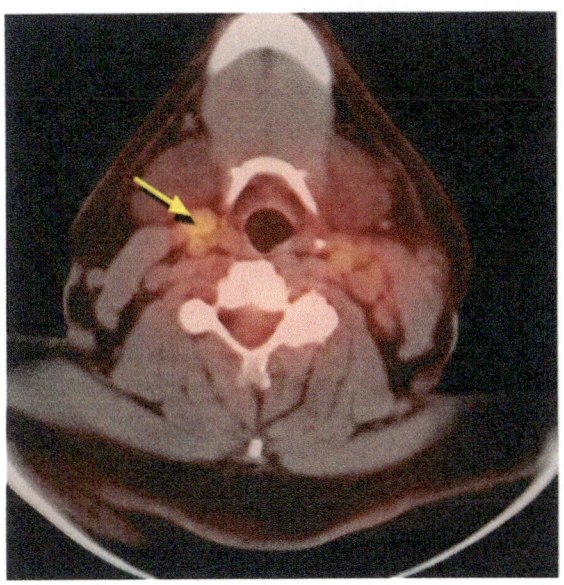

Image 2. Fused axial image demonstrating small, hypermetabolic lymph node (arrow).

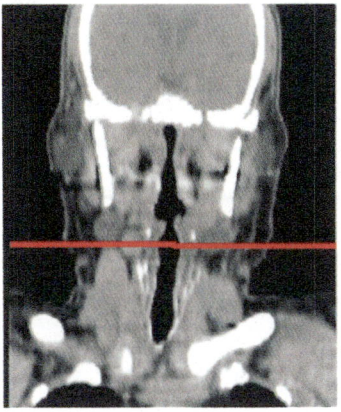

Image 2 (axial)

Localizer

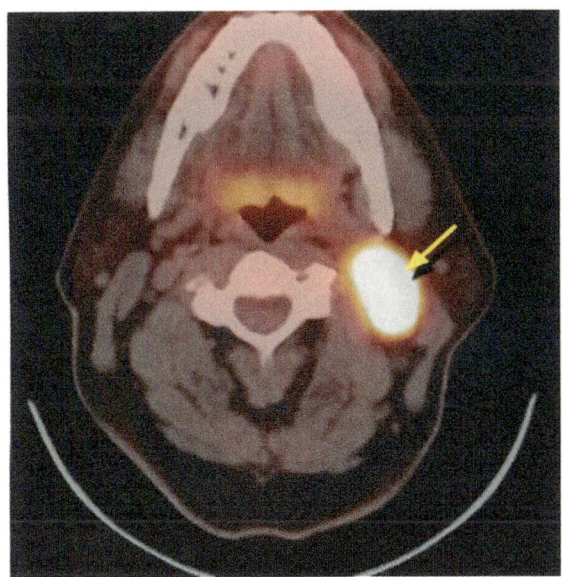

Image 3. Fused axial image with the large hypermetabolic left neck mass (arrow).

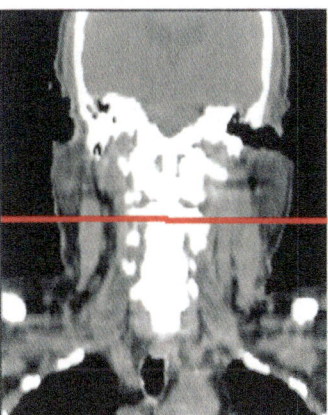

Image 3 (axial)

Localizer

Contrast PET/CT of Hodgkin's Disease

Clinical History

14 year-old male with relapsed Hodgkin's Disease who underwent autologous stem cell transplant 4 weeks ago.

PET/CT indication: Restaging.

Findings

A small focus of increased glycolytic activity is identified in the right upper lung lobe. Given the patient's immuno-suppression this is more likely to represent infection/inflammation than residual lymphoma.

Teaching Point

1) The PET/CT study was performed during intravenous contrast administration. Intravenous contrast can cause "pseudo FDG uptake". However, this is rarely a source of misinterpretation if CT studies are inspected carefully and if non-corrected PET images are also reviewed. In the current case and in many others, contrast did not induce an artifact.

2) A small focus of increased uptake was identified in the right upper lung lobe. This is most likely consistent with benign inflammatory changes in this immuno-suppressed patient.

Image 1

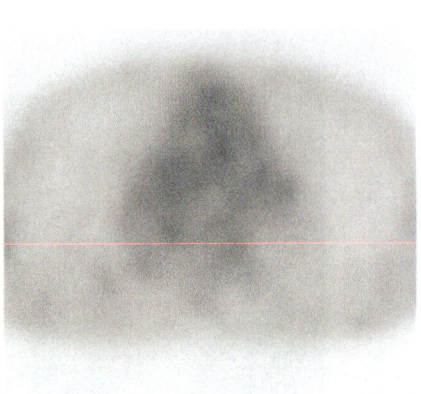

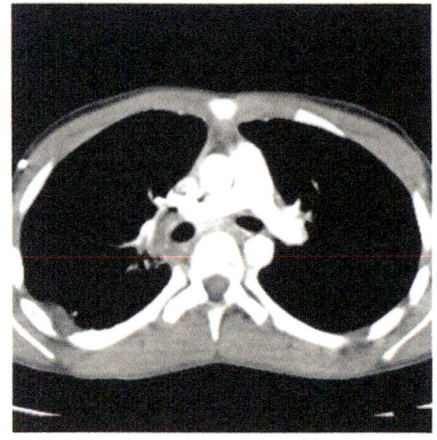

PET (axial)   CT (axial)

Image 1. Axial PET image (left) reveals normal mediastinal blood pool activity. Axial contrast CT showing the corresponding contrast-enhanced mediastinal vessels (right).

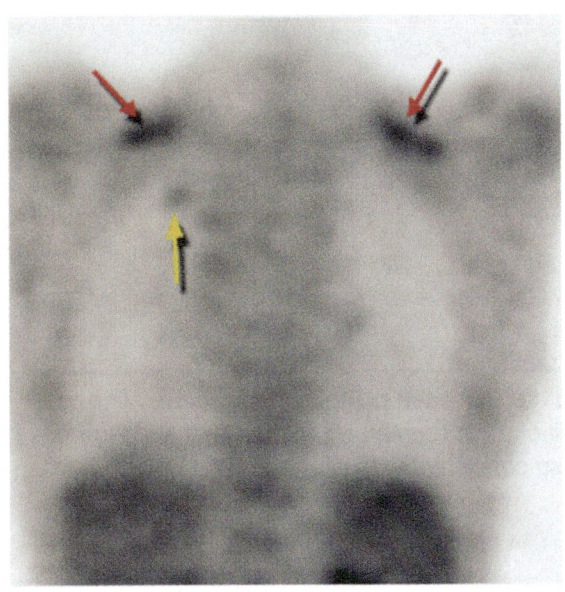

Image 2 (coronal)

Image 2. Coronal PET image with small hypermetabolic focus in the right upper lung (yellow arrow). Also note the symmetrically increased supraclavicular tracer activity consistent with brown fat (red arrows).

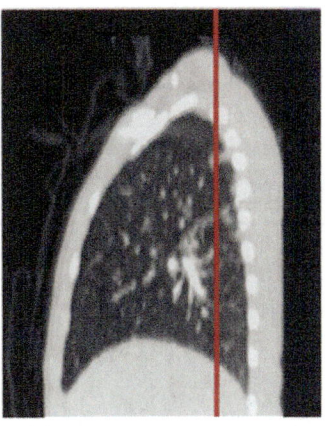

Localizer

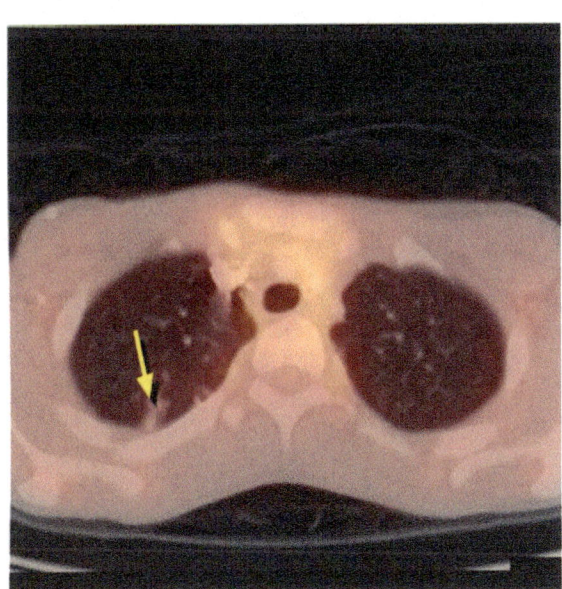

Image 3 (axial)

Image 3. Fused PET/contrast CT image showing mildly increased glycolytic activity corresponding to the ground glass opacity (arrow). This is likely consistent with inflammation in this immuno-supressed patient.

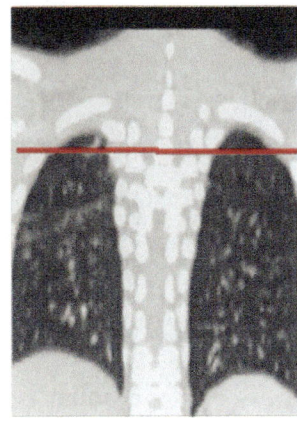

Localizer

Hodgkin's Lymphoma

Clinical History

Young patient with recently diagnosed Hodgkin's lymphoma.

PET/CT indication: Staging.

Findings

Moderately increased metabolic uptake is noted along the left posterior neck, correlating to a chain of enlarged cervical lymph nodes. In addition, some enlarged mediastinal lymph nodes exhibit mildly increased FDG uptake. This is also consistent with lymphoma.

Teaching Point

PET/CT studies of the head and neck and mediastinum frequently benefit from intravenous contrast application. This allows better visualization of lymph nodes on CT and permits to differentiate FDG- blood pool from lymph node activity.

Image 1

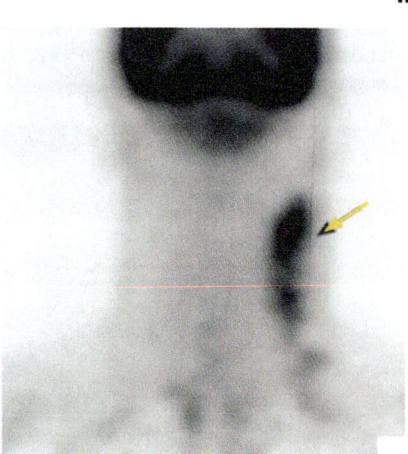
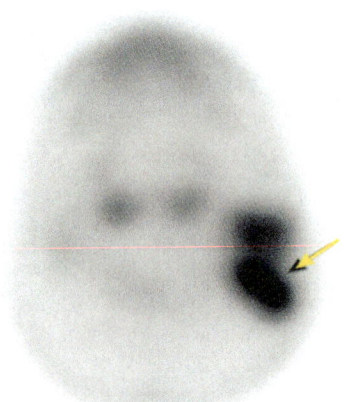

coronal   **axial**

Image 1. Coronal (left) and axial (right) PET images with intense glucose metabolic activity in the left neck (arrows).

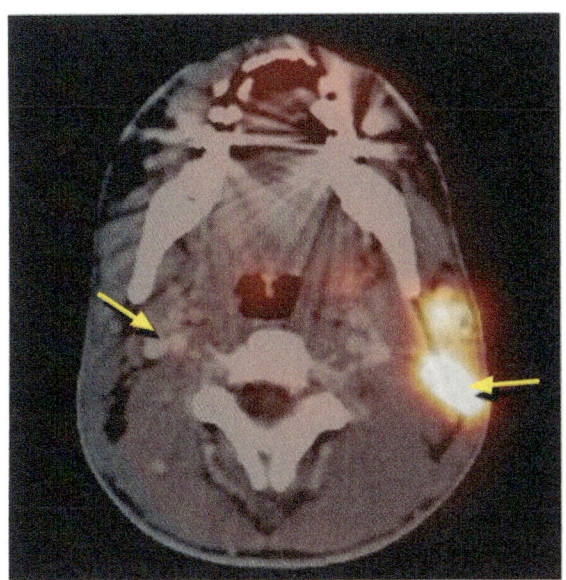

Image 2 (coronal)

Image 2. Fused axial images localizing the hypermetabolic activity to left cervical nodes (right arrow). Left arrow shows contrast-enhanced neck vessels.

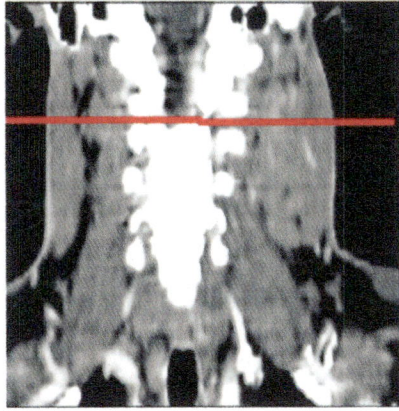

Localizer

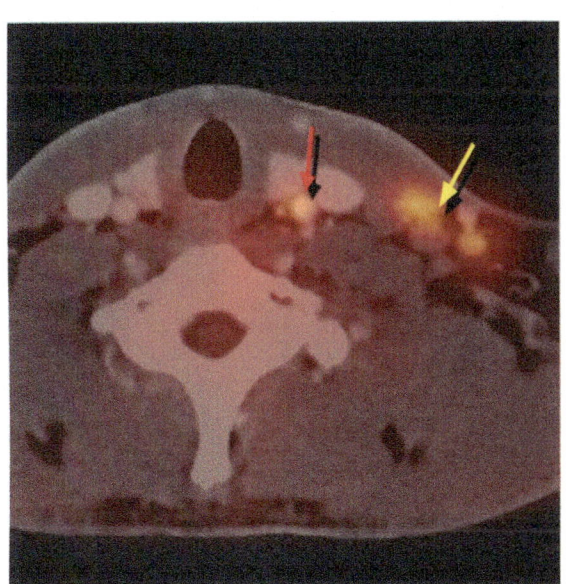

Image 3 (axial)

Image 3. The lower cervical area of increased FDG uptake (red arrow) represents blood pool activity, the yellow arrow points to metastatic lymph nodes.

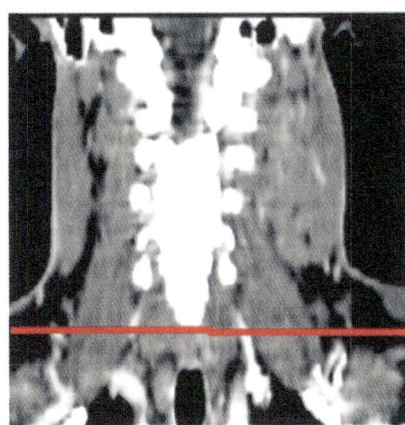

Localizer

Chapter 9

Cancers
of the Skin

Cases:

Chapter 9

Cancers of the Skin

Melanoma causes more than 75% of all skin cancer deaths with an estimated 44,000 new cases of melanoma in the United States in the year 2000. Melanoma exhibits the highest FDG uptake of all malignancies. FDG-PET is therefore used to stage and restage the disease. Treatment options are limited in melanoma. However, the molecular information provided by PET is of particular importance if experimental treatments are contemplated or if surgery for removing "isolated" metastases is considered.

No data are thus far available to determine the additional value of PET/CT over PET alone.

Key Indications: Staging and Restaging

Suggested Reading

Steinert HC, Huch Böni RA, Buck A, Böni R, Berthold T, Marincek B, Burg G, von Schulthess GK. Malignant melanoma: staging with whole-body positron emission tomography and 2-[F-18]-fluoro-2-deoxy-D-glucose. Radiology. 1995;195(3):705-709.

Macfarlane DJ, Sondak V, Johnson T, Wahl RL. Prospective evaluation of 2-[18F]-2-deoxy-D-glucose positron emission tomography in staging of regional lymph nodes in patients with cutaneous malignant melanoma. J Clin Oncol. 1998;16(5):1770-1776.

Rinne D, Baum RP, Hör G, Kaufmann R. Primary staging and follow-up of high risk melanoma patients with whole-body 18F-fluorodeoxyglucose positron emission tomography: results of a prospective study of 100 patients. Cancer. 1998;82(9):1664-1671.

Eigtved A, Andersson AP, Dahlstrom K, Rabol A, Jensen M, Holm S, Sorensen SS, Drzewiecki KT, Hojgaard L, Friberg L. Use of fluorine-18 fluorodeoxyglucose positron emission tomography in the detection of silent metastases from malignant melanoma. Eur J Nucl Med. 2000;27(1):70-75.

Jadvar H, Johnson DL, Segall GM. The effect of fluorine-18 fluorodeoxyglucose positron emission tomography on the management of cutaneous malignant melanoma. Clin Nucl Med. 2000;25(1):48-51.

Schwimmer J, Essner R, Patel A, Jahan SA, Shepherd JE, Park K, Phelps ME, Czernin J, Gambhir SS. A review of the literature for whole-body FDG PET in the management of patients with melanoma. Q J Nucl Med. 2000;44(2):153-167.

Crippa F, Leutner M, Belli F, Gallino F, Greco M, Pilotti S, Cascinelli N, Bombardieri E. Which kinds of lymph node metastases can FDG PET detect? A clinical study in melanoma. J Nucl Med. 2000;41(9):1491-1494.

Wong C, Silverman DH, Seltzer M, Schiepers C, Ariannejad M, Gambhir SS, Phelps ME, Rao J, Valk P, Czernin J. The Impact of 2-deoxy-2[18F] fluoro-D-glucose whole body positron emission tomography for managing patients with melanoma: the referring physician's perspective. Mol Imaging Biol. 2002;4(2):185-190.

Melanoma

Clinical History

50-year-old female with history of metastatic melanoma with new swelling in right sub-mandibular region.

PET/CT indication: Restaging.

Findings

Increased activity in the right submandibular gland is consistent with recurrent disease.

Teaching Point

Interpretation of PET images of the head/neck is complicated by the complex anatomy of this region. PET alone can be difficult to interpret because of variable patterns of glycolytic activity ascribed to striated muscle and brown fat (in younger patients). Additional problems can arise in patients who are imaged after surgery or radiation that can lead to asymmetric FDG distribution. In this case, CT provided lesion localization and differentiation from normal muscle activity.

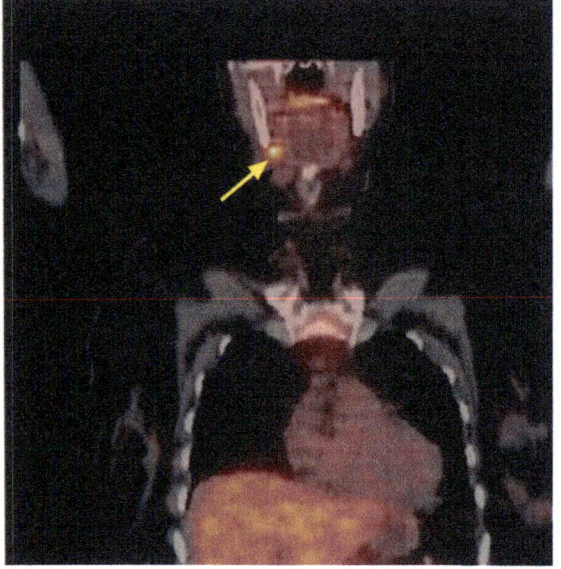

Image 1. Fused coronal image revealing a focus of increased glycolytic activity in the right submandibular region (arrow).

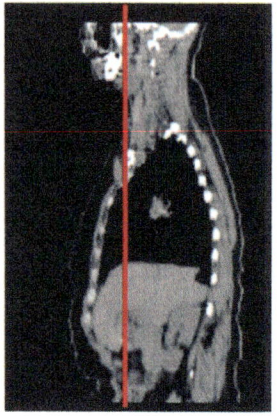

Image 1 (coronal)

Localizer

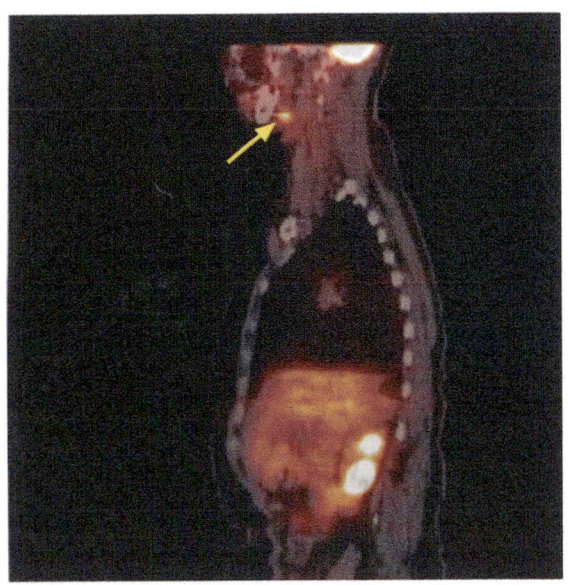

Image 2 (sagittal)

Image 2. Right-sided submandibular lymph node shown in a sagittal view (arrow).

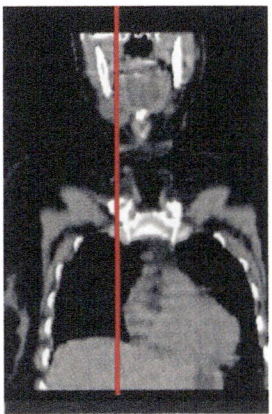

Localizer

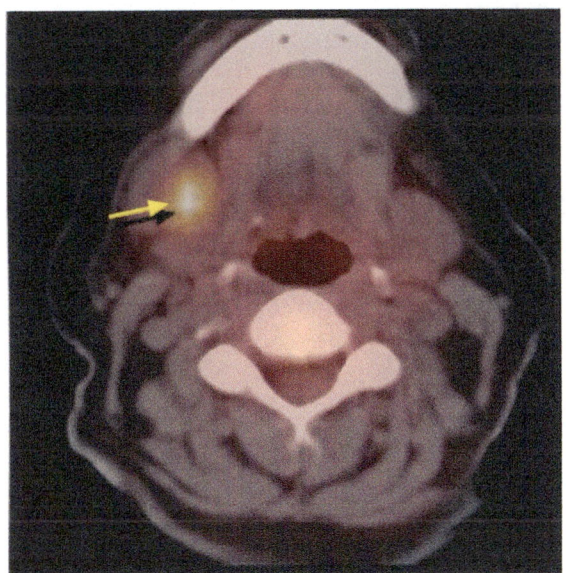

Image 3 (axial)

Image 3. Axial image demonstrating enlarged right-sided lymph node.

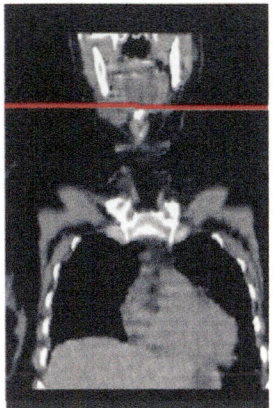

Localizer

Melanoma

Clinical History

67-year-old female diagnosed with melanoma of digit 5 of the left foot.

PET/CT indication: Staging.

Findings

A focus of abnormally increased tracer uptake in the small toe of the left foot is consistent with the patient's known primary site of malignancy.

Pathology: Malignant melanoma.

Teaching Point

PET stages melanoma with a high accuracy. Melanoma exhibits high glucose metabolic activity.

Image 1

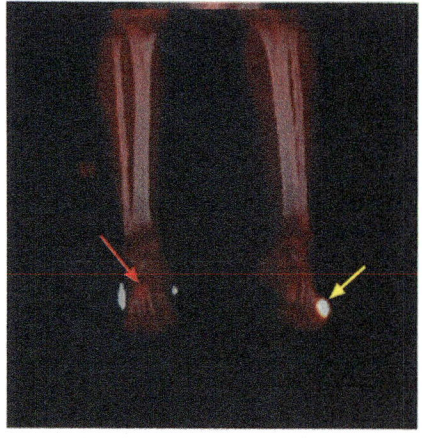
coronal

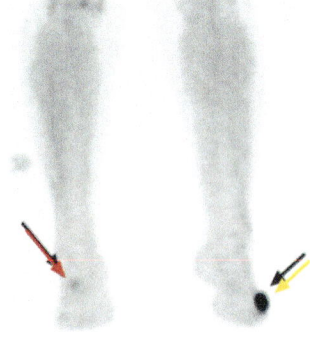
axial

Image 1. Intense hyper-metabolic activity in digit 5 of the left foot is consistent with primary melanoma site (yellow arrow) on fused (left) and PET projection (right) images. Note the mildly increased FDG uptake in the contralateral foot (red arrow). This is an unspecific finding and can be explained by inflammation, trauma or degenerative disease.

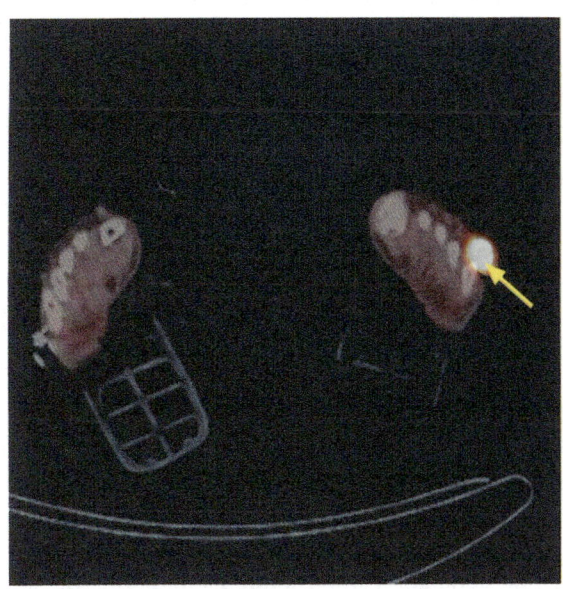

Image 2. Fused axial image demonstrating the primary melanoma site in the soft tissue above the 5th digit (arrow).

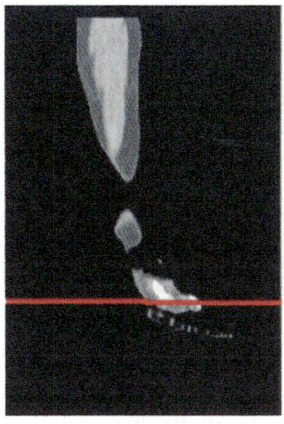

Image 2 (axial)

Localizer

Image 3. Fused coronal image affording exact lesion localization (arrow).

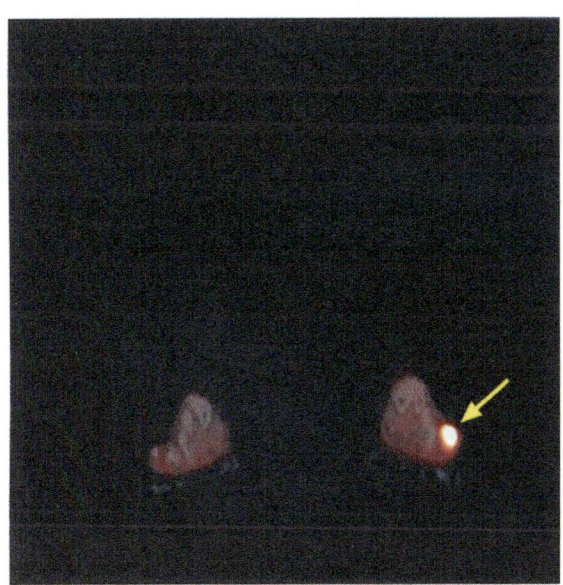

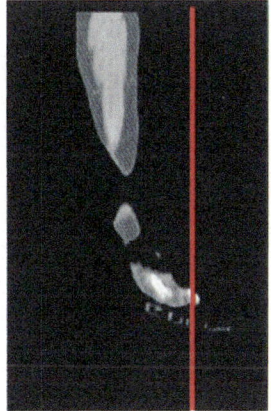

Image 3 (coronal)

Localizer

Restaging Melanoma

Clinical History

41-year-old male patient with melanoma who is status post surgery and radiation. He is currently undergoing interferon treatment.

PET/CT indication: Restaging.

Findings

Two large and two moderately sized foci of intensely increased FDG uptake are located in the superior and medial aspects of the spleen. These surround an area of photopenia on PET and hypodensity on CT and corresponding to tumor necrosis.
In addition multiple hypermetabolic liver lesions are consistent with metastases.

Histological Verification: Total splenectomy: findings consistent with metastatic melanoma.

Teaching Point

Melanoma is a systemic disease that can metastasize to any organ. The splenic involvement in this case was an unexpected finding.

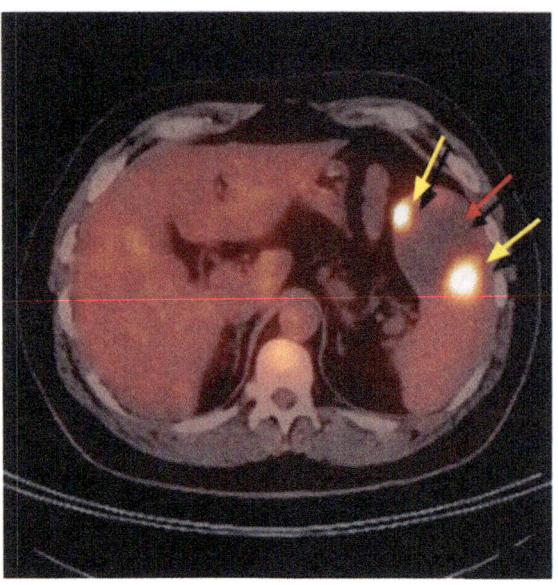

Image 1 (axial)

Image 1. Fused axial image with hypermetabolic activity (yellow arrows) surrounding an ametabolic, hypodense lesion (red arrow) in the spleen.

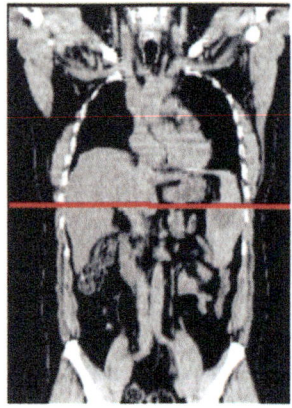

Localizer

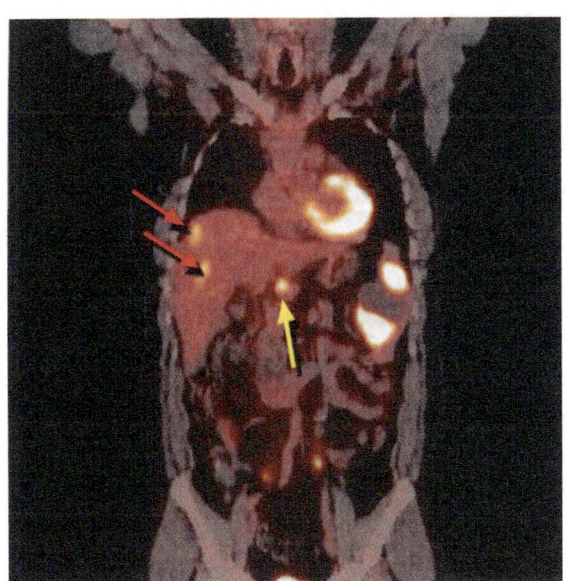

Image 2 (coronal)

Image 2. Fused coronal image with two hypermetabolic liver lesions (red arrows) and focally increased uptake corresponding to a metastatic celiac node (yellow arrow).

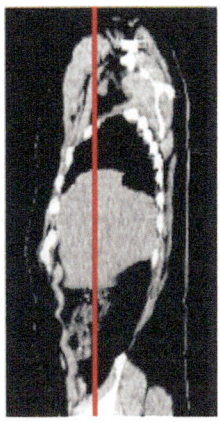

Localizer

Metastatic Melanoma

Clinical History

62-year-old male with metastatic melanoma and a recently discovered large abdominal mass.

PET/CT indication: Restaging.

Findings

A large and irregular focus of very intense tracer uptake is identified in the right lower quadrant of the abdomen extending through the right ilium. An additional small focus of increased FDG uptake is identified medial to the right ureter. These lesions are consistent with metastatic disease.

Teaching Point

PET alone cannot determine tumor extension into the bone and cannot localize small hypermetabolic foci to distinct anatomic structures.

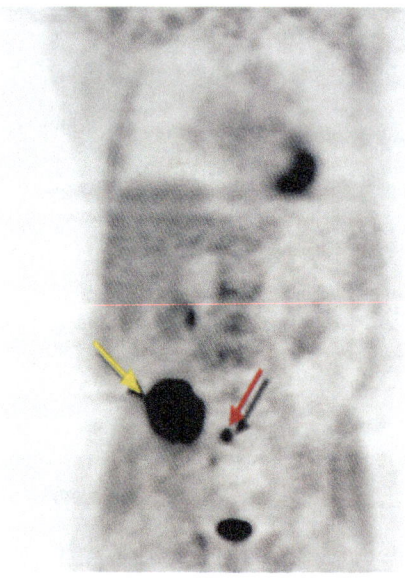

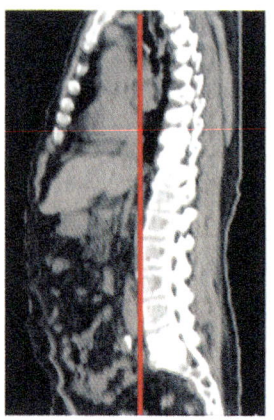

Image 1. Coronal PET image demonstrating large hypermetabolic focus (yellow arrow) and a small, more medially located lesion (red arrow). Exact lesion localization is not possible.

Image 1 (coronal)

Localizer

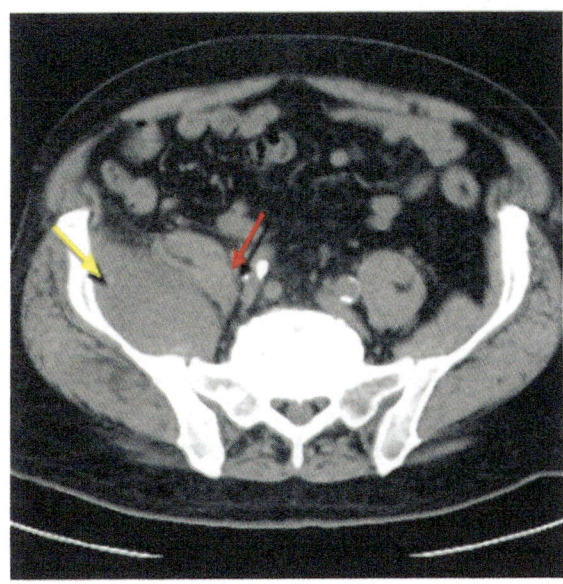

Image 2 (axial)

Image 2. Axial CT images demonstrating the large right pelvic mass (yellow arrow) and a small more medially located lymph node (red arrow).

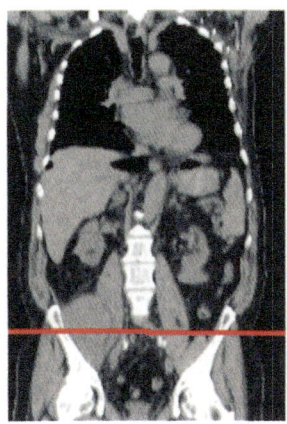

Localizer

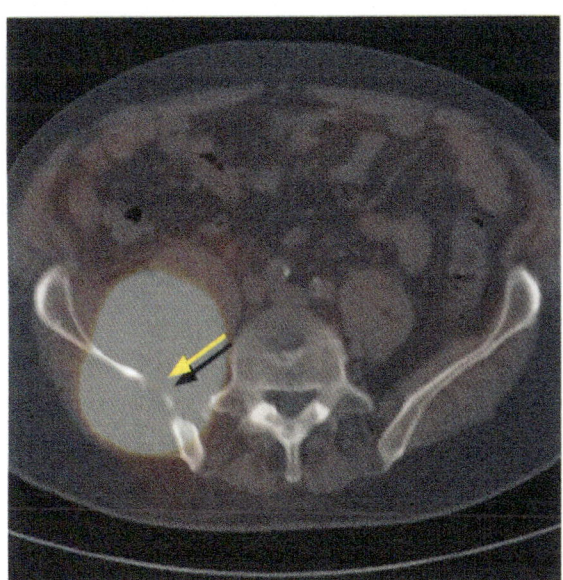

Image 3 (axial)

Image 3. Fused PET/CT image (bone window) demonstrating bone destruction (arrow).

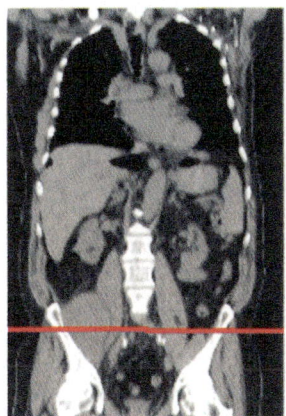

Localizer

Ocular Melanoma

Clinical History

Female patient with a history of left ocular melanoma. PET/CT was acquired after surgical resection, radiation therapy and interferon treatment.

PET/CT indication: Restaging.

Findings

Three hypermetabolic foci are identified in the liver that are suspicious for metastases. One is located at the dome of the liver measuring 2.5 x 2.8 cm. Two other foci are seen in the anterior segment and the posterior segment of the right hepatic lobe. No abnormal focus is identified in the left orbit.

Teaching Point

Coronal PET images demonstrate increased FDG uptake at the interface of lung and liver. CT provided accurate location of the metastatic lesion to the liver.

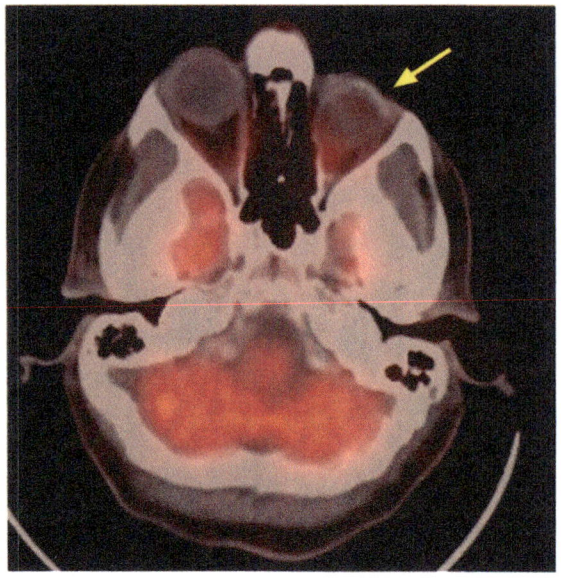

Image 1 (axial)

Image 1. Fused axial images demonstrating post-surgical changes in the left orbit (arrow). No abnormal activity was present to suggest local disease recurrence.

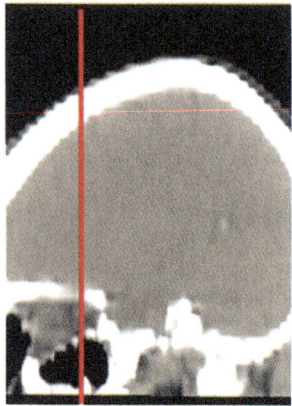

Localizer

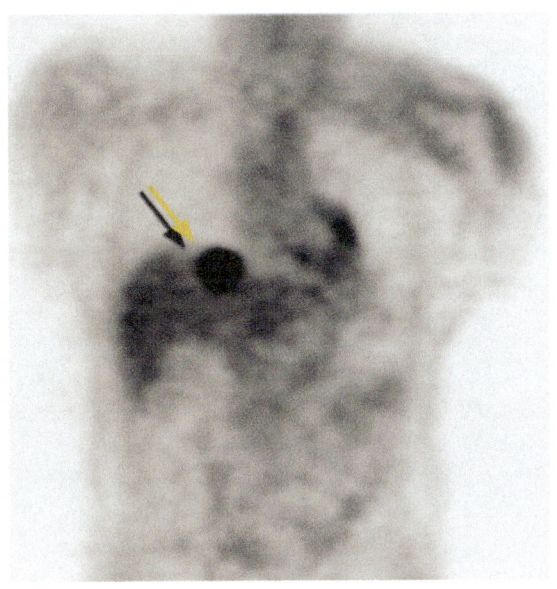

Image 2. Coronal PET image with intense hypermetabolic focus at the interface between liver and lung (arrow).

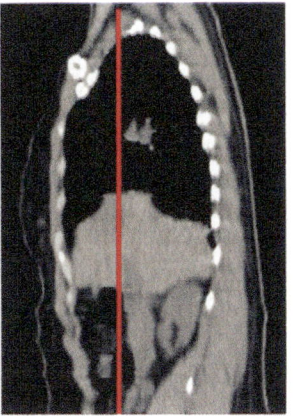

Image 2 (coronal)

Localizer

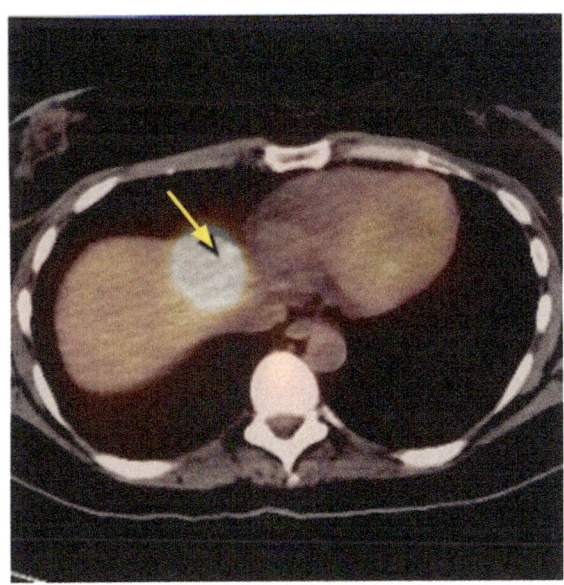

Image 3. Fused axial image demonstrating the hypermetabolic liver focus (arrow). Thus PET/CT provided lesion localization.

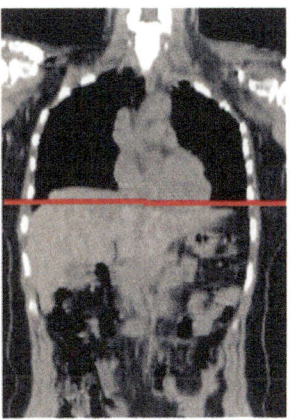

Image 3 (axial)

Localizer

Chapter 10

Breast Cancer

Cases:

Chapter 10

Breast Cancer

Approximately 183,000 women are diagnosed with breast cancer each year in the United States. Breast cancer is the leading cancer and the second leading cause of mortality in women. Limitations of mammography with regards to breast cancer detection in women with dense breasts have prompted a considerable interest in FDG-PET for diagnosing breast cancer.

As a whole body technique, PET stages not only axillary and internal mammary nodes but also the whole body for unexpected sites of disease.

The value of FDG-PET for predicting patient outcome has been established.

The role of PET/CT for primary diagnosis and axillary lymph node involvement has not been studied. Most frequently, PET and PET/CT are used to restage breast cancer, identify sites of disease recurrence and to characterize equivocal anatomical "abnormalities". Finally, treatment monitoring is another important indication for PET or PET/CT.

Key Indications: Staging, Restaging, Treatment Monitoring, "Problem Solver" for cancer detection in women with "difficult to image breasts"

Suggested Reading

Wahl RL, Zasadny K, Helvie M, Hutchins GD, Weber B, Cody R. Metabolic monitoring of breast cancer chemohormonotherapy using positron emission tomography: initial evaluation. J Clin Oncol. 1993;11(11):2101-2111.

Crippa F, Agresti R, Donne VD, Pascali C, Bogni A, Chiesa C, De Sanctis V, Schiavini M, Decise D, Bombardieri E. The contribution of positron emission tomography (PET) with 18F-fluorodeoxyglucose (FDG) in the preoperative detection of axillary metastases of breast cancer: the experience of the National Cancer Institute of Milan. Tumori. 1997;83(2):542-543.

Smith IC, Welch AE, Hutcheon AW, Miller ID, Payne S, Chilcott F, Waikar S, Whitaker T, Ah-See AK, Eremin O, Heys SD, Gilbert FJ, Sharp PF. Positron emission tomography using [18F]-fluorodeoxy-D-glucose to predict the pathologic response of breast cancer to primary chemotherapy. J Clin Oncol. 2000;18(8):1676-1688.

Schelling M, Avril N, Nährig J, Kuhn W, Römer W, Sattler D, Werner M, Dose J, Janicke F, Graeff H, Schwaiger M. Positron emission tomography using [18F] fluorodeoxyglucose for monitoring primary chemotherapy in breast cancer. J Clin Oncol. 2000;18(8):1689-1695.

Mandelson MT, Oestreicher N, Porter PL, White D, Finder CA, Taplin SH, White E. Breast density as a predictor of mammographic detection: comparison of interval- and screen-detected cancers. J Natl Cancer Inst. 2000;92(13):1081-1087.

Avril N, Rosé CA, Schelling M, Dose J, Kuhn W, Bense S, Weber W, Ziegler S, Graeff H, Schwaiger M. Breast imaging with fluorine-18 fluorodeoxyglucose: use and limitations. J Clin Oncol. 2000;18(20):3495-3502.

Schirrmeister H, Kühn T, Guhlmann A, Santjohanser C, Hörster T, Nussle K, Koretz K, Glatting G, Rieber A, Kreienberg R, Buck AC, Reske SN. Fluorine-18 2-deoxy-2-fluoro-D-glucose PET in the preoperative staging of breast cancer: comparison with the standard staging procedures. Eur J Nucl Med. 2001;28(3):351-358.

Yap CS, Seltzer MA, Schiepers C, Gambhir SS, Rao J, Phelps ME, Valk PE, Czernin J. Impact of whole-body 18F-FDG PET on staging and managing patients with breast cancer: the referring physician's perspective. J Nucl Med. 2001;42(9):1334-1337.

Vranjesevic D, Filmont JE, Meta J, Silverman DH, Phelps ME, Rao J, Valk PE, Czernin J. Whole-body 18F-FDG PET and conventional imaging for predicting outcome in previously treated breast cancer patients. J Nucl Med. 2002;43(3):325-329.

Extensive Metastatic Disease

Clinical History

44-year-old female with history of breast cancer status post radical mastectomy with right pectoralis sparing mastectomy and axillary node dissection.

Findings

Diffuse metastatic disease involving the lungs, mediastinum, possibly the right anterior chest wall as well as multiple bony structures.

A bony metastasis in the right femoral neck which corresponds to a lytic lesion seen on CT is concerning for impending fracture.

Teaching Point

PET/CT imaging is very useful for detecting bone involvement and might obviate the need for additional bone scans.

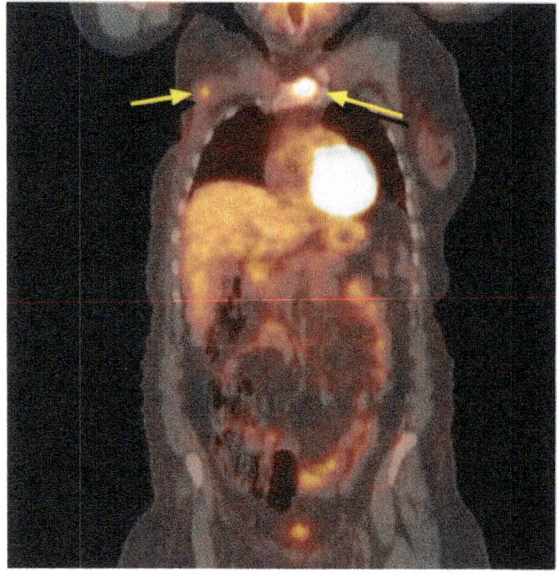

Image 1 (coronal)

Image 1. Fused coronal image demonstrating increased uptake in the sternum and right pectoralis muscle. Both are consistent with metastatic disease (arrows).

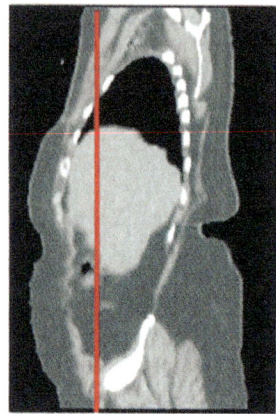

Localizer

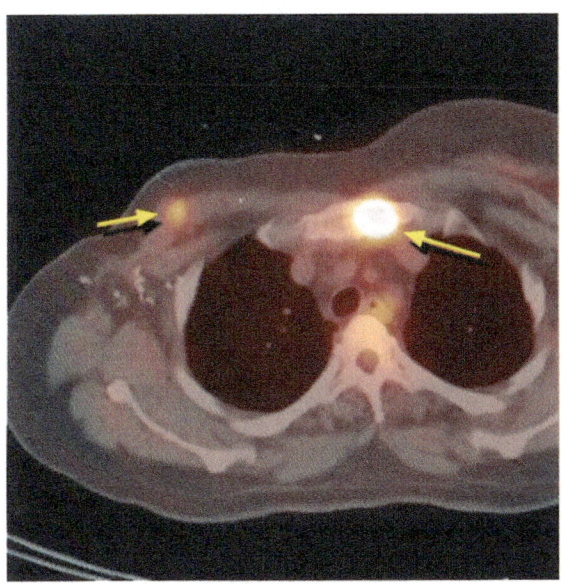

Image 2 (axial)

Image 2. Small focus of increased activity in the region of the right pectoralis muscle consistent with soft tissue recurrence (arrow). Intensely increased glycolytic activity consistent with metastatic disease is present in the sternum (arrow).

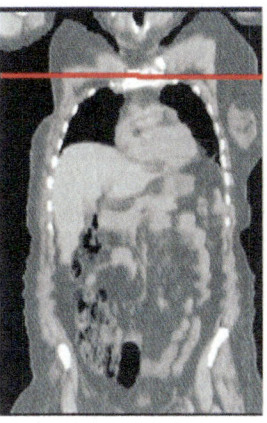

Localizer

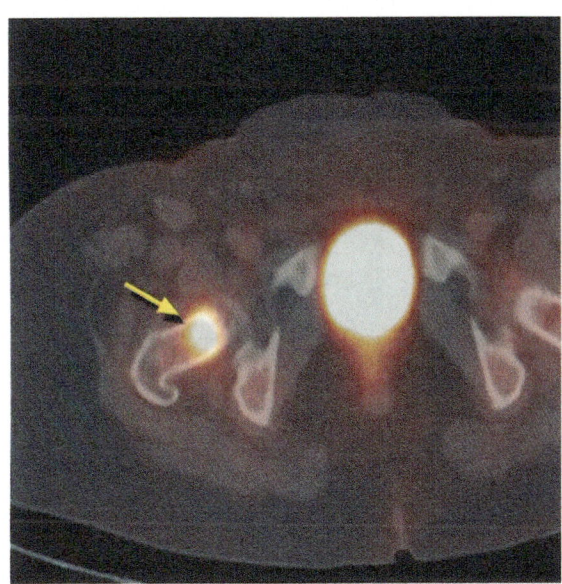

Image 3 (axial)

Image 3. Fused axial image demonstrating intense hyper-metabolic activity in the right femoral neck (arrow). The extent of the lytic lesion by CT was worrisome for impending fracture.

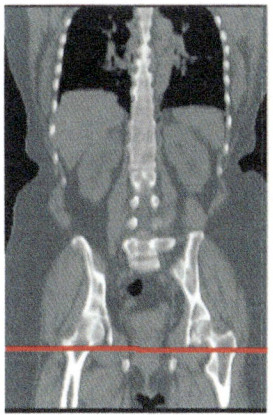

Localizer

Lung and Bone Metastases

Clinical History

This 33-year-old breast cancer patient is status post mastectomy. A recent biopsy of a right supraclavicular lymph node revealed recurrent disease.

PET/CT indication: Restaging.

Findings

Multiple areas of hypermetabolic activity throughout the skeleton are consistent with metastatic disease.

Focal areas of hypermetabolic activity in the right mid-lung and liver are also highly suspicious for metastatic disease.

Teaching Point

PET/CT provided accurate localization of bone, soft tissue and lung metastases while PET imaging alone can still provide accurate staging and prognostic information in breast cancer patients.

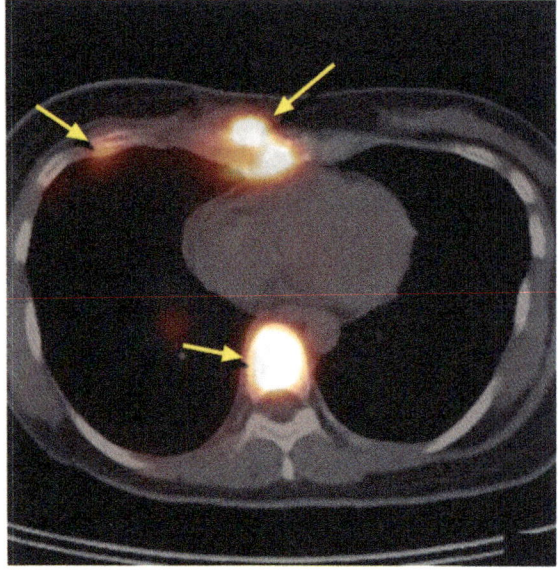

Image 1. Fused axial image with bone involvement including sternum (arrow), rib (arrow) and vertebral body (arrow).

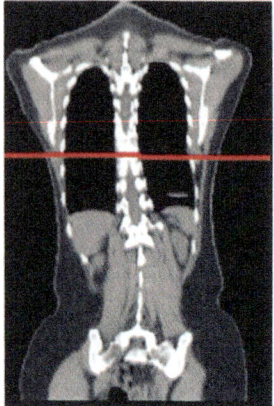

Image 1 (axial)

Localizer

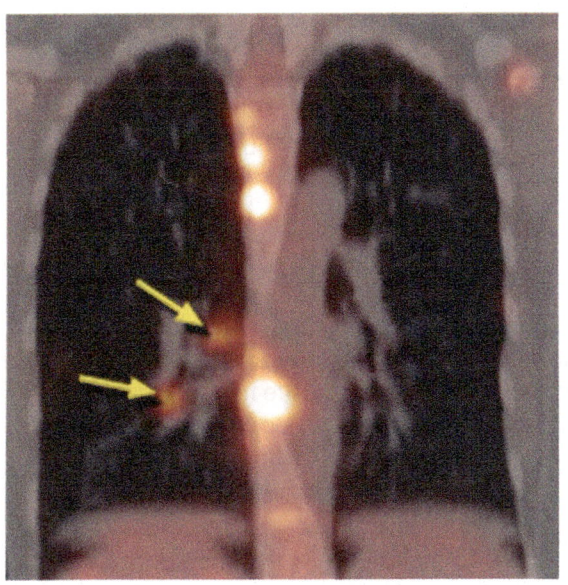

Image 2 (coronal)

Image 2. Fused coronal image revealing multiple metastatic spine lesions as well as posterior right hilar lymph node involvement (arrows).

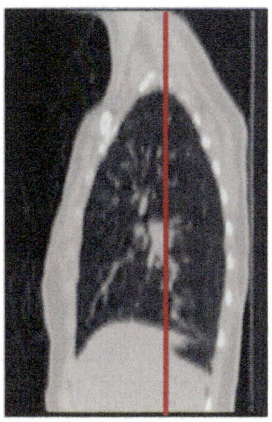

Localizer

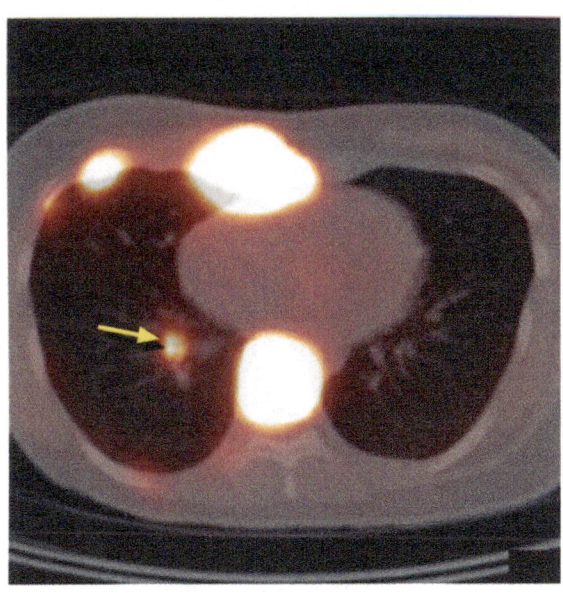

Image 3 (axial)

Image 3. Small right-sided lung metastasis (arrow) and several bone lesions are depicted on fused axial image (arrows).

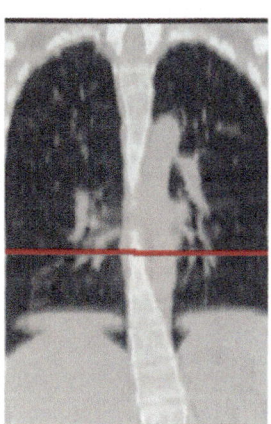

Localizer

Metastatic Breast Cancer

Clinical History

45-year old female patient status post left mastectomy for breast cancer. She subsequently had a left chest wall recurrence and has known metastatic disease to liver, lung, brain and colon. She is currently undergoing chemotherapy.

PET/CT indication: Restaging.

Findings

Diffusely increased bone marrow activity is consistent with regenerating bone marrow. A focal area of increased activity in the left chest wall corresponds to a soft tissue mass in the pectoralis muscle and is consistent with known chest wall recurrence.

Increased glucose metabolic activity in the right lower extremity is consistent with an additional soft tissue metastatic focus. In addition, several other metastatic lesions involving lung, mediastinum, peritoneum and soft tissue were identified (not shown in the images below).

Teaching Point

Obviously, the PET/CT study had no impact on managing this patient with widespread metastatic disease. Rather, this study points to the improved lesion localization afforded by PET/CT. PET alone failed to accurately localize the hypermetabolic foci. The importance of a whole body molecular tumor survey is emphasized by the unexpected metastasis of the right thigh.

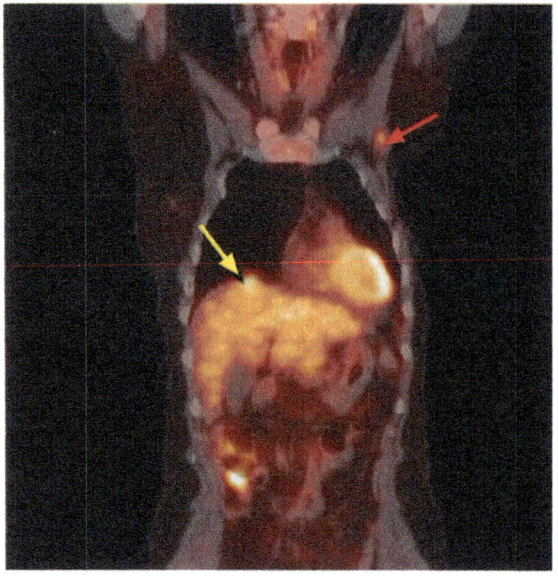

Image 1 (coronal)

Image 1. Metastatic disease of the liver (yellow arrow) and the left-sided chest wall recurrence (red arrow) are depicted on this fused coronal image.

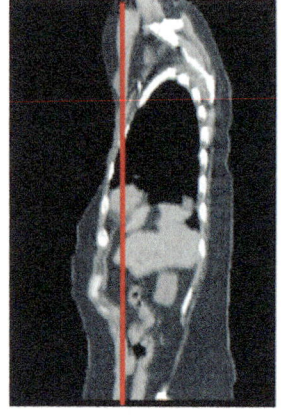

Localizer

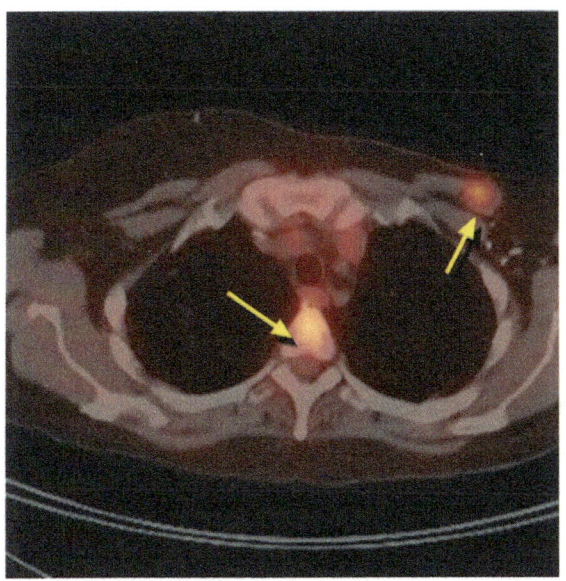

Image 2. Fused axial image demonstrating increased bone marrow activity due to ongoing chemotherapy (arrow) and hypermetabolic focus in the left chest wall consistent with the site of chest wall recurrence (arrow).

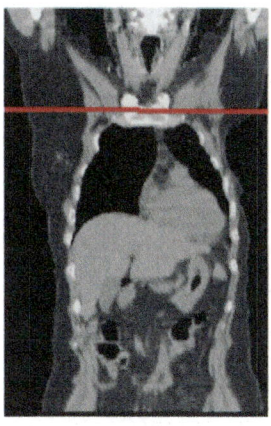

Image 2 (axial)

Localizer

Image 3. Fused axial image demonstrating the unexpected soft tissue metastasis in the lateral aspect of the right thigh (arrow).

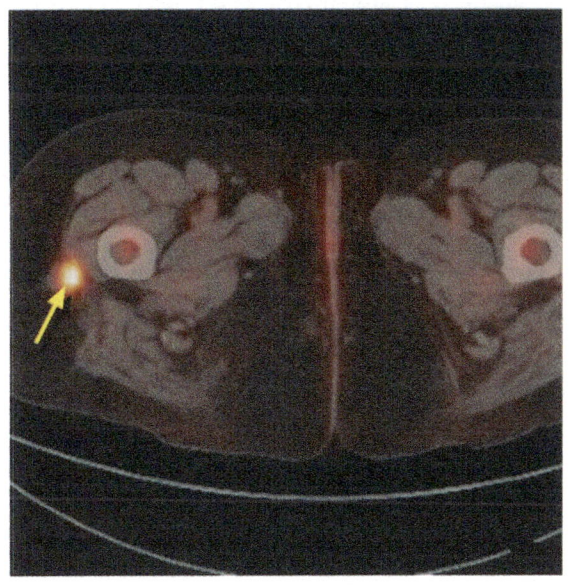

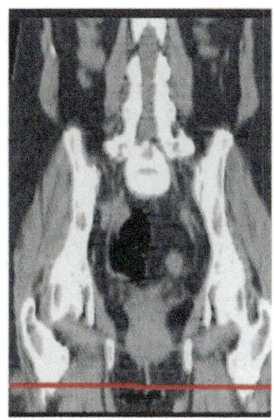

Image 3 (axial)

Localizer

Internal Mammary Lymph Nodes

Clinical History

44-year-old patient with infiltrating ductal carcinoma of the left breast.

PET/CT indication: Restaging.

Findings

Two intense hypermetabolic foci in the left internal mammary lymph node chain are consistent with metastatic disease.

Teaching Point

FDG-PET is an excellent technique for assessing internal mammary node involvement in breast cancer patients. Sometimes, hypermetabolic foci in this region can be erroneously assigned to bony structures or chest wall. PET/CT correctly differentiated internal mammary node from bone involvement.

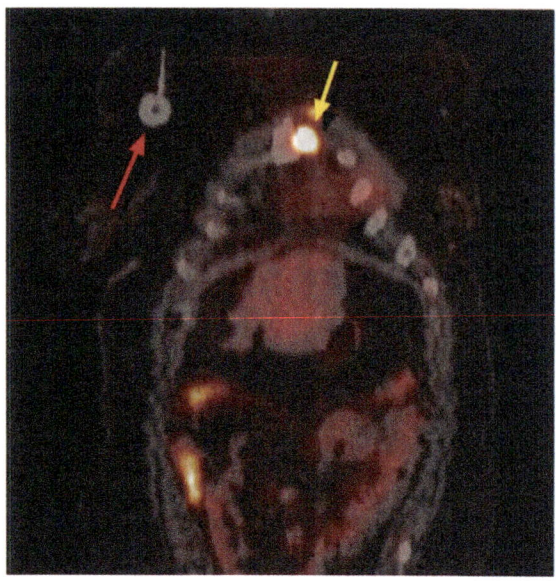

Image 1 (coronal)

Image 1. Intense hypermetabolic focus in the mid-anterior chest wall is shown on fused coronal image (yellow arrow). Note the port-A-cath (red arrow).

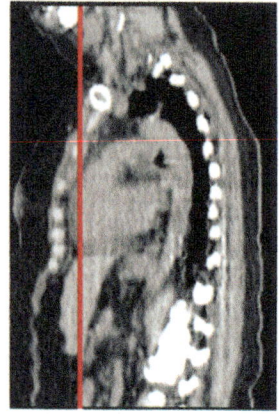

Localizer

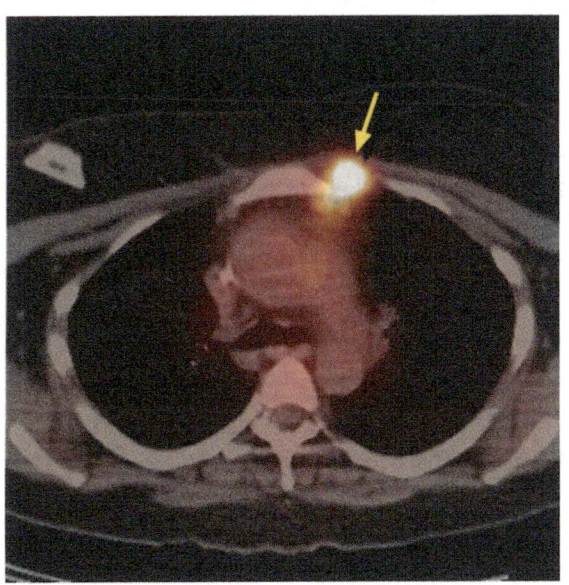

Image 2 (axial)

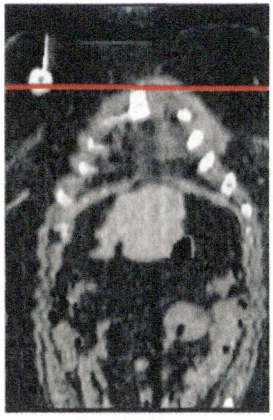

Localizer

Image 2. Fused PET/CT axial image allowed differentiation between bone and soft-tissue involvement (arrow).

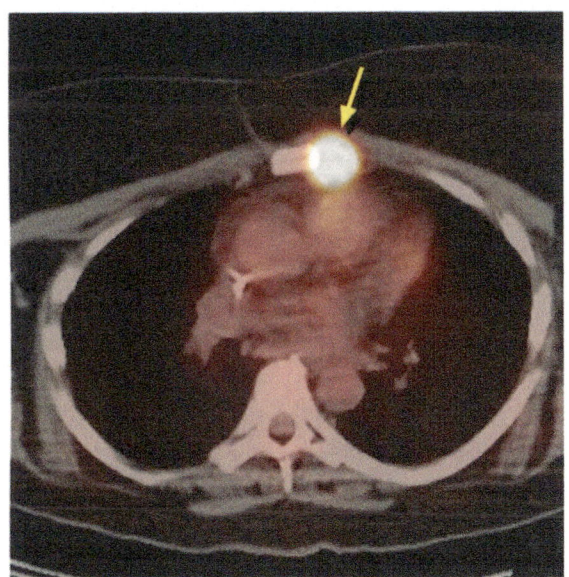

Image 3 (axial)

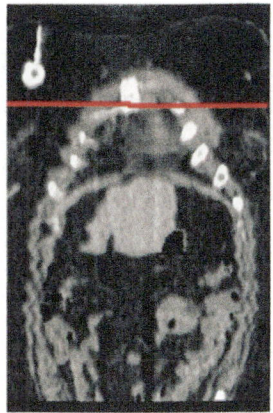

Localizer

Image 3. Fused axial PET/CT image shows a second soft tissue lesion corresponding to an internal mammary lymph node (arrow).

Breast Implants

Clinical History

This 69-year-old patient with breast implants recently noticed a left breast mass.

PET/CT indication: Tissue Characterization.

Findings

Abnormal glycolytic activity in the left breast, left axilla and left supraclavicular region strongly suggesting primary breast cancer and metastatic lymph node involvement.

Teaching Point

FDG-PET is very useful as a problem solver in women with difficult to image breasts. These include women with very dense breasts, scars or implants. Mammography frequently fails to provide the correct answer in these patients.

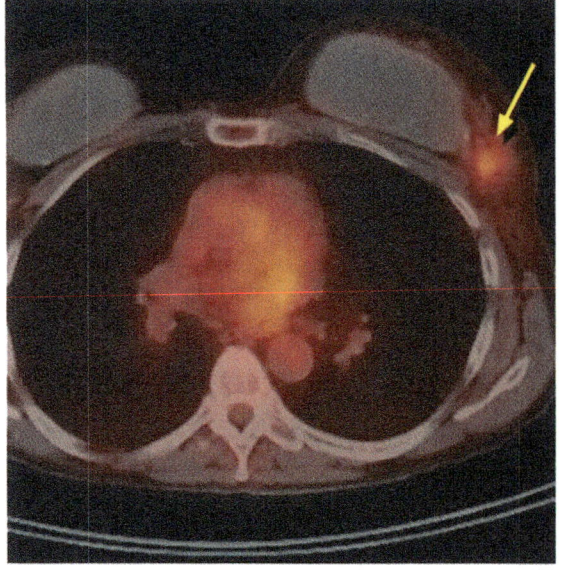

Image 1 (axial)

Image 1. The hypermetabolic primary breast cancer lesion was located lateral to the breast implant (arrow).

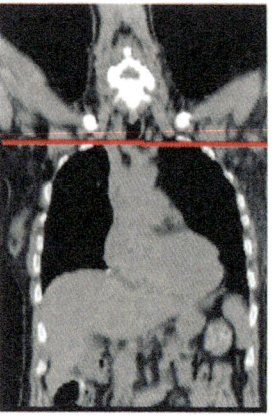

Localizer

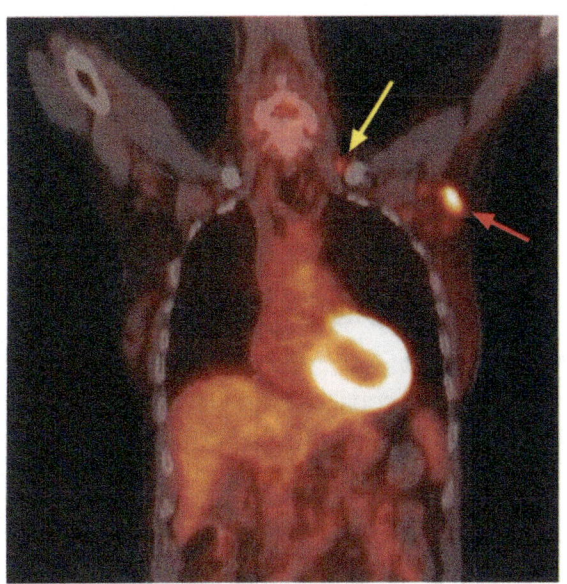

Image 2 (coronal)

Image 2. Intensely increased FDG uptake in the left axillar area (red arrow). Note also the small hyperglycolytic left-sided supraclavicular lymph node (yellow arrow).

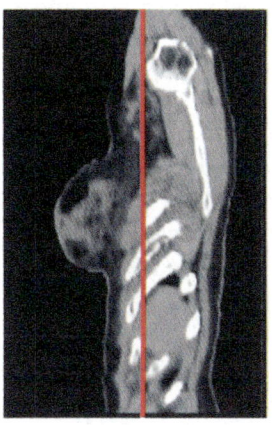

Localizer

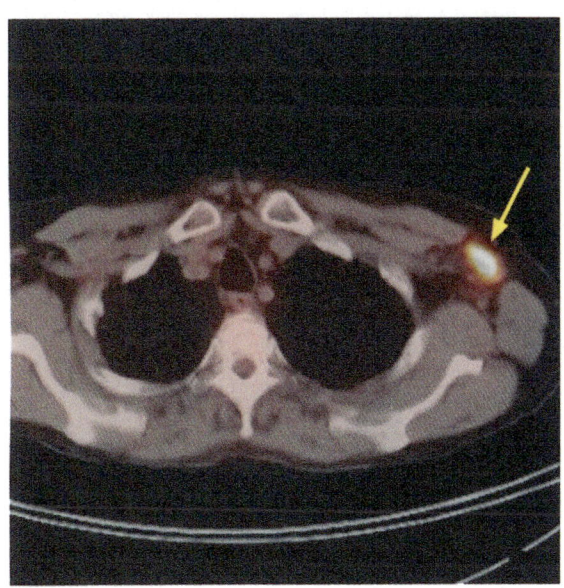

Image 3 (axial)

Image 3. Fused axial image demonstrating a large hypermetabolic left axillary lymph node.

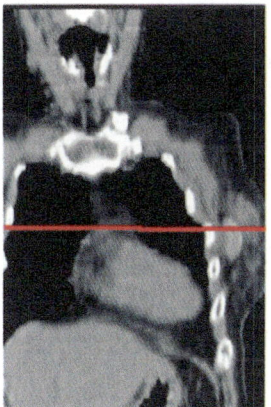

Localizer

Inflammatory Breast Cancer

Clinical History

76-year-old female with inflammatory breast cancer who is status post radiation treatment.

PET/CT indication: Restaging.

Findings

Diffusely increased cutaneous FDG uptake in the left breast consistent with inflammatory cancer. Increased FDG uptake in several left internal mammary lymph nodes strongly suggests metastatic disease.

Teaching Point

FDG-PET/CT diagnoses, stages and re-stages breast cancer with a high diagnostic accuracy. As shown in this example, internal mammary node involvement, an important prognostic marker, can be readily identified.

Image 1. Markedly increased glycolytic activity in the retro-sternal region (arrow). In addition, diffusely increased glycolytic activity is noted in the periphery of the left breast (red arrow).

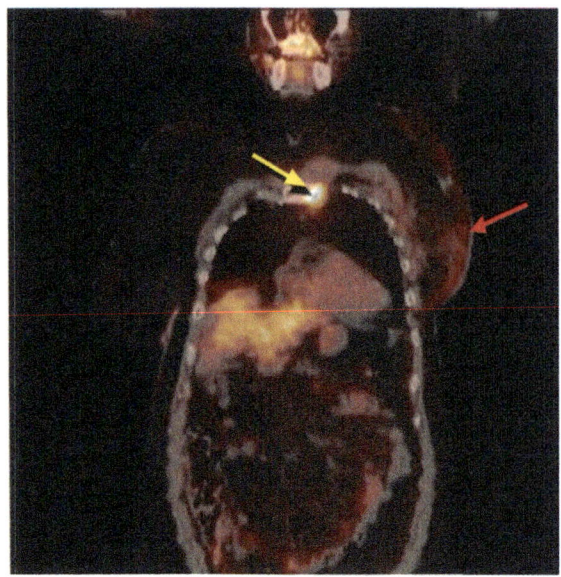

Image 1 (coronal)

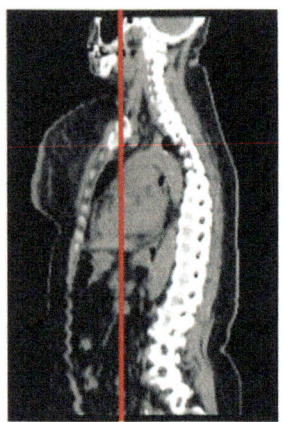

Localizer

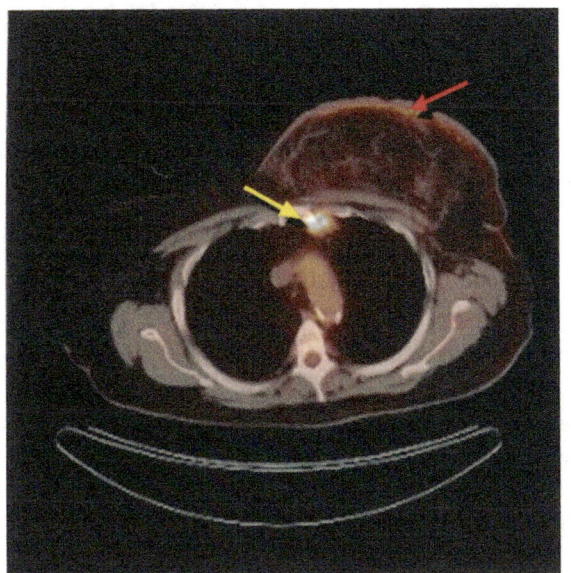

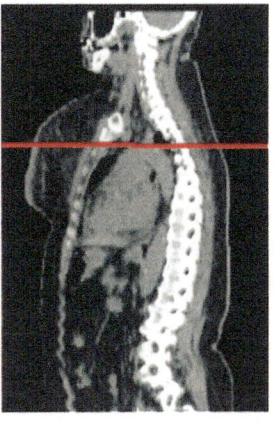

Image 2. Fused axial image clearly reveals retro-sternal node involvement (yellow arrow). Note, the increased FDG uptake in the skin of the left breast (red arrow).

Image 2 (axial)

Localizer

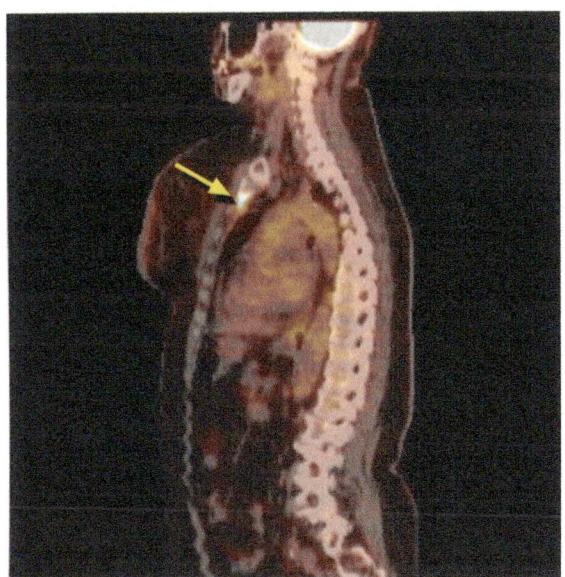

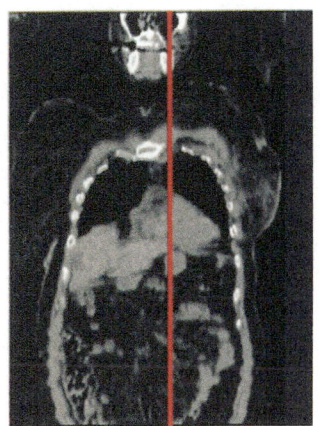

Image 3. Fused sagittal image showing internal mammary lymp node involvement (arrow).

Image 3 (sagittal)

Localizer

Benign and Malignant Masses

Clinical History

50-year-old female recently diagnosed with left breast cancer.

PET/CT indication: Staging.

Findings

A large focus of intense tracer activity in the left breast is consistent with the primary tumor. A hypodense lesion seen on CT inferior and lateral to the primary lesion does not show increased FDG uptake and is therefore consistent with a cyst.

Histological Verification: Poorly-differentiated infiltrating ductal carcinoma.

Teaching Point

CT demonstrated a hypodense breast mass without increased FDG uptake. PET accurately distinguishes malignant from benign masses.

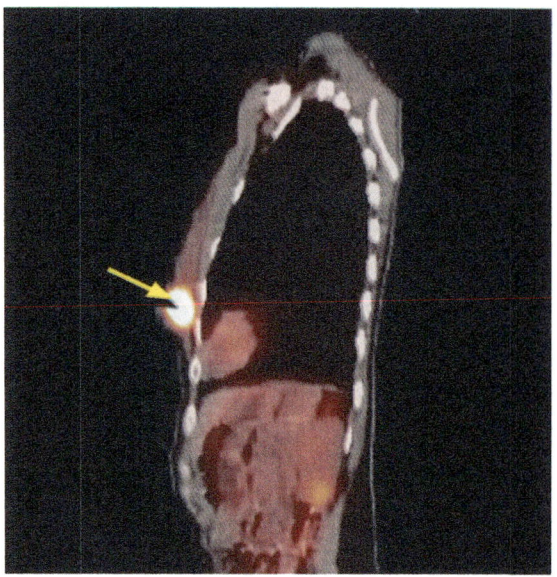

Image 1 (sagittal)

Image 1. Fused sagittal image demonstrating the intensely hypermetabolic primary infiltrating ductal carcinoma (arrow).

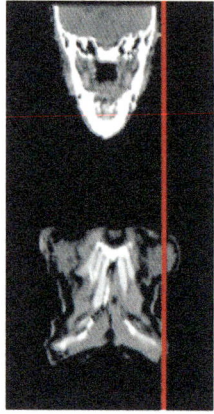

Localizer

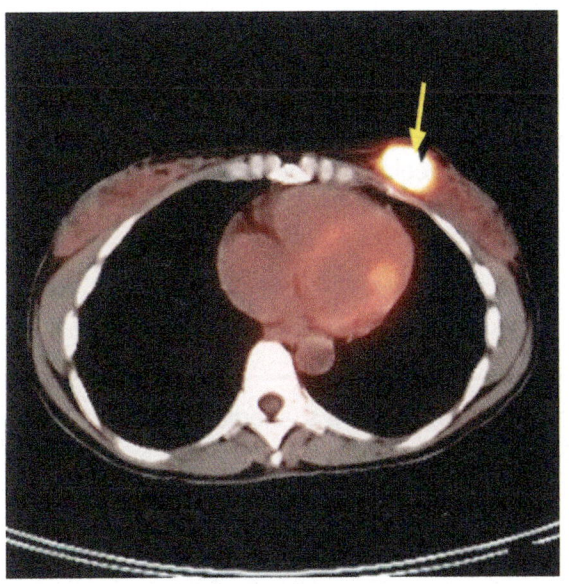

Image 2. Fused axial image showing the hypermetabolic primary tumor (arrow).

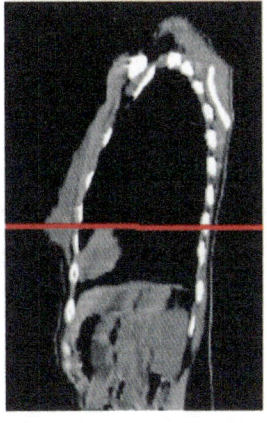

Image 2 (axial)

Localizer

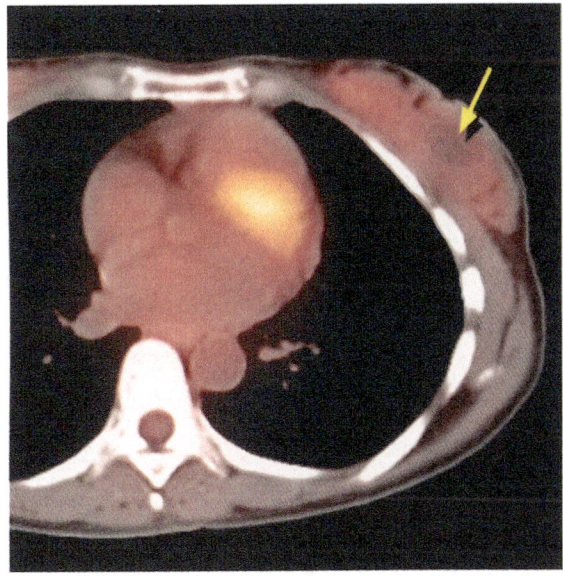

Image 3. Fused axial image depicting the hypodense breast lesion without increased FDG uptake (arrow). This is consistent with a benign cyst.

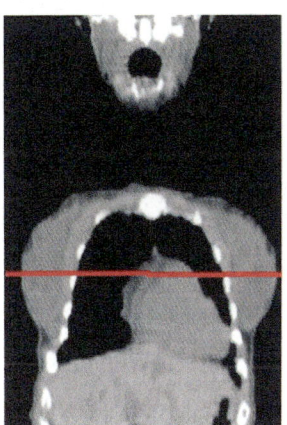

Image 3 (axial)

Localizer

Two Primary Cancers

Clinical History

87-year-old female with history of right breast cancer and colon cancer status-post right hemicolectomy.

PET/CT indication: Restaging.

Findings

Multiple foci of moderately increased glucose metabolic activity are scattered throughout the body and are consistent with metastatic disease.

Teaching Point

In patients with multiple primary cancers the source of metastatic disease cannot be identified. In the current case multiple metastatic lesions can originate from either breast cancer or colon cancer or from both cancers.
Exact lesion localization was only possible by PET/CT.

Image 1

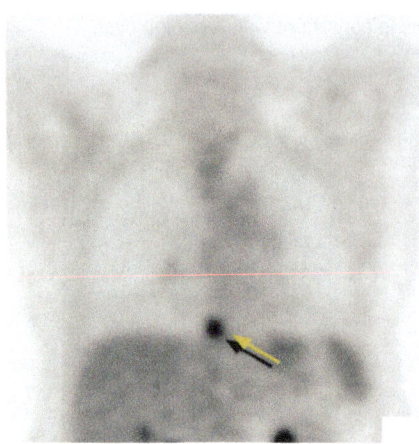 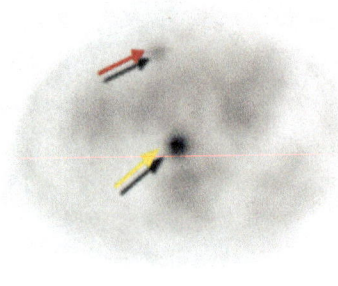

coronal   **axial**

Image 1. Coronal (left) and axial (right) PET images with focally increased FDG uptake in the region of the gastro-esophageal junction (yellow arrows). An additional small focus of increased uptake (red arrow on axial PET image) that cannot be assigned to a specific anatomical structure by PET is also consistent with metastatic disease.

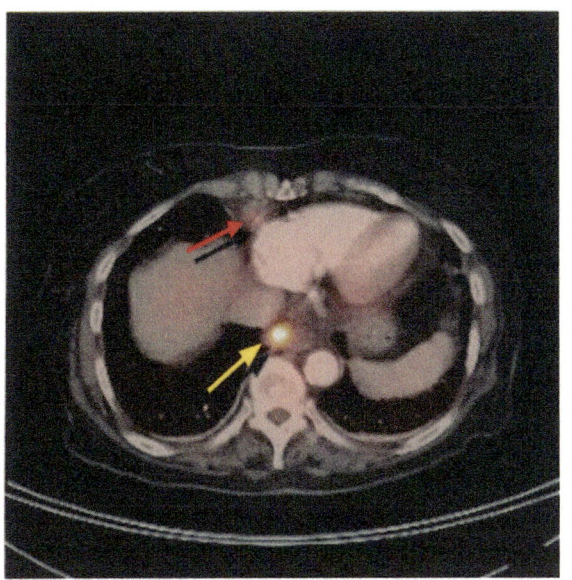

Image 2. Fused axial image demonstrates an enlarged, hypermetabolic peri-aortic lymph node (arrow). The anterior hypermetabolic lesion (arrow) is also consistent with metastatic disease.

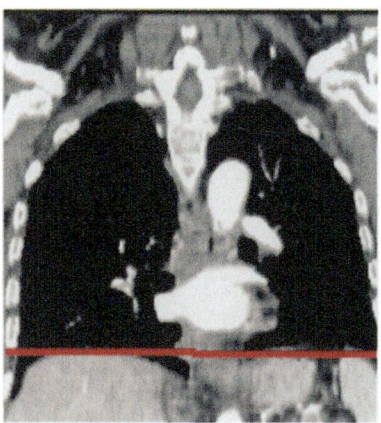

Image 2 (axial)

Localizer

Image 3. Fused axial image assigns another hypermetabolic focus to an enlarged hilar lymph node (arrow).

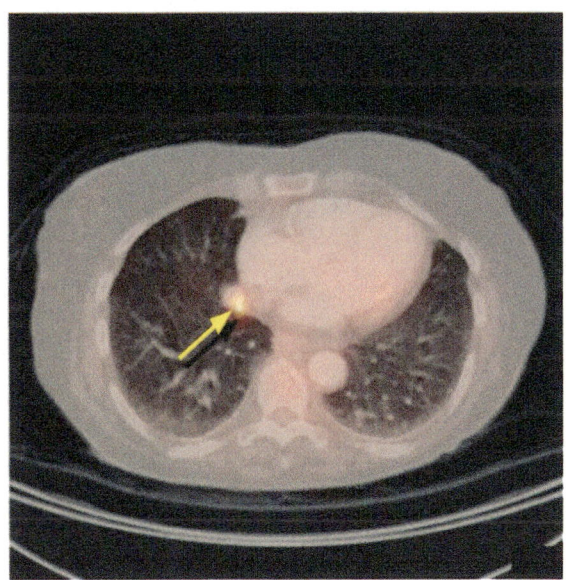

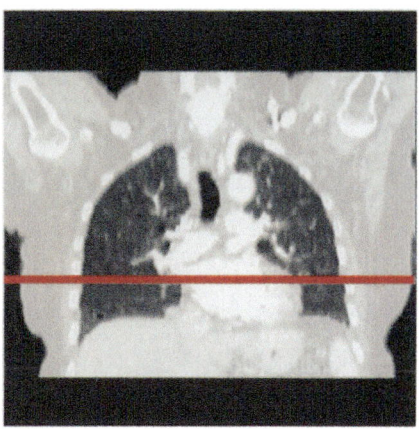

Image 3 (axial)

Localizer

Chapter 11

Gynecological Cancers

Cases:

Chapter 11

Gynecological Cancers

Cancers of the ovaries account for 4% of all cancers and 5% of all cancer deaths. Approximately 28,000 new cases of ovarian cancer occur annually in the United States. There is increasing evidence that FDG-PET is useful for staging and restaging of cervical cancer. Less promising results were published regarding the ability of FDG-PET to diagnose or stage ovarian cancer. This is because the apparent glucose metabolic activity of most ovarian cancers is relatively low. Several specific features of these cancers might account for this finding. First, tumors are frequently cystic and lack the tumor bulk required for imaging. Secondly, mucin production, frequently occurring in ovarian cancer is associated with low glycolytic tumor cell activity. FDG-PET has mainly been used to determine sites of tumor recurrence in women with rising tumor markers. This is sometimes complicated because the peritoneum is a frequent site of recurrence and physiological bowel activity can limit the ability to clearly differentiate between tumor and physiological activity. Whether PET/CT offers diagnostic advantages over PET alone has not been established.

Key Indications: Staging, Restaging

Suggested Reading

Hubner KF, McDonald TW, Niethammer JG, Smith GT, Gould HR, Buonocore E. Assessment of primary and metastatic ovarian cancer by positron emission tomography (PET) using 2-[18F]deoxyglucose (2-[18F]FDG). Gynecol Oncol. 1993;51(2):197-204.

Bromley B, Goodman H, Benacerraf BR. Comparison between sonographic morphology and Doppler waveform for the diagnosis of ovarian malignancy. Obstet Gynecol. 1994;83(3):434-437.

Shalev E, Eliyahu S, Peleg D, Tsabari A. Laparoscopic management of adnexal cystic masses in postmenopausal women. Obstet Gynecol. 1994;83(4):594-596.

Parker WH, Levine RL, Howard FM, Sansone B, Berek JS. A multicenter study of laparoscopic management of selected cystic adnexal masses in postmenopausal women. J Am Coll Surg. 1994;179(6):733-737.

Römer W, Avril N, Dose J, Ziegler S, Kuhn W, Herz M, Janicke F, Schwaiger M. Metabolic characterization of ovarian tumors with positron-emission tomography and F-18 fluorodeoxyglucose. Rofo Fortschr Geb Rontgenstr Neuen Bildgeb Verfahr. 1997;166(1):62-68.

Zimny M, Schröder W, Wolters S, Cremerius U, Rath W, Bull U. 18F-fluorodeoxyglucose PET in ovarian carcinoma: methodology and preliminary results. Nuklearmedizin. 1997;36(7):228-233.

Fenchel S, Kotzerke J, Stöhr I, Grab D, Nüssle K, Rieber A, Kreienberg R, Brambs HJ, Reske SN. Preoperative assessment of asymptomatic adnexal tumors by positron emission tomography and F 18 fluorodeoxyglucose. Nuklearmedizin. 1999;38(4):101-107.

Grab D, Flock F, Stöhr I, Nüssle A, Fenchel A, Brambs HJ, Reske SN, Kreienberg R. Classification of asymptomatic adnexal masses by ultrasound, magnetic resonance imaging, and positron emission tomography. Gynecol Oncol. 2000;77(3):454-459.

Kubich-Huch RA, Dörffler W, von Schulthess GK, Marincek B, Köchli OR, Seifert B, Haller U, Steinert HC. Value of 18F-FDG positron emission tomography, computed tomography, and magnetic resonance imaging in diagnosing primary and recurrent ovarian carcinoma. Eur Radiol. 2000;10(5):761-767.

Fallopian Tube Carcinoma

Clinical History

49-year-old woman with fallopian tube carcinoma who is status post hysterectomy in 1996 and had a tumor recurrence in 1999. Radiation therapy was continued until 2000 and the last chemotherapy was administered 6 months prior to the current PET/CT study.

PET/CT indication: Restaging.

Findings

A retroperitoneal focus of moderately increased FDG uptake close to the midline at the level of L5 is consistent with metastatic lymph node involvement.

Teaching Point

Two foci of increased FDG uptake are identified in two adjacent areas in the abdomen. One is consistent with an enlarged lymph node, the other one represents normal urine activity in the ureter. PET images alone were difficult to interpret because both areas of increased uptake were focal. PET/CT provided the anatomic information for appropriate image interpretation and differentiation between normal and abnormal FDG uptake.

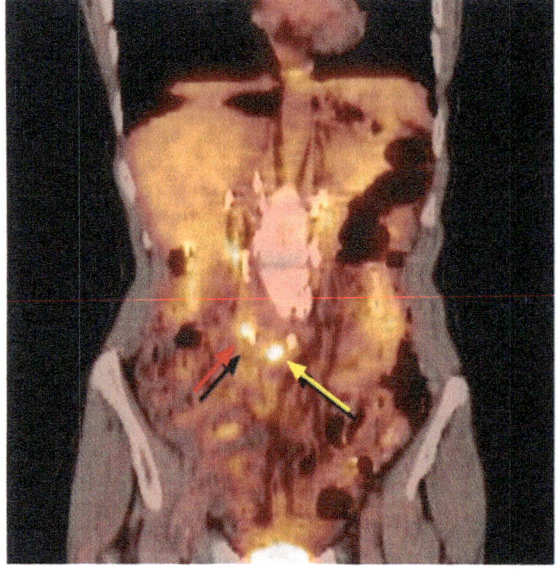

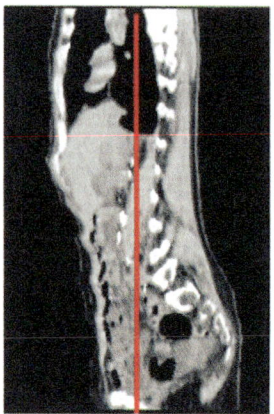

Image 1. Coronal PET/CT view showing two abnormal foci of FDG uptake; lymph node (yellow arrow) and ureter (red arrow).

Image 1 (coronal)

Localizer

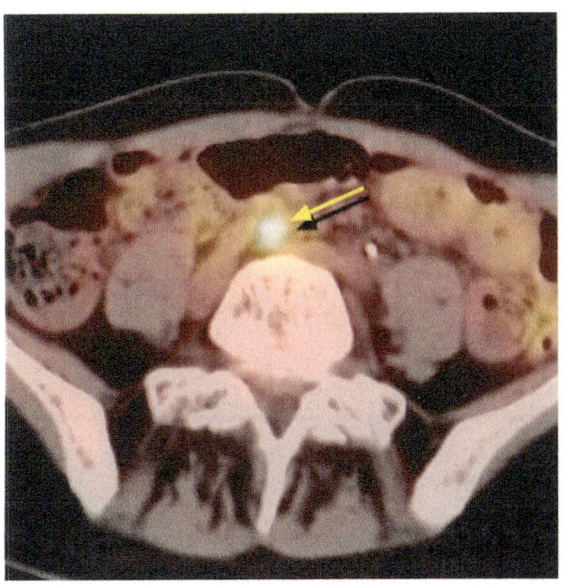

Image 2 (axial)

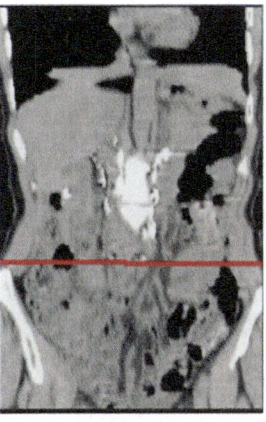

Localizer

Image 2. Focus of increased FDG uptake is present just anterior to L5 vertebral body. CT revealed a corresponding enlarged lymph node consistent with metastatic lymph node involvement.

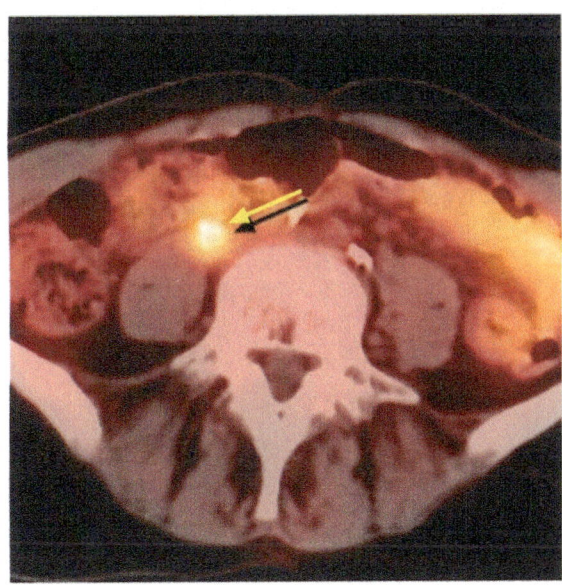

Image 3 (axial)

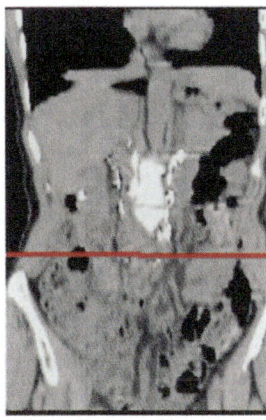

Localizer

Image 3. Fused axial image demonstrates another focus of increased uptake in the antero-medial aspect of the psoas muscle consistent with normal ureteral FDG activity.

Widespread Metastatic Ovarian Cancer

Clinical History

A 64-year-old female patient with history of ovarian carcinoma presents with rising tumor markers. She is status post hysterectomy and chemotherapy more than 6 months prior to this study.

PET/CT indication: Restaging.

Findings

Multiple foci of hypermetabolic activity in the right inguinal, left external iliac, left common iliac, pre-vertebral and retro-crural regions are consistent with metastatic disease.

Teaching Point

This study revealed widespread metastatic disease that can be documented by PET alone, CT alone or PET/CT. CT provided exact lesion localization for PET. In many cases, exact lesion localization is of little clinical significance because it does not affect patient management.

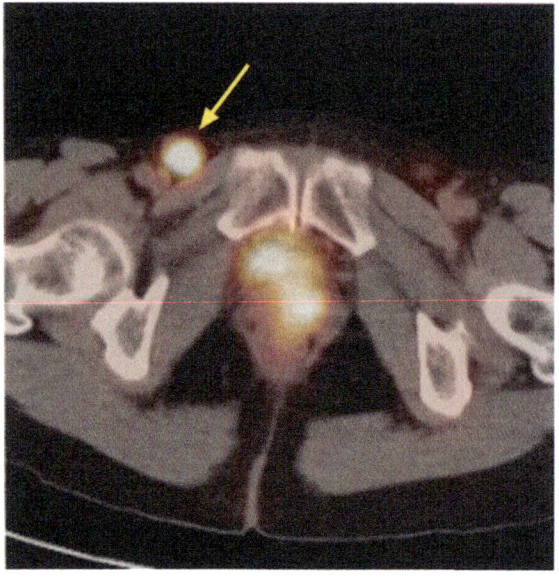

Image 1. Fused axial image reveals increased tracer uptake of a right inguinal lymph node (arrow). Normal bladder activity is noted.

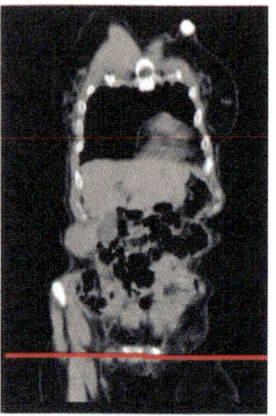

Image 1 (axial)

Localizer

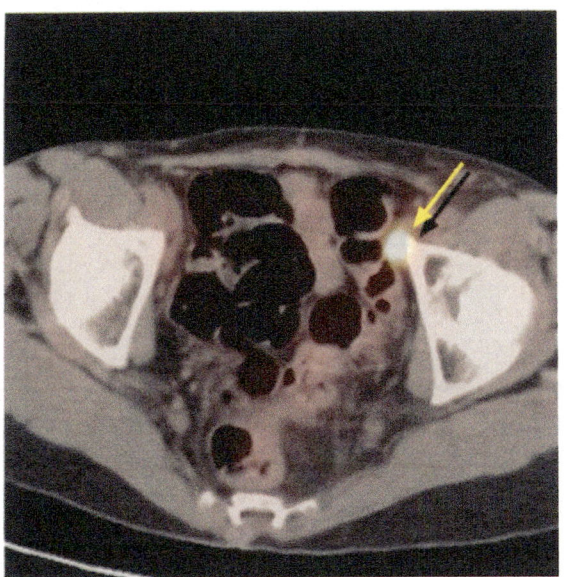

Image 2 (axial)

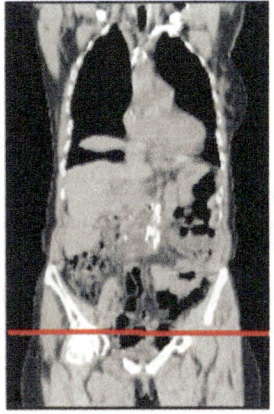

Localizer

Image 2. Fused axial image reveals increased tracer uptake of a mesenteric lymph node (arrow).

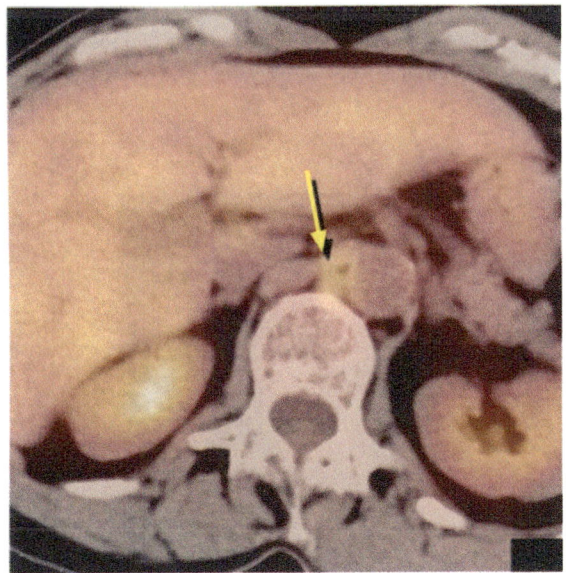

Image 3 (axial)

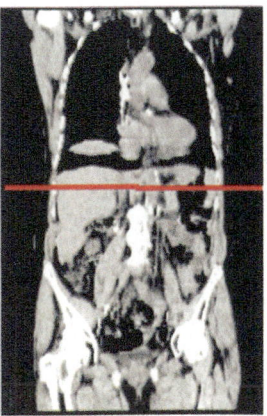

Localizer

Image 3. Fused axial image reveals pathological para-aortic lymphadenopathy (arrow).

Metastatic Ovarian Cancer

Clinical History

68-year-old female with metastatic ovarian cancer who is status post chemotherapy and resection.

PET/CT indication: Restaging.

Findings

A large and irregularly shaped area of increased FDG uptake is consistent with metastasis of the T12 vertebral body. Two additional lesions located in the right and left lung with increased metabolic activity were also identified and are also consistent with metastatic disease.

Teaching Point

PET/CT facilitates the localization and identification of recurrent and metastatic ovarian cancer.

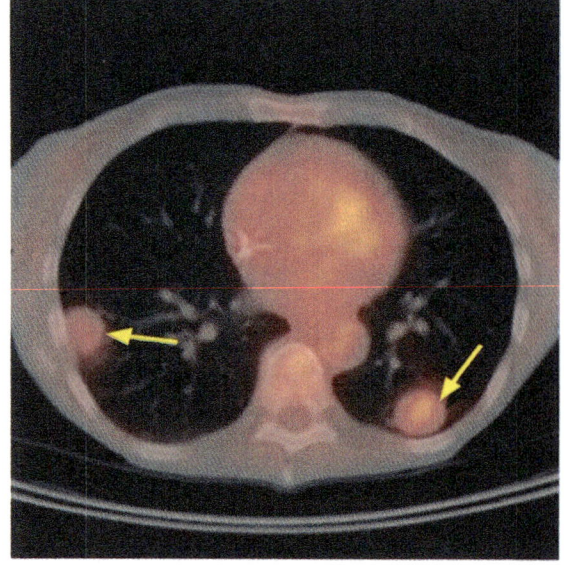

Image 1. Fused axial image shows two metabolically active lung lesions (arrows).

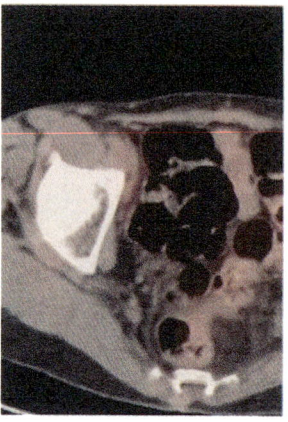

Image 1 (axial)

Localizer

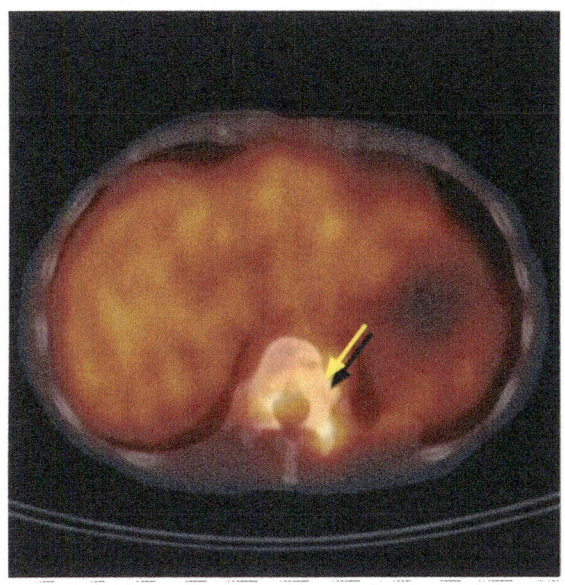

Image 2 (sagittal)

Image 2. Fused sagittal image showing the metastatic T12 lesion (arrow).

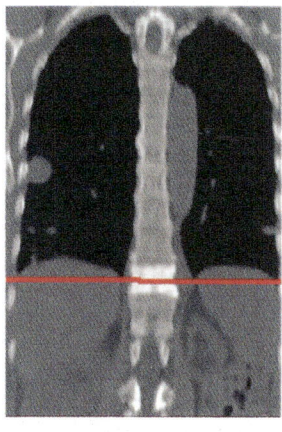

Localizer

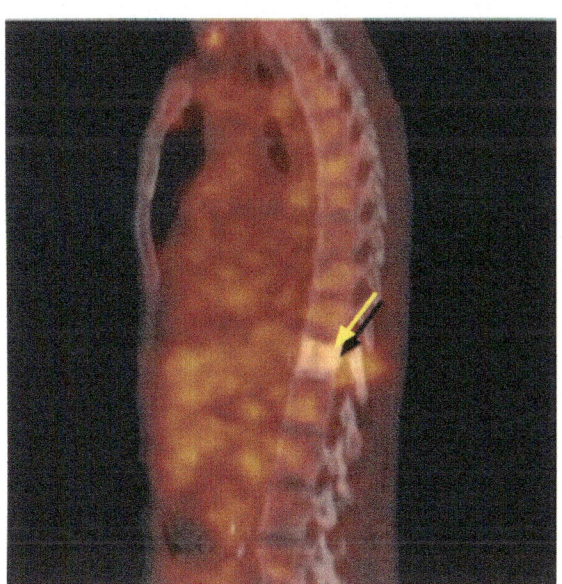

Image 3 (axial)

Image 3. Hypermetabolic lesion at the level of T12 consistent with metabolically active metastasis (arrow).

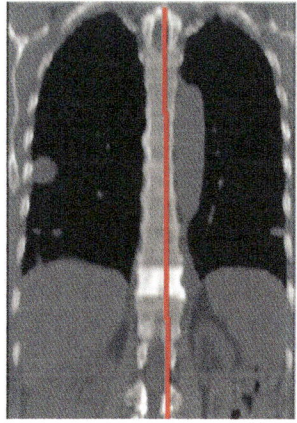

Localizer

Cervical Cancer

Clinical History

36-year-old female recently diagnosed with cervical cancer.

PET/CT indication: Staging.

Findings

A focus of intense tracer activity is noted in the uterus corresponding to a solid tissue mass on CT representing tumor extension into the uterus.

Histological Verification: Tumor measures 4 cm in maximum horizontal width. No evidence for lymph node involvement.

Teaching Point

PET and PET/CT diagnose and stage cervical cancer with a high accuracy. Image fusion facilitates the differentiation of tumor versus prominent bowel activity.

Image 1. Axial PET image demonstrating prominent bowel activity (anterior arrow). A large medial mass (posterior arrow) and a small focus of activity to the left (arrow to the right) are consistent with primary tumor and focal bowel activity..

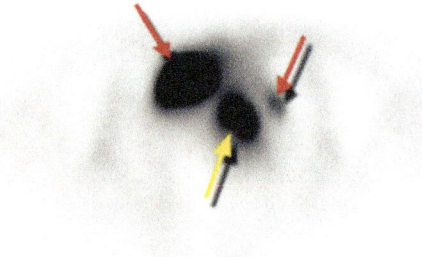

Image 1 (axial)

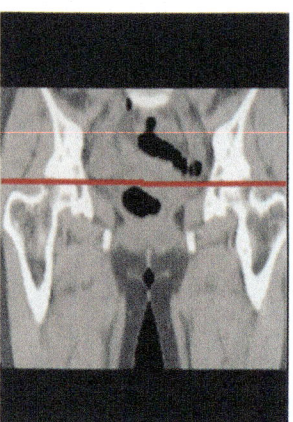

Localizer

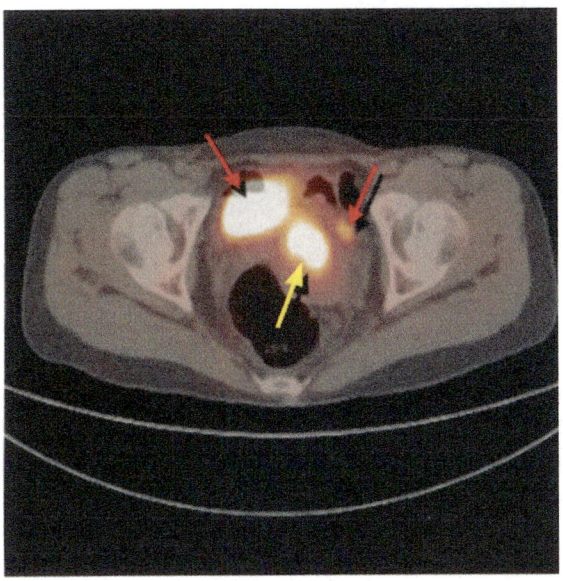

Image 2 (axial)

Image 2. Fused axial image demonstrating three areas of increased FDG uptake. The large right anterior focus represents bowel activity (arrow). The focus in the middle signifies the uterine malignancy (middle arrow) and the small left-sided focus represents bowel activity (arrow).

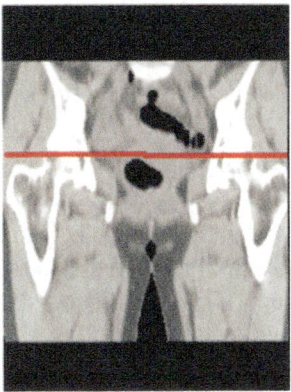

Localizer

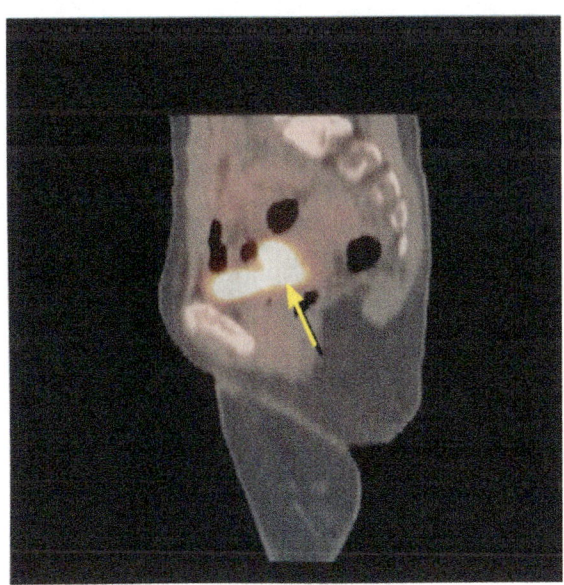

Image 3 (sagittal)

Image 3. Fused sagittal images showing a large area of increased FDG uptake corresponding to the uterine malignancy (arrow).

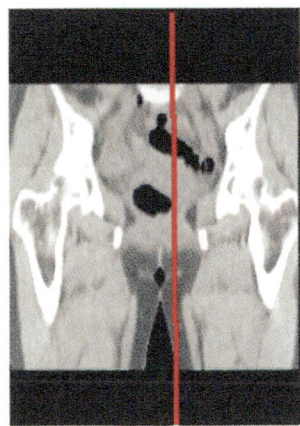

Localizer

Ovarian Cancer

Clinical History

42-year-old female with ovarian carcinoma, status post hysterectomy and bilateral salpingo-oophorectomy.

PET/CT indication: Restaging.

Findings

Two foci of increased activity in the pelvis correspond to an approximately 2 cm soft tissue mass adjacent to the distal sigmoid colon and to increased activity along the anterior wall of the rectum. These are consistent with peritoneal metastases.

Histological Verification: Bowel metastases.

Teaching Point

PET and PET/CT allow accurate diagnosis and staging of cervical cancer with a high accuracy in determination of tumoral tissue extension. Fused images facilitate the determination of tumor versus prominent bowel activity.

Image 1. Sagittal PET with two foci of increased uptake (arrows). This might represent tumor versus physiological bowel activity.

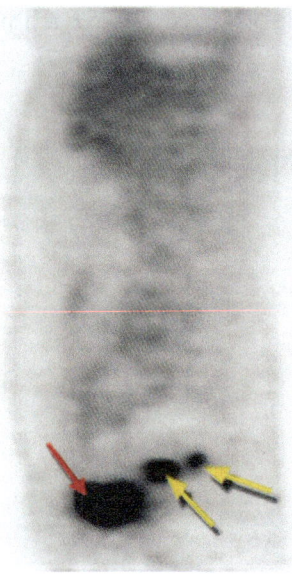

Image 1 (sagittal)

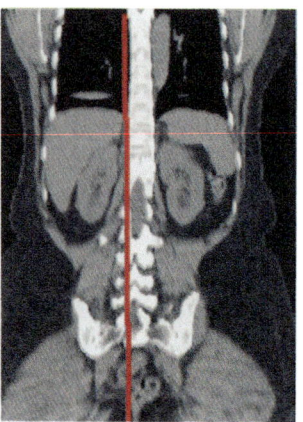

Localizer

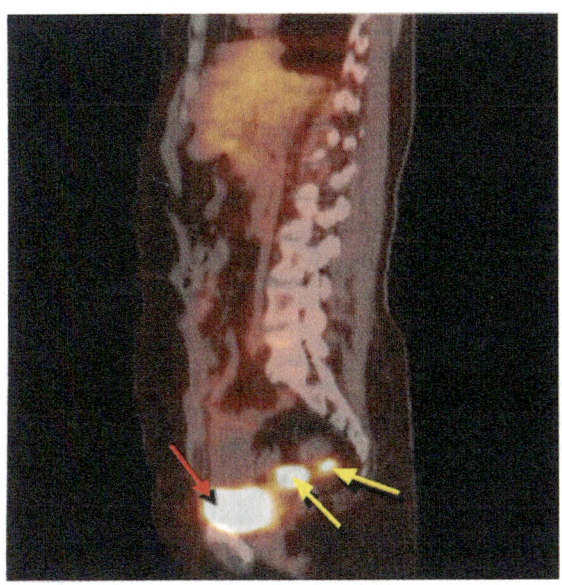

Image 2 (sagittal)

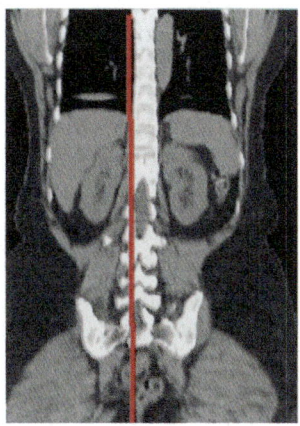

Localizer

Image 2. Fused sagittal image demonstrating tumor involved bowel in the posterior pelvic area (yellow arrows). The anterior area of high intensity tracer uptake (red arrow) corresponds to FDG concentration in the bladder.

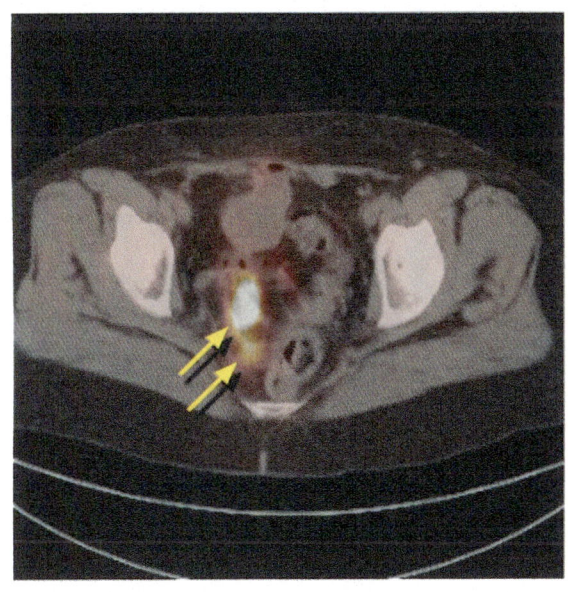

Image 3 (axial)

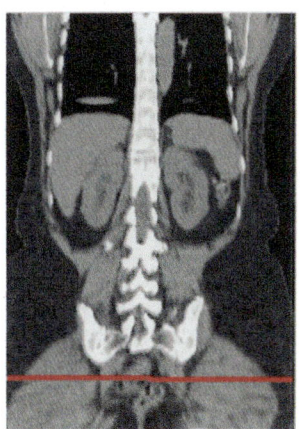

Localizer

Image 3. Axial PET/CT demonstrating tumor involved bowel (arrows).

Uterine Cancer

Clinical History

57-year-old female with newly diagnosed uterine cancer.

PET/CT indication: Staging.

Findings

A large and irregularly shaped focus of increased tracer uptake is noted in the medial aspect of the uterus. This measures approximately 1.5 x 3.0 cm in size and correlates with a soft tissue mass seen on CT. This is consistent with the primary malignancy.

Teaching Point

Uterine cancer exhibits high glucose metabolic rates and is imaged well with PET. False positive findings for cancer can occur with uterine fibroids, menstrual blood and inflammation.

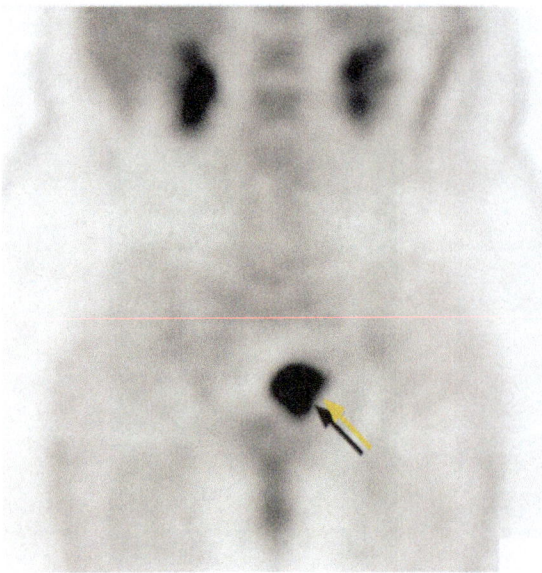

Image 1. Coronal PET image demonstrating a large hypermetabolic pelvic focus (arrow).

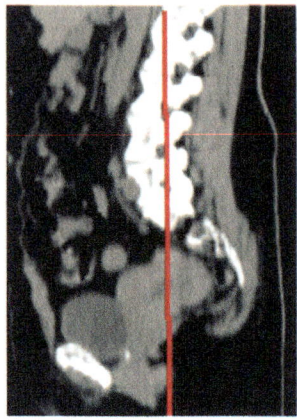

Image 1 (coronal)

Localizer

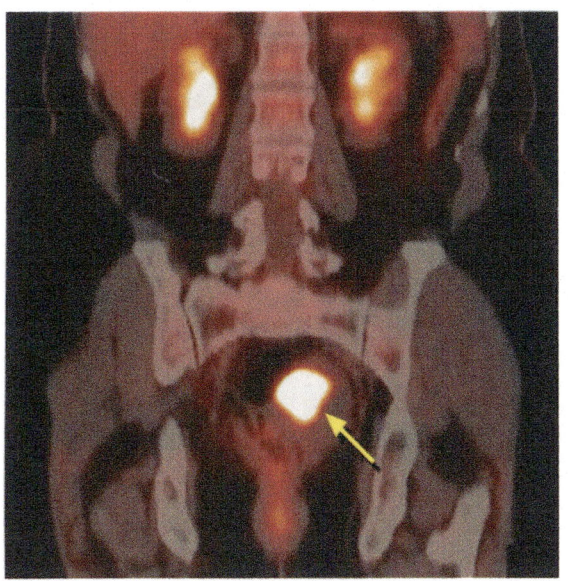

Image 2 (coronal)

Image 2. Fused coronal image demonstrating large hypermetabolic lesion corresponding to a uterine mass (arrow).

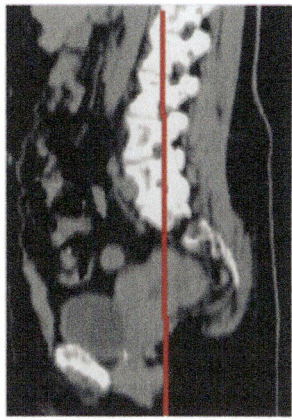

Localizer

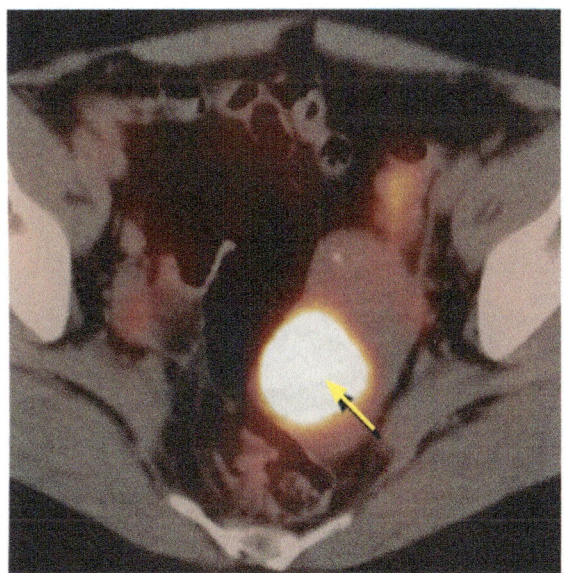

Image 3 (axial)

Image 3. Fused axial image denoting normal and abnormal (arrow) uterine tissue.

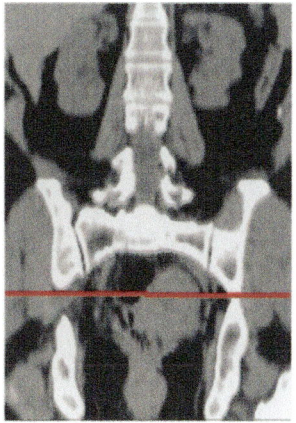

Localizer

Chapter 12

Cancers of the Genito-Urinary System

Cases:

Chapter 12

Cancers of the Genito-Urinary System

Renal Cell Cancer

Renal Cell Cancer is diagnosed in about 30,000 patients/year and accounts for 3% of the malignancies in adults in the United States. Advanced Renal Cell Cancer carries a poor prognosis. New treatment strategies such as immuno-therapy are being employed in an attempt to delay the progression of disease but remain controversial. Non-invasive tests for diagnosing, staging and monitoring the course of disease would be desirable. The current procedures for staging and re-staging of patients with renal cell cancer consist primarily of anatomic imaging modalities.

A small number of studies have addressed the potential role of FDG-PET for staging of renal cell cancer.

Key Indications: Staging and Restaging

Testicular Cancer

Cancer of the testis are the most common solid tumor in men between the ages of 20 and 35 years. Testicular cancer is a diverse group of cancers with seminoma accounting for about 50%. Other testicular cancers include seminoma, embryonal carcinoma and teratoma.

FDG-PET can improve the staging and restaging of patients with testicular cancer. However, both PET and CT may fail to identify small retroperitoneal lymp nodes.

Key Indications: Staging and Restaging

Prostate Cancer

Prostate cancer is the most commonly diagnosed cancer in American men and is the second leading cause of cancer death in men. The existing literature suggests that, because of tracer accumulation in the bladder, FDG-PET has a limited role for detecting primary prostate cancer. FDG-PET can be useful for detecting metastatic disease, for characterizing anatomical bone lesions as malignant or benign, and to detect lymph node metastases.

Thepresent data suggest that FDG-PET provides only limited diagnostic and staging information in patients with prostate cancer.

Key Indications: Staging and Restaging

Bladder Cancer

Limited information regarding FDG-PET performance to stage bladder cancer is available. However, bladder cancer exhibits markedly increased rates of glycolysis, and hence, FDG-PET might be useful for staging and restaging.

Key Indications: Staging and Restaging

Suggested Reading

Renal Cell Cancer

Kocher F, Grimmel S, Hautmann R, Reske SN. Positron emission tomography. Introduction of a new procedure in diagnosis of urologic tumors and initial clinical results. J Nucl Med. 1994;35:223P.

Bachor R, Kotzerke J, Gottfried HW, Brandle E, Reske SN, Hautmann R. Positron emission tomography in diagnosis of renal cell carcinoma. Urologe A. 1996;35(2):146-150.

Miyauchi T, Brown RS, Grossman HB, Wojno K, Wahl RL. Correlation between visualization of primary renal cancer by FDG-PET and histopathological findings. J Nucl Med. 1996;37(5 Suppl):64P.

Goldberg MA, Mayo-Smith WW, Papanicolaou N, Fischman AJ, Lee MJ. FDG PET characterization of renal masses: preliminary experience. Clin Radiol. 1997;52(7):510-515.

Montravers F, Grahek D, Kerrou K, Younsi N, Doublet JD, Gattegno B, Rossert J, Costa de Beauregard MA, Thibault P, Talbot JN. Evaluation of FDG uptake by renal malignancies (primary tumor or metastases) using a coincidence detection gamma camera. J Nucl Med. 2000;41(1):78-84.

Safaei A, Figlin R, Hoh CK, Silverman DH, Seltzer M, Phelps ME, Czernin J. The usefulness of F-18 deoxyglucose whole-body positron emission tomography (PET) for re-staging of renal cell cancer. Clin Nephrol. 2002;57(1):56-62.

Testicular Cancer

Cremerius U, Effert PJ, Adam G, Sabri O, Zimny M, Wagenknecht G, Jakse G, Buell U. FDG PET for detection and therapy control of metastatic germ cell tumor. J Nucl Med. 1998;39(5):815-822.

Cremerius U, Wildberger H, Borchers H, Zimny M, Jakse G, Gunther RW, Buell U. Does positron emission tomography using 18-fluoro-2-deoxyglucose improve clinical staging of testicular caner?--Results of a study in 50 patients. Urology. 1999;54(5):900-904.

Prostrate Cancer

Effert PJ, Bares R, Handt S, Wolff JM, Büll U, Jakse G. Metabolic imaging of untreated prostate cancer by positron emission tomography with [18]fluorine-labeled deoxyglucose. J Urol. 1996;155(3):994-998.

Shreve PD, Grossman HB, Gross MD, Wahl RL. Metastatic prostate cancer: initial findings of PET with 2-deoxy-2-[F-18]fluoro-D-glucose. Radiology. 1996;199(3):751-756.

Yeh SD, Imbiraco M, Larson SM, Garza D, Zhang JJ, Kalaigian H, Finn RD, Reddy D, Horowitz SM, Goldsmith SJ, Scher HI. Detection of bony metastases of androgen-independent prostate cancer by PET-FDG. Nucl Med Biol. 1996;23(6):693-697.

Seltzer MA, Barbaric Z, Belldegrun A, Naitoh J, Dorey F, Phelps ME, Gambhir SS, Hoh CK. Comparison of helical computerized tomography, positron emission tomography and monoclonal antibody scans for evaluating lymph node metastases in patients with prostate specific antigen relapse after treatment for localized prostate cancer. J Urol. 1999;162(4):1322-1328.

Liu IJ, Zafar MB, Lai YH, Segall GM, Terris MK. Fluorodeoxyglucose positron emission tomography studies in diagnosis and staging of clinically organ-confined prostate cancer. Urology. 2001;57(1):108-111.

Bladder Cancer

Kosuda S, Kison PV, Greenough R, Grossman HDB, Wahl RL. Preliminary assessment of fluorine-18 fluorodeoxyglucose positron emission tomography in patients with bladder cancer. Eur J Nucl Med. 1997;24(6):615-620.

Prostate Cancer

Clinical History

This 72-year-old patient with prostate cancer who is status post prostatectomy presented with rising PSA levels.

PET/CT indication: Restaging.

Findings

Hypermetabolic focus in the prostate bed is highly suggestive of local tumor recurrence. Hypermetabolic focus in the right transverse process of T7 corresponds to a lytic lesion identified on CT. This is consistent with bone metastasis.

Teaching Point

PET alone is limited in its ability to determine local recurrence in patients after prostatectomy. This is because considerable activity in the urinary bladder obscures the prostate bed. PET/CT helps to delineate anatomically the prostate bed from the bladder and in the current case provided evidence for local recurrence and bone metastasis (localized to a transverse process).

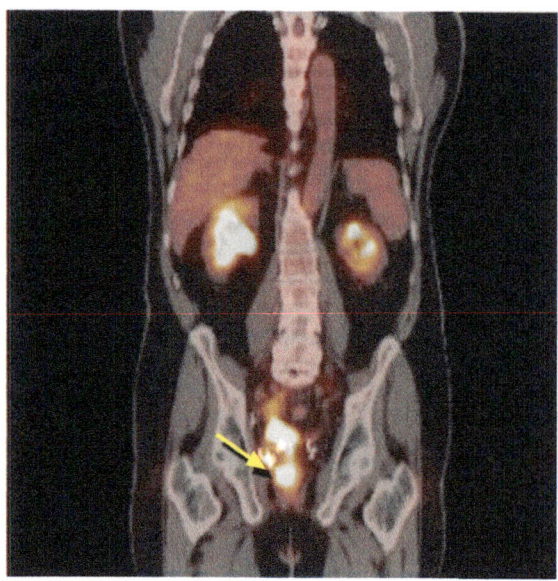

Image 1 (coronal)

Image 1. Abnormal FDG uptake is seen in the lower pelvis (arrow).

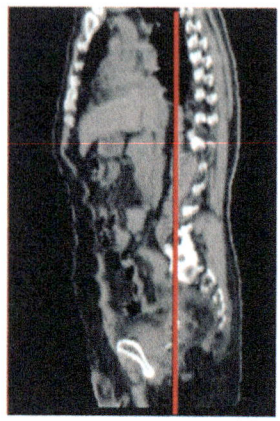

Localizer

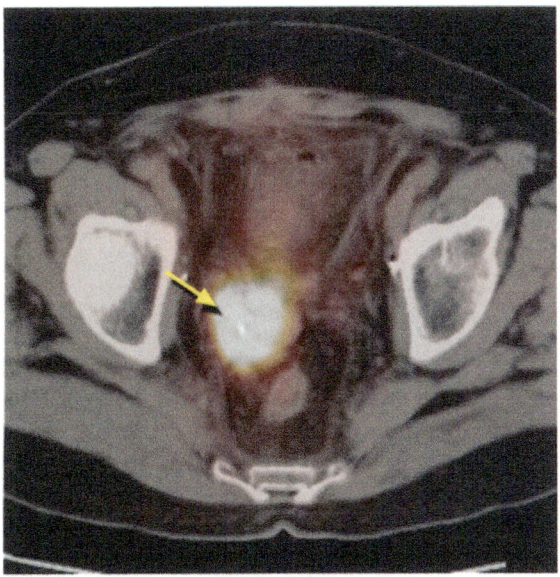

Image 2 (axial)

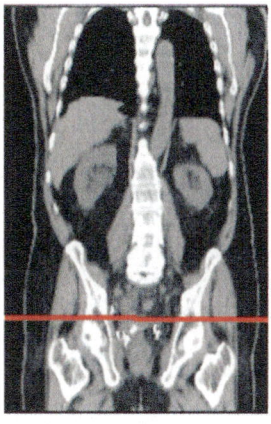

Localizer

Image 2. Increased FDG uptake in the prostate bed is consistent with increased glycolysis of recurrent prostate cancer (arrow).

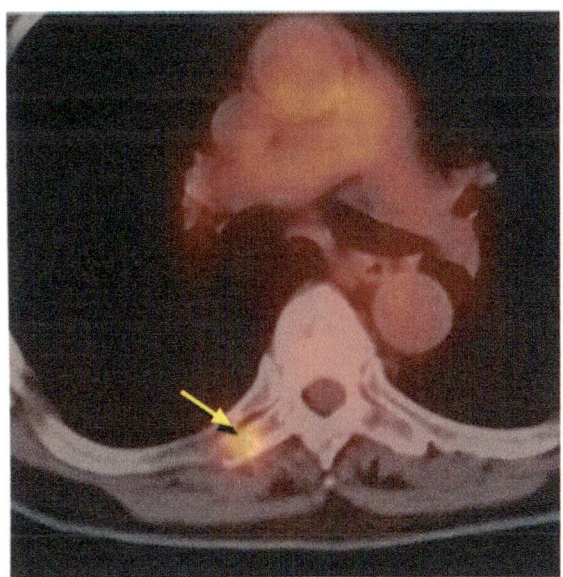

Image 3 (axial)

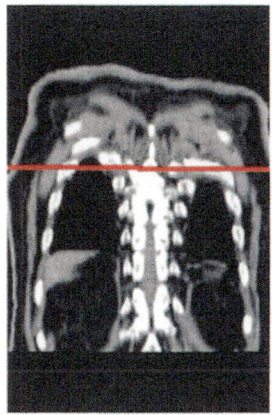

Localizer

Image 3. Increased glycolytic activity in a right transverse process corresponds to lytic metastatic lesion on CT (arrow).

Renal Cell Carcinoma

Clinical History

34-year-old female with history of metastatic renal cell carcinoma and right nephrectomy.

PET/CT indication: Restaging.

Findings

Intense hypermetabolic foci corresponding to a para-aortic lymph node at the level of the left renal artery and another one at the level of L3-L4 just anterior to the right psoas muscle. These are consistent with metastatic disease.

Teaching Point

Focal FDG uptake could not be assigned to a specific anatomic structure on FDG images alone. The hypermetabolic lymph nodes were below the critical size criteria on CT images. PET/CT provided accurate localization and diagnosis.

Image 1. Fused coronal image demonstrating right para-aortic lymph node metastasis (arrow).

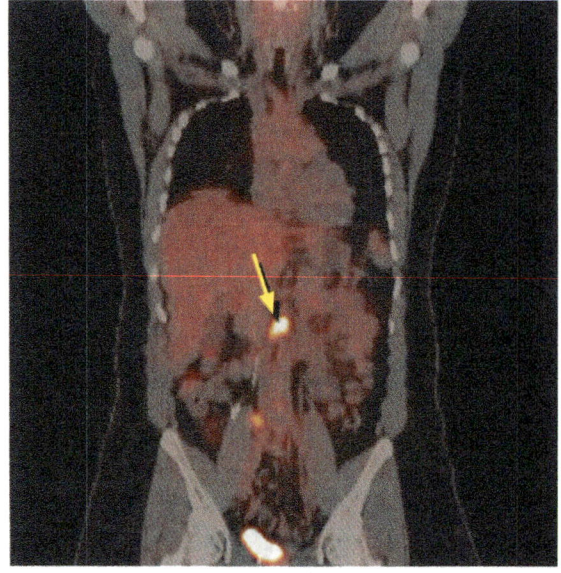

Image 1 (coronal)

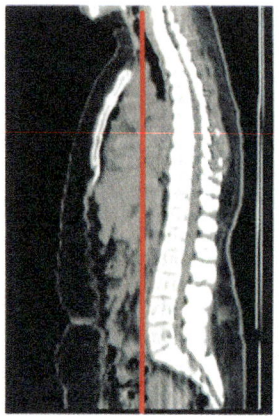

Localizer

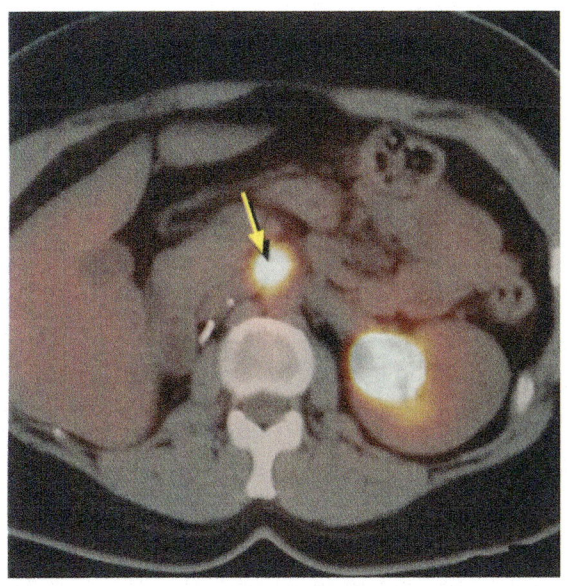

Image 2 (axial)

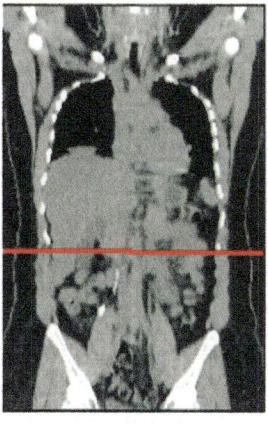

Localizer

Image 2. Fused axial cut showing intense physiological tracer accumulation in the left renal pelvis and a pre-aortic lymph node (arrow).

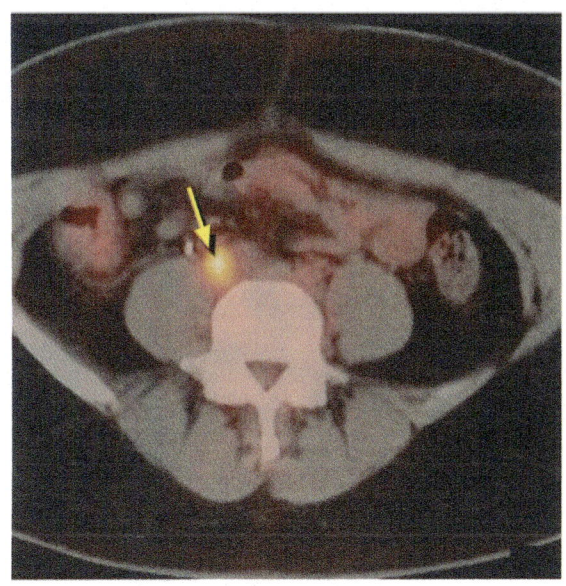

Image 3 (axial)

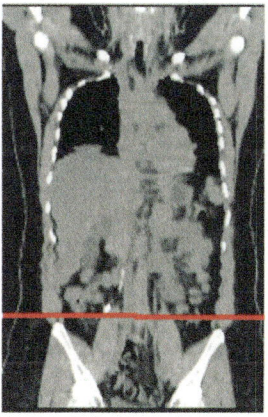

Localizer

Image 3. Fused axial cut at the level of L3/L4 demonstrating sub-centimeter hypermetabolic lymph node on the right side (arrow).

Renal Cell Carcinoma

Clinical History

56 year-old male with newly diagnosed left renal cancer.

PET/CT indication: Staging.

Findings

Diffuse tracer activity of moderate intensity in the region of the left kidney and corresponding to a left renal mass on CT is consistent with malignancy.

Small lung lesion without increased glucose metabolic activity is present.

Teaching Point

Note the difference between renal mass on CT and tumor viability by PET. The small right lung base nodule was not metabolically active. It measured less than 5 mm and malignancy cannot be ruled out.

Image 1. Large left renal mass with eccentric glycolytic activity suggesting a large necrotic core (red arrow) of the tumor surrounded by viable tumor tissue (yellow arrows).

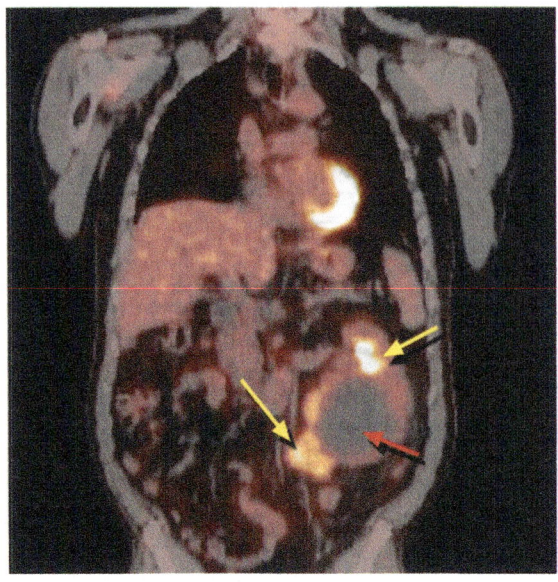

Image 1 (coronal)

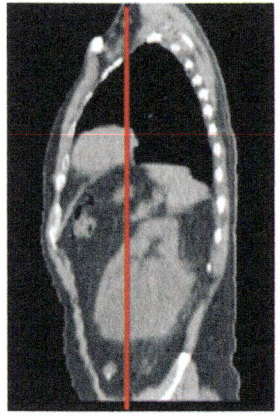

Localizer

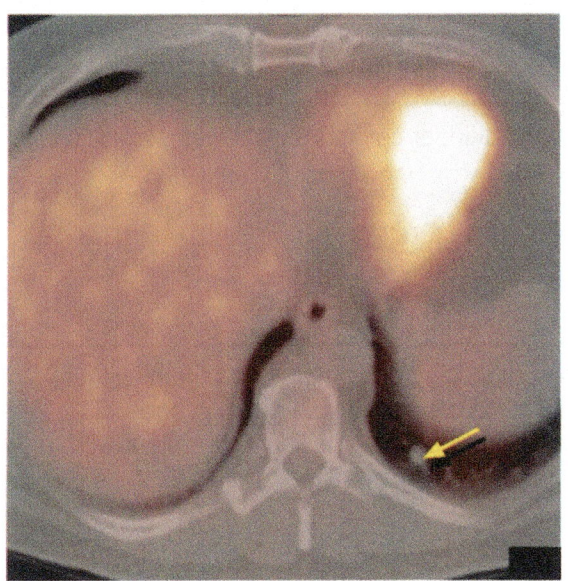

Image 2 (axial)

Image 3. Small lung nodule on CT without increased metabolic activity. Because of the small lesions size metastasis cannot be ruled out.

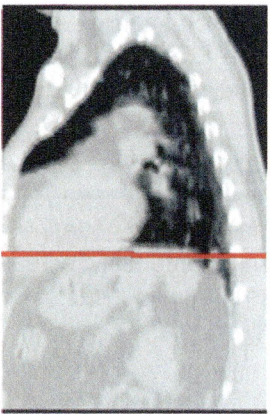

Localizer

Bladder Cancer

Clinical History

64-year-old male patient with a history of metastatic bladder carcinoma that was surgically removed. The patient also underwent chemotherapy.

PET/CT indication: Restaging.

Findings

A para-aortic lymph node, postero-lateral to the right of the abdominal aorta at the level of L1/L2, shows intensely increased FDG uptake. This is consistent with a lymph node metastasis. A mild focus of increased uptake in the right shoulder is likely consistent with fibrous dysplasia.

Teaching Point

1) Primary bladder carcinoma is difficult to be imaged with FDG PET because of normal tracer accumulation in the bladder. Metastatic bladder cancer is metabolically very active and PET (PET/CT) can therefore be used to stage and restage the disease.

2) A small lesion in the right scapula was identified in this study. By CT, this lesion was most consistent with fibrous dysplasia that is known to exhibit increased FDG uptake. CT was helpful in identifying the etiology for increased FDG uptake.

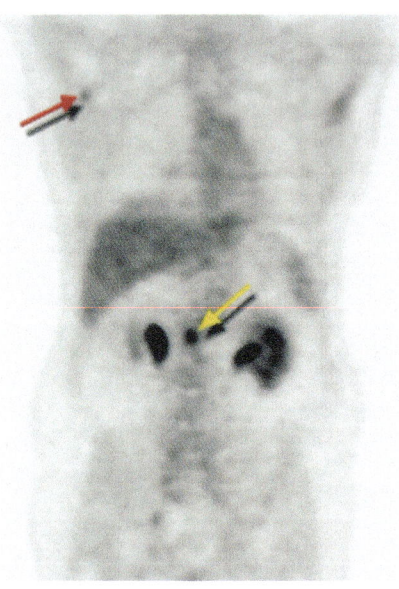

Image 1 (coronal)

Image 1. Coronal PET image demonstrating a hypermetabolic focus in the mid-abdomen (yellow arrow) and a small focus in the posterior right chest wall (red arrow), exact lesion localization of this lesion was not possible with PET alone.

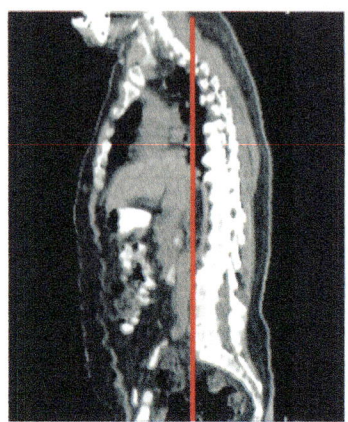

Localizer

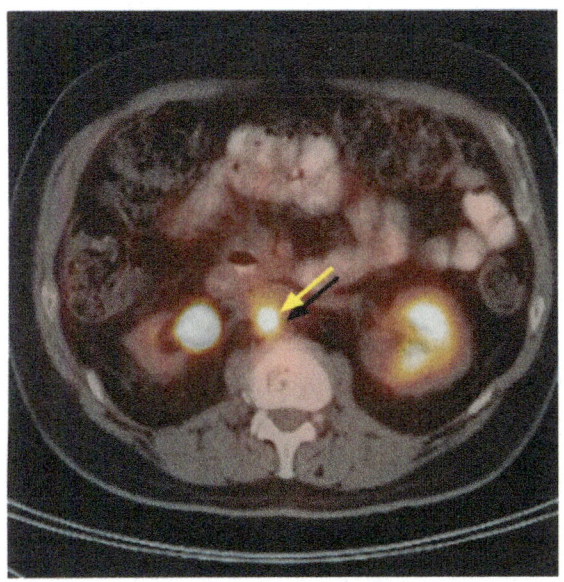

Image 2 (axial)

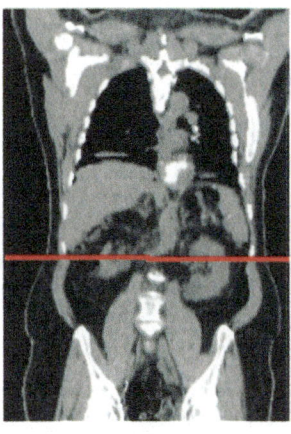

Localizer

Image 2. Fused axial image denoting normal renal activity and identifying hypermetabolism related to a metastatic peri-aortic lymph node (arrow).

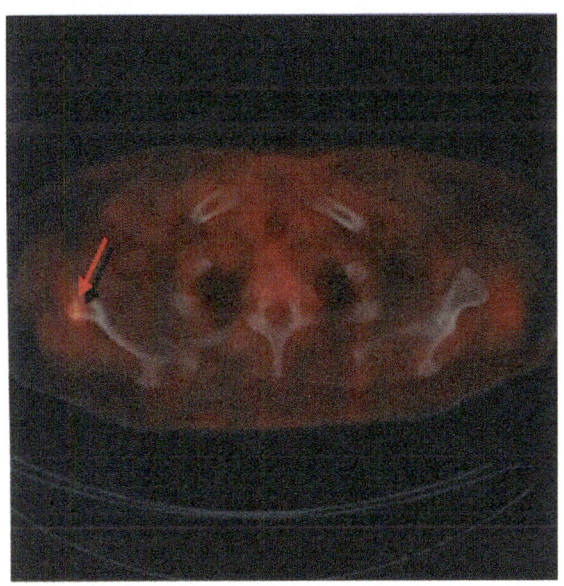

Image 3 (axial)

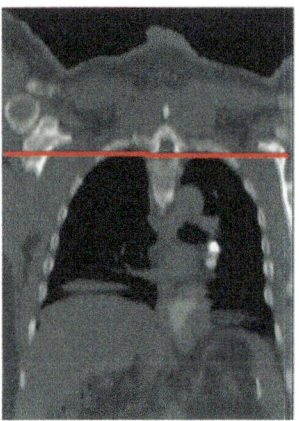

Localizer

Image 3. Fused axial image showing the focal FDG uptake in the right scapula consistent with fibrous dysplasia (arrow).

Testicular Cancer

Clinical History

Patient with metastatic testicular cancer (embryonal cell type). The PET/CT study was obtained post right groin dissection, left radical orchiectomy and chemotherapy.

PET/CT indication: Restaging.

Findings

Increased tracer activity in the right hemi-scrotum. Malignancy in the right testicle cannot be excluded. However, this finding appears relatively stable since the previous examination. Mildly increased activity in the right inguinal region likely represents post-surgical changes.

Teaching Point

Testicular cancers frequently exhibit intensely increased glucose metabolic activity. Mildly to moderately increased testicular FDG uptake can represent a normal finding or might be consistent with testicular malignancy.

Therapeutic interventions such as surgery or radiation treatment can result in mildly increased FDG uptake for many months.

Image 1

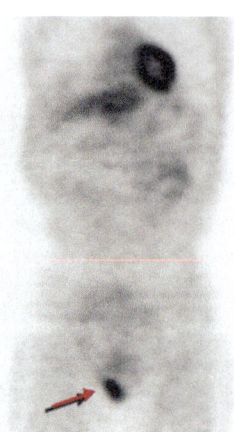

PET (coronal)

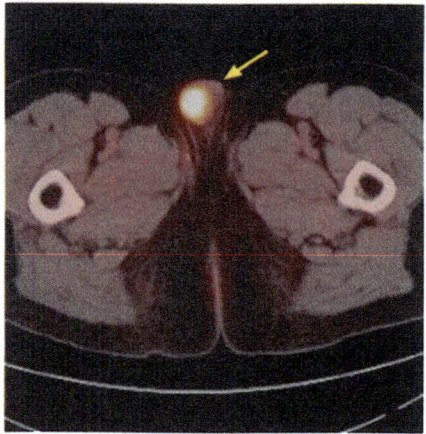

PET/CT (axial)

Image 1. Increased FDG uptake in the right hemi-scrotum (red arrow) is demonstrated on this coronal PET image. Fused axial image showing hypermetabolism of the right hemi-scrotum (yellow arrow) which might also be a normal variant; however, malignancy cannot be excluded.

Image 2

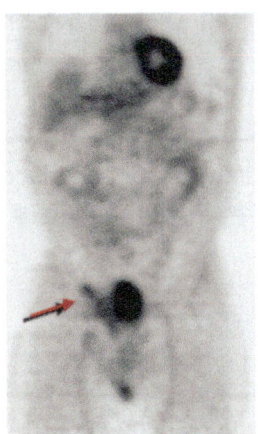

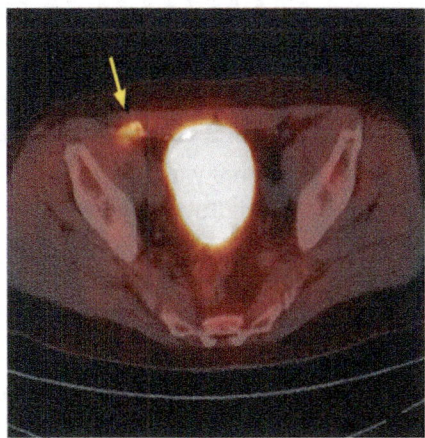

PET (coronal)   **PET/CT (axial)**

Image 2. Coronal PET image with mildly and linearly increased FDG uptake in the right groin (red arrow). This is an unspecific finding and can occur after radiation treatment or for several months after surgery. Increased FDG uptake in the region of the previous surgery (yellow arrow) shown on fused axial image. CT demonstrates surgical clips and post-surgical fibrous tissue. The increased uptake can be explained by post-surgical and post-radiation changes.

Transitional Cell Cancer

Clinical History

69-year-old male patient with transitional cell cancer of kidney, ureter and bladder who is status post left radical uretero-nephrectomy. The patient was free of symptoms and in clinical remission at the time of the PET/CT study.

PET/CT indication: Restaging.

Findings

One left-sided and one right-sided para-aortic lymph node measuring about 1 cm exhibit increased glucose metabolic activity.

Mildly increased FDG uptake is present in the right anterior lower lung lobe corresponding to a lung nodule on CT.

Teaching Point

PET alone was interpreted as negative for metastatic lung involvement. Image co-registration revealed mildly increased FDG uptake in the lung lesion. Two intense foci of increased glucose metabolic activity were present in the posterior mid abdomen and corresponded to two lymph nodes measuring about 1 cm. Thus, the nodes were equivocal/negative for tumor involvement by CT size criteria. PET/CT converted false-negative/equivocal CT findings into a positive result while CT helped to identify a lung metastisis.

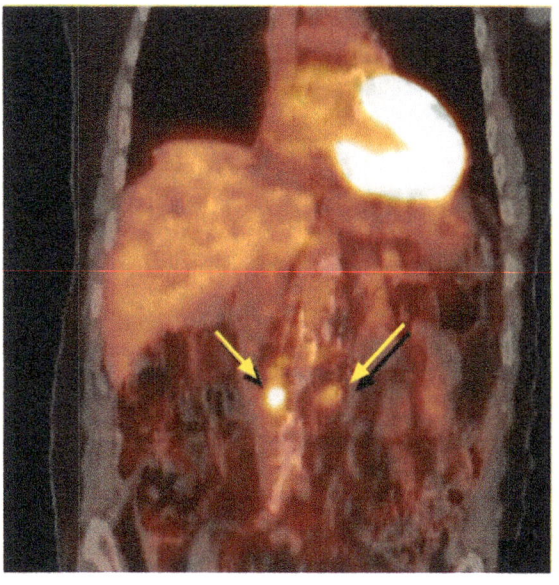

Image 1 (coronal)

Image 1. Fused coronal image of abdomen and pelvis with increased FDG uptake in bilateral para-aortic lymph nodes (see arrows).

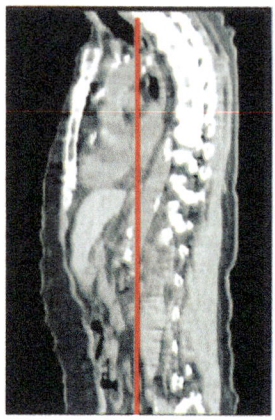

Localizer

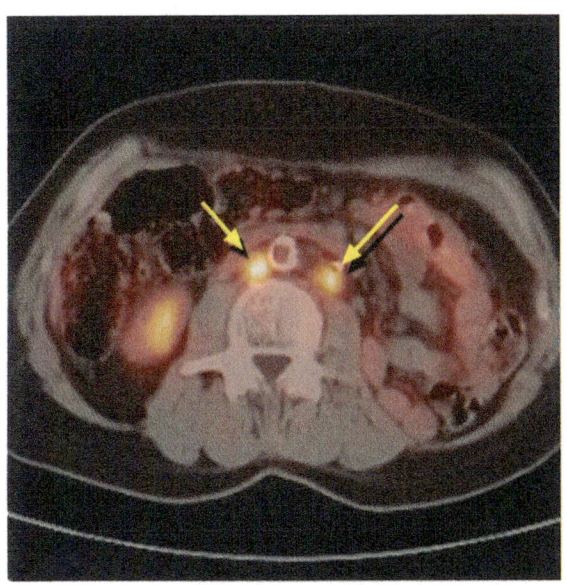

Image 2 (axial)

Image 2. Axial image demonstrating increased glycolytic activity in the para-aortic nodes (arrows). Axial CT image revealed two para-aortic lymph nodes measuring approximately 1 cm (see arrows).

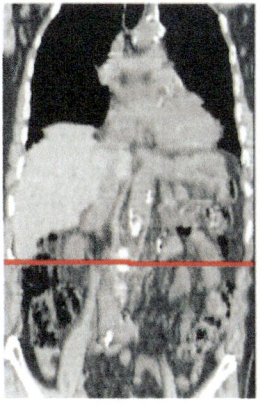

CT Image

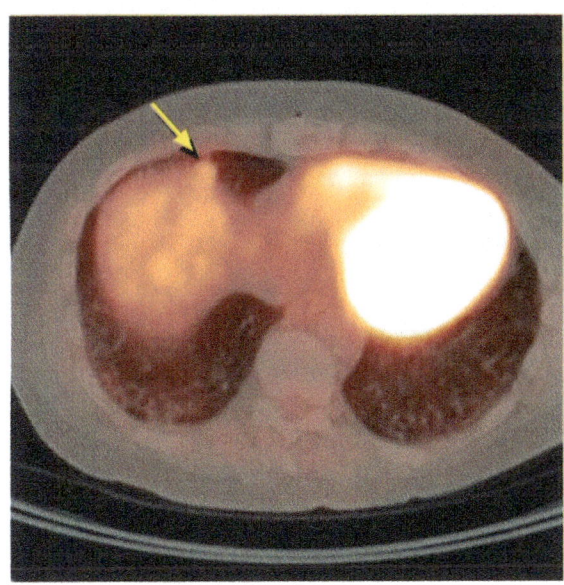

Image 3 (axial)

Image 3. Small focus of mildly increased FDG uptake in the anterior aspect of the right lower lung lobe (arrow) corresponding to small lung nodule on CT.

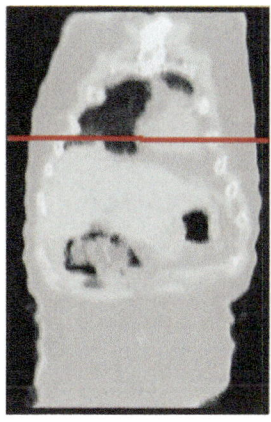

Localizer

Chapter 13

Benign Diseases

Cases:

Chapter 13

Benign Diseases

Benign tumors and inflammatory tissue can exhibit considerably increased glucose metabolism due to glycolytic activity of fibroblasts, macrophages, and acute inflammatory cells.

This can result in "false" positive PET/CT findings. However, inflammatory diseases can be diagnosed and monitored with FDG-PET.

Suggested Reading

Shreve PD, Anzai Y, Wahl RL. Pitfalls in oncologic diagnosis with FDG PET imaging: physiologic and benign variants. Radiographics. 1999;19(1):61-77.

Bakheet SM, Powe J, Kandil A, Ezzat A, Rostom A, Amartey J. F-18 FDG uptake in breast infection and inflammation. Clin Nucl Med. 2000;25(2):100-103.

Alavi A, Gupta N, Alberini JL, Hickeson M, Adam LE, Bhargava P, Zhuang H. Positron emission tomography imaging in nonmalignant thoracic disorders. Semin Nucl Med. 2002;32(4):293-321.

Keidar Z, Engel A, Nitecki S, Bar Shalom R, Hoffman A, Israel O. PET/CT using 2-deoxy-2-[18F]fluoro-D-glucose for the evaluation of suspected infected vascular graft. Mol Imaging Biol. 2003;5(1):23-25.

Chacko TK, Zhuang H, Nakhoda KZ, Moussavian B, Alavi A. Applications of fluorodeoxyglucose positron emission tomography in the diagnosis of infection. Nucl Med Commun. 2003;24(6):615-624.

Shimizu A, Oriuchi N, Tsushima Y, Higuchi T, Aoki J, Endo K. High [18F] 2-fluoro-2-deoxy-D-glucose (FDG) uptake of adrenocortical adenoma showing subclinical Cushing's syndrome. Ann Nucl Med. 2003;17(5):403-406.

Bhargava P, Reich P, Alavi A, Zhuang H. Radiation-induced esophagitis on FDG PET imaging. Clin Nucl Med. 2003;28(10):849-850.

Roivainen A, Parkkola R, Yli-Kerttula T, Lehikoinen P, Viljanen T, Mottonen T, Nuutila P, Minn H. Use of positron emission tomography with methyl-11C-choline and 2-18F-fluoro-2-deoxy-D-glucose in comparison with magnetic resonance imaging for the assessment of inflammatory proliferation of synovium. Arthritis Rheum. 2003;48(11):3077-3084.

Bleeker-Rovers CP, De Kleijn EM, Corstens FH, Van Der Meer JW, Oyen WJ. Clinical value of FDG PET in patients with fever of unknown origin and patients suspected of focal infection or inflammation. Eur J Nucl Med Mol Imaging. 2004;31(1):29-37.

Osteopoikilosis

Clinical History

39-year-old female with a history of breast cancer status post resection and chemotherapy now found to have rising tumor markers.

PET/CT indication: Restaging.

Findings

Mildly increased FDG uptake in the L-spine consistent with prior lumbar spine surgery. No other focus of abnormally increased tracer uptake is identified.

CT images reveal extensive sclerotic lesions associated with known osteopoikilosis.

Teaching Point

Rare case of a patient with osteopoikilosis demonstrated on CT. None of the sclerotic lesions exhibited increased glycolytic activity.

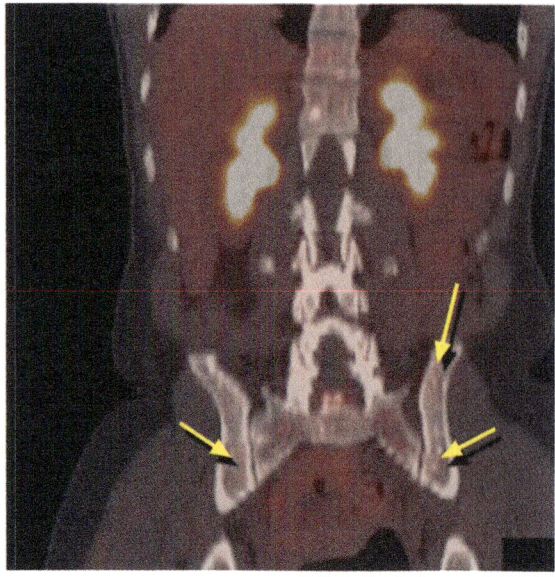

Image 1. Coronal PET/CT image with extensive sclerotic lesions consistent with osteopoikilosis and absence of abnormal FDG uptake (arrows).

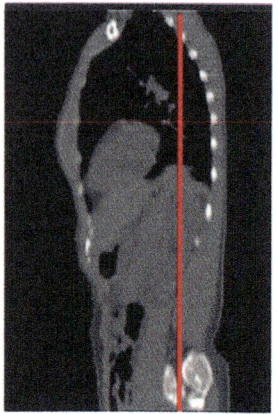

Image 1 (coronal)

Localizer

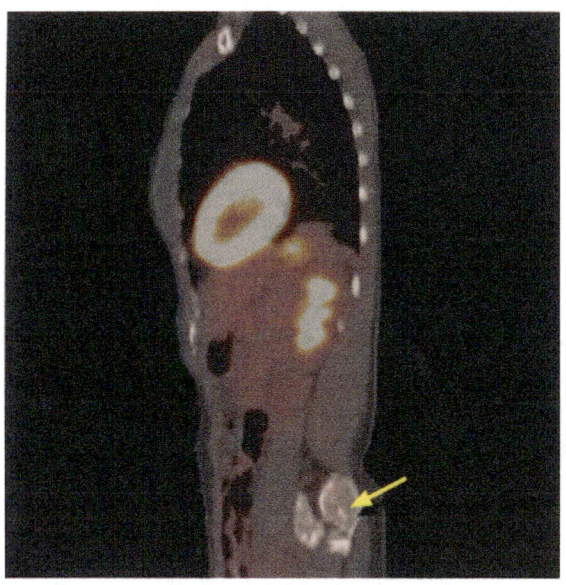

Image 2 (sagittal)

Image 2. Sagittal PET/CT image with extensive sclerotic lesions consistent with osteopoikilosis and absence of abnormal FDG uptake (arrow).

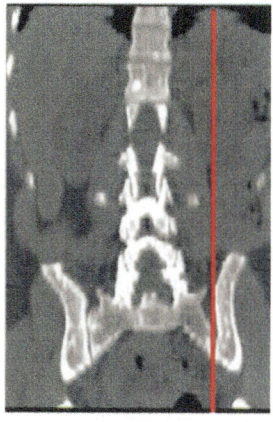

Localizer

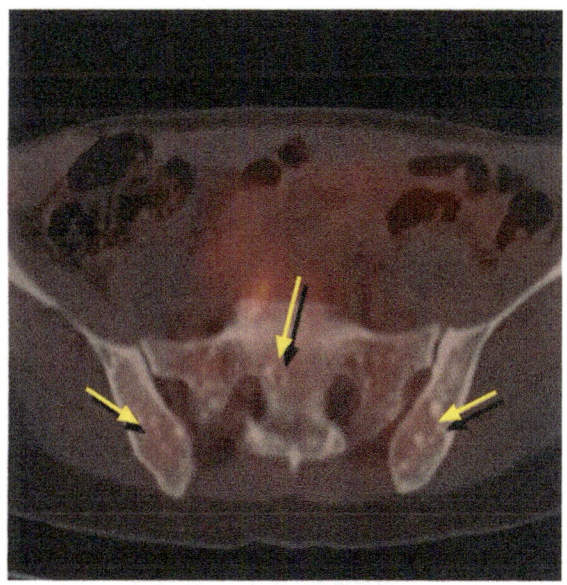

Image 3 (axial)

Image 3. Axial PET/CT image with extensive sclerotic lesions consistent with osteopoikilosis (arrows). These lesions were not hypermetabolic.

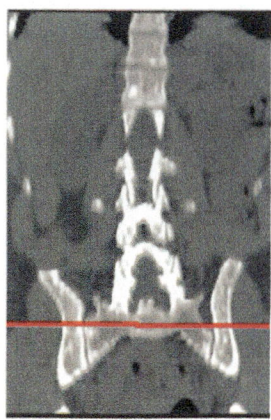

Localizer

Inflammation, Infection

Clinical History

Patient with suspicious pelvic mass on CT.

PET/CT indication: Tissue characterization.

Findings

A soft tissue mass adjacent to the ilio-psoas encompasses the acetabulum, displacing the femoral vessels medially and extending inferiorly down to the level of the lesser trochanter. It has a central low density lesion (15 Hounsfield units) with a thin soft tissue rim exhibiting increased glycolytic activity. This might represent inflammation, infection or malignancy. Biopsy is strongly recommended.

Verification: Benign inflammatory mass.

Teaching Point

Increased FDG uptake is not specific for malignancy. Infectious and inflammatory tissue also exhibit increased rates of glycolytic activity. Thus, false positive findings can occur with PET and PET/CT. Nevertheless, focally increased FDG uptake demands a biopsy for definitive diagnosis.

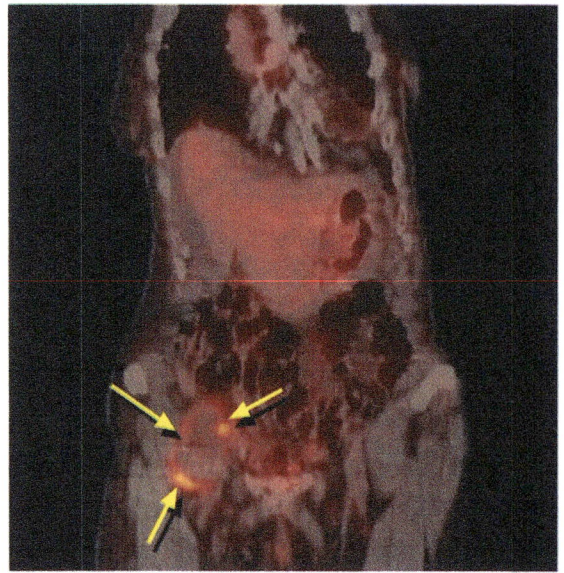

Image 1 (coronal)

Image 1. Fused coronal image depicting the soft tissue mass with an excentric and "incomplete" hypermetabolic rim (arrows).

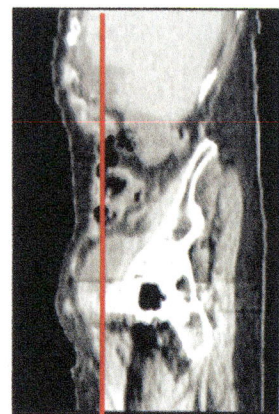

Localizer

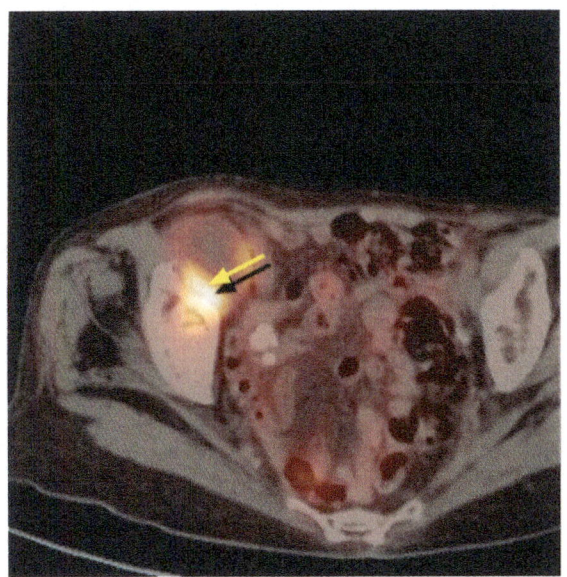

Image 2. Axial image demonstrating the partially hypermetabolic mass (arrow).

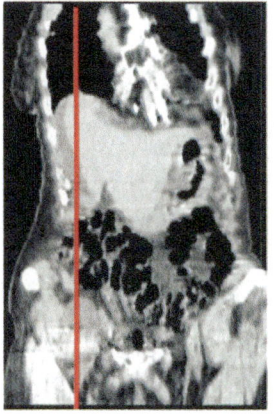

Image 2 (axial)

Localizer

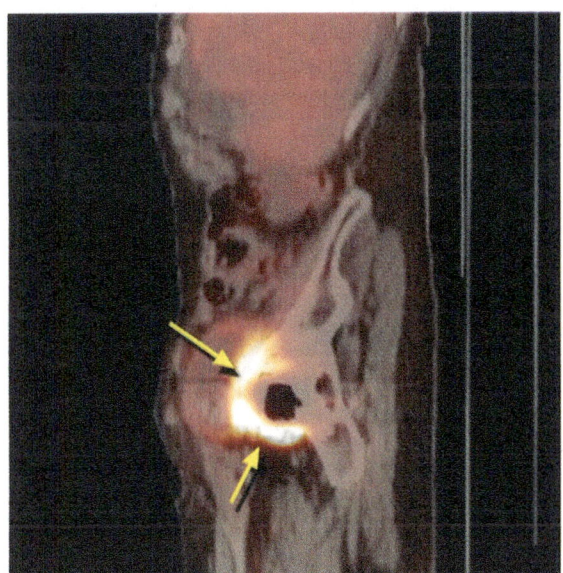

Image 3. Fused sagittal image reveal intense hypermetabolism involving soft-tissue surrounding the femoral head and the acetabulum (arrows). Biopsy revealed benign reactive inflammatory process.

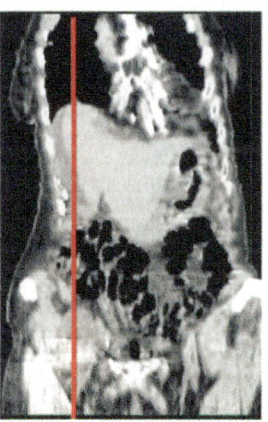

Image 3 (sagittal)

Localizer

Foreign Body Reaction

Clinical History

55-year-old patient with infiltrating ductal carcinoma of the left breast treated with lumpectomy and chemotherapy.

PET/CT indication: Restaging.

Findings

Two hypermetabolic foci corresponding to small lymph nodes on CT are identified in the left axilla. The more medial lymph node measures 7 mm and the larger one 1.2 cm. Diffusely increased bone marrow activity is consistent with regenerating marrow after chemotherapy.

Pathology verification: Focal fat necrosis with histiocytic inflammation including foreign-body type giant cell reaction.

Teaching Point

Most common false positives encountered with PET and PET/CT are due to inflammatory and infectious processes.

Image 1. Fused coronal image with two hypermetabolic foci in the left axilla (arrows). Biopsy revealed a benign etiology.

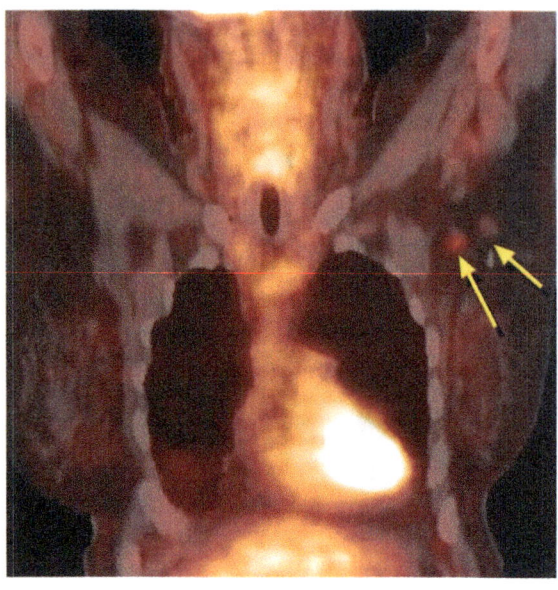

Image 1 (coronal)

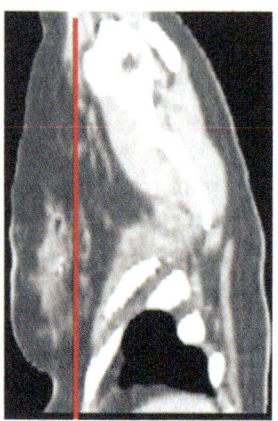

Localizer

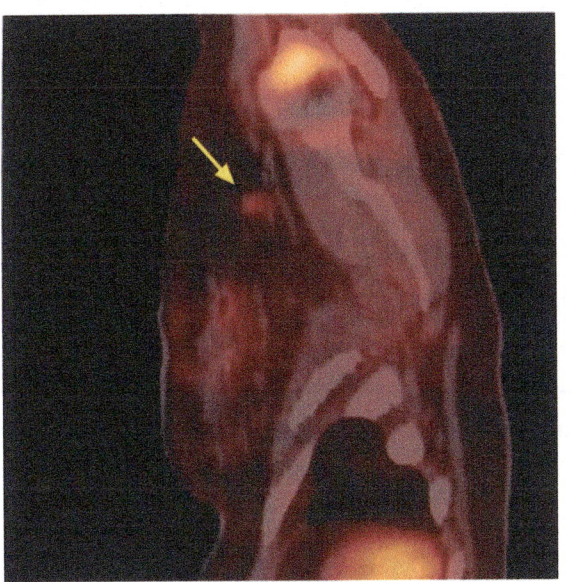

Image 2 (sagittal)

Image 2. Fused sagittal image with hypermetabolic focus in the left axilla (arrow).

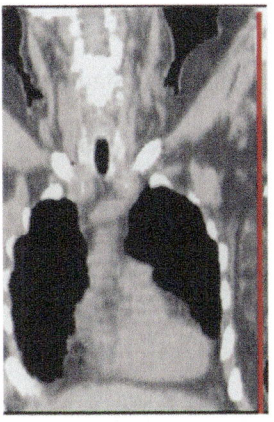

Localizer

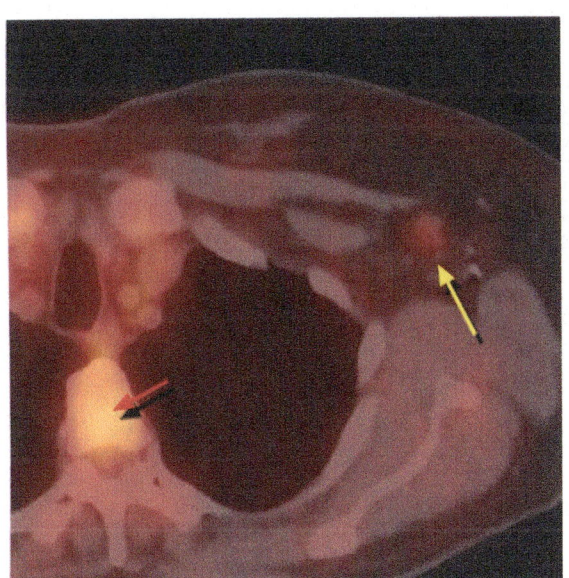

Image 3 (axial)

Image 3. Fused axial image denoting left axillary lymph nodes with increased glycolytic activity (yellow arrow). Increased bone marrow activity is due to regenerating bone marrow after chemotherapy (red arrow).

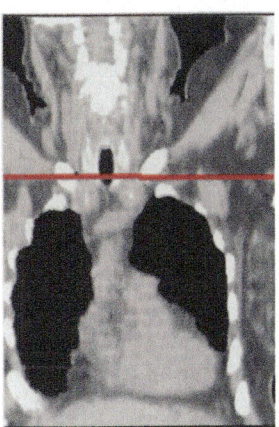

Localizer

Uterine Fibroid

Clinical History

36-year-old female patient with a history of right breast cancer and a history of uterine fibroids.

PET/CT indication: Staging.

Findings

A large focus of increased tracer uptake is identified in the uterus. This is likely consistent with uterine fibroids.

Teaching Point

Uterine fibroids can exhibit markedly increased FDG uptake. Uptake is usually well circumscribed. Benign etiologies of increased uterine FDG uptake should be considered in cancer patients.

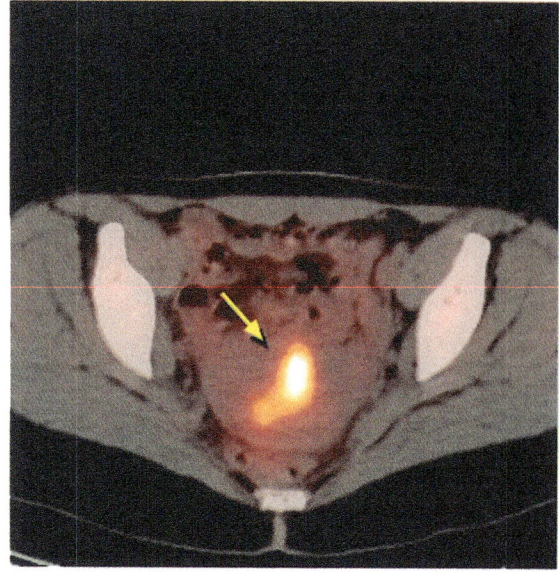

Image 1. Fused axial PET/CT image demonstrating increased FDG uptake in the uterus (arrow). This is consistent with the known history of uterine fibroids in this patient with breast cancer.

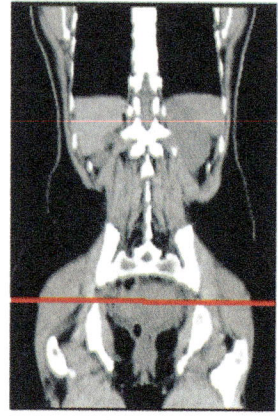

Image 1 (axial)   **Localizer**

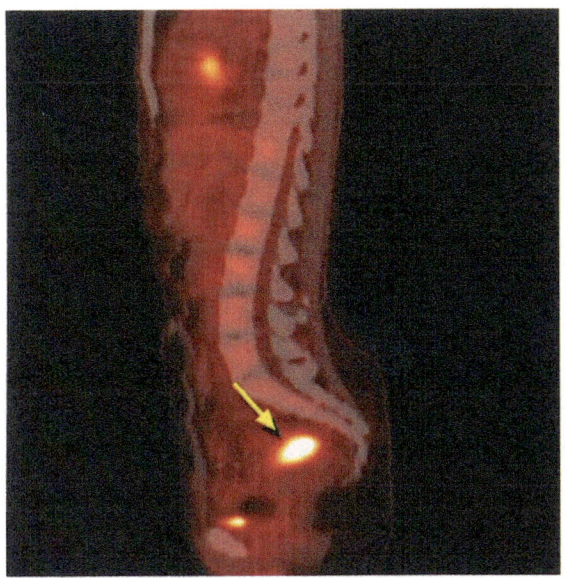

Image 2 (sagittal)

Image 2. Sagittal PET/CT view demonstrating increased FDG uptake in the uterus (arrow).

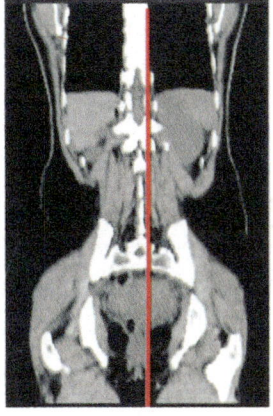

Localizer

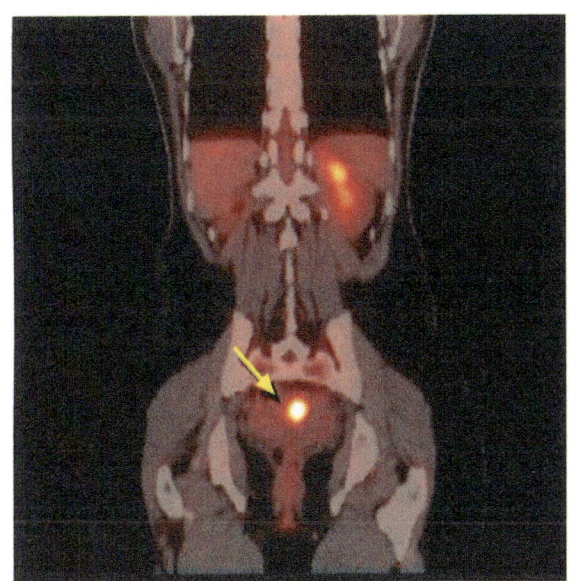

Image 3 (coronal)

Image 3. Fused coronal image of chest, abdomen and pelvis demonstrating focally increased FDG uptake corresponding to a uterine fibroid (arrow).

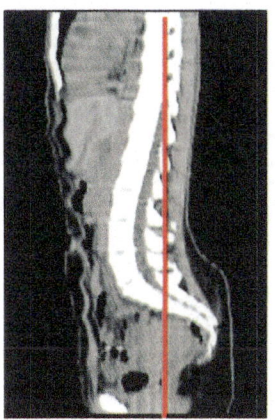

Localizer

Fistula

Clinical History

55-year-old patient with history of right nephrectomy for renal cell carcinoma who subsequently developed a draining fistula from the right renal fossa to the dorsal skin surface.

PET/CT indication: Restaging.

Findings

Mildly increased FDG uptake in the right renal fossa. These findings are consistent with chronic inflammation.

Teaching Point

The case emphasizes the difficulty in distinguishing recurrent cancer from chronic inflammation. Follow up scans revealed further decreasing glycolytic activity after antibiotic treatment in the patient with known draining fistula.

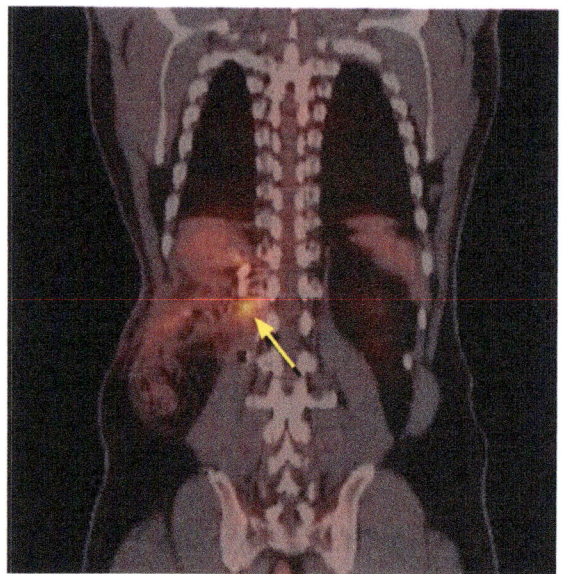

Image 1 (coronal)

Image 1. Fused coronal PET/CT image with mildly increased FDG uptake in the right posterior paraspinal region (arrow).

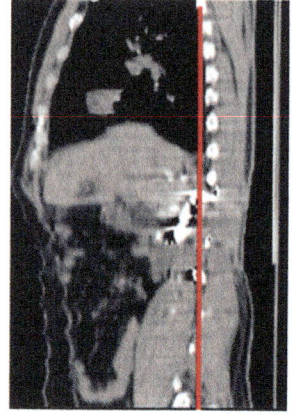

Localizer

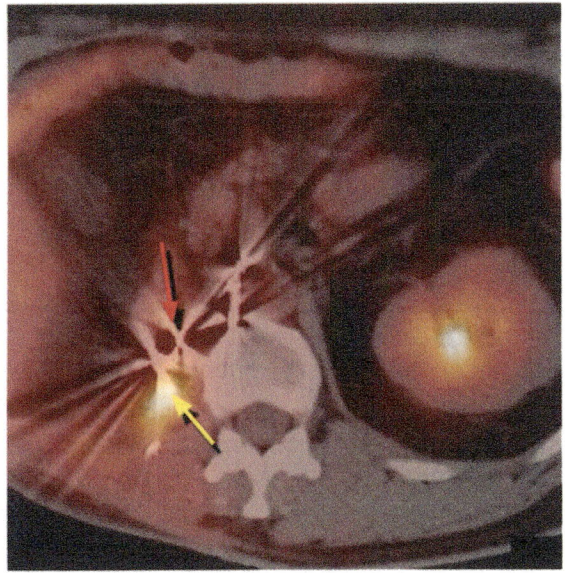

Image 2 (axial)

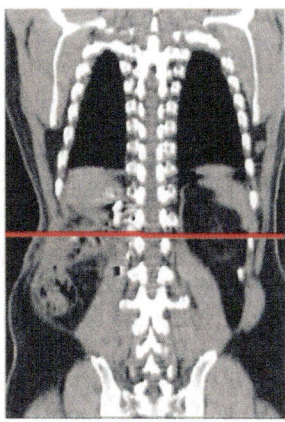

Localizer

Image 2. Axial image demonstrating increased FDG uptake in the region of the right posterior para-spinal region (arrow). The CT artifact is explained by a metal-containing mesh (arrow).

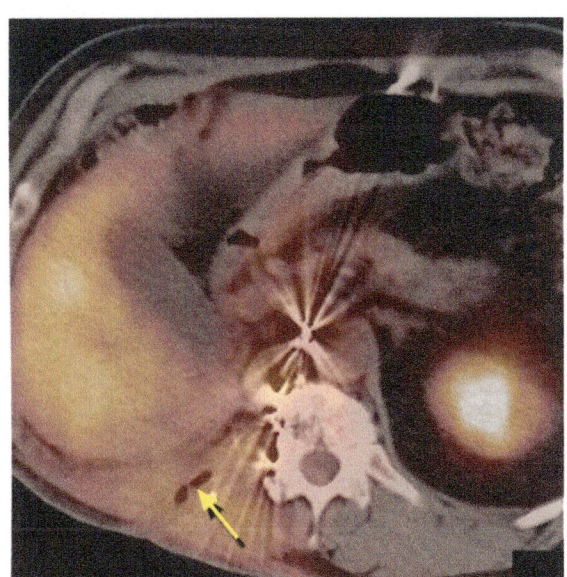

Image 3 (axial)

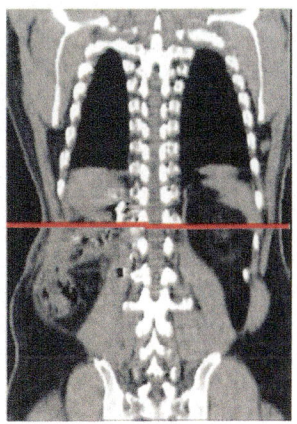

Localizer

Image 3. Fused axial images demonstrating the fistula track (arrow) after antibiotic treatment.

Sarcoidosis

Clinical History

42-year-old asymptomatic patient with three-year history of enlarging left testicular mass.

PET/CT indication: Lesion characterization.

Findings

Highly abnormal whole body PET/CT scan with multiple intense hypermetabolic foci involving the mediastinum, bilateral hilar regions, para-aortic nodes, and multiple vertebral bodies in the T-spine and L-spine, and the right ilium.
These findings, together with the patient's history of enlarging left testicular mass, strongly suggest metastatic testicular cancer.

Mediastinoscopy and biopsy: Findings consistent with sarcoidosis.

Teaching Point

Granuloma frequently exhibits moderate to intense FDG uptake. In this particular case, the abnormalities were involving soft tissue as well as bone and given the patient's history of an enlarging testicular mass, testicular cancer was suspected. Mediastinoscopy however revealed sarcoidosis. Thus, PET/CT allowed lesion localization but did not improve PET specificity.

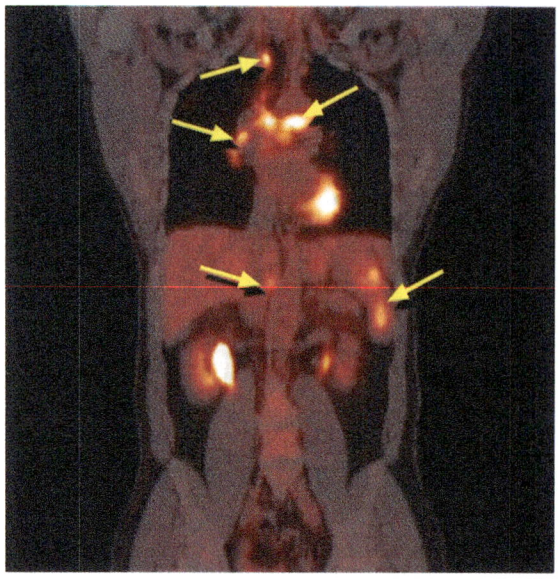

Image 1. Axial fused image with increased FDG uptake in the mediastinum (arrow), bilateral hilar region (arrow), spleen (arrow) and a para-aortic lymph node (arrow) on the right side.

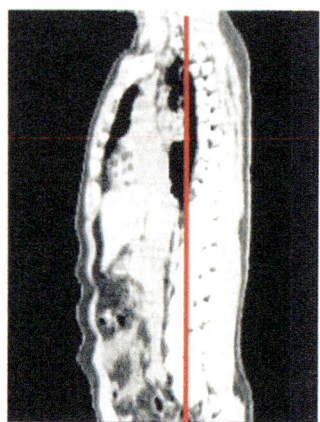

Image 1 (axial)   **Localizer**

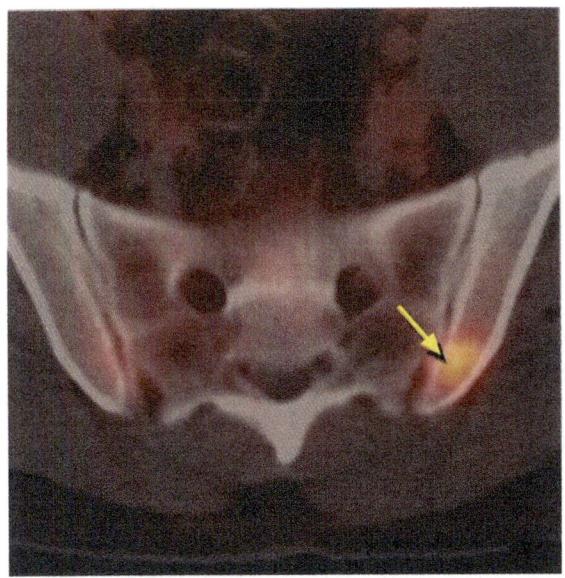

Image 2. Abnormal focus of hypermetabolic activity in the left iliac bone (arrow).

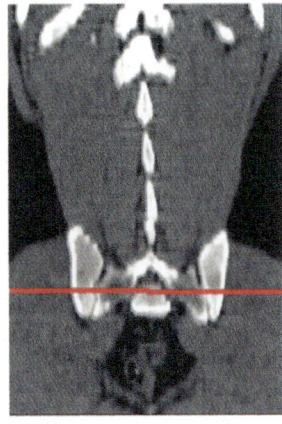

Image 2 (axial)

Localizer

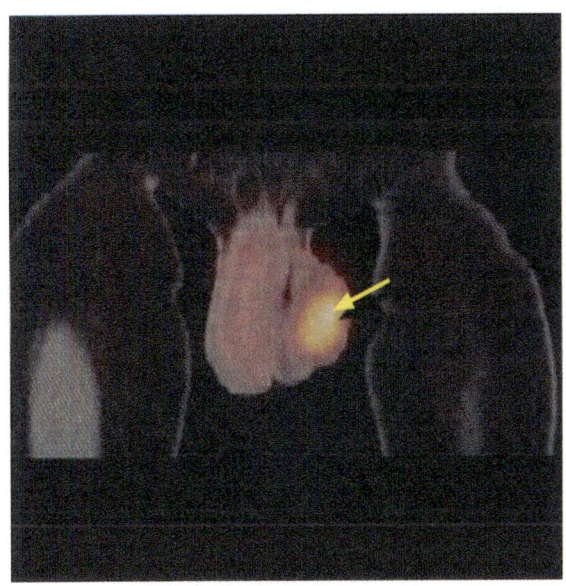

Image 3. Increased FDG uptake in the left testicle (arrow).

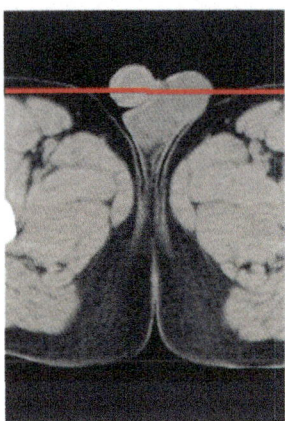

Image 3 (coronal)

Localizer

Tubular Adenoma

Clinical History

76-year-old male who is status post left upper lobectomy for non-small cell lung cancer.

Findings

Normal tracer activity is identified within the lungs, mediastinum, liver, kidneys, bladder, and bowel. Intense FDG uptake in the recto-sigmoid region is due to a normal variant of bowel activity. There is no evidence of recurrent or metastatic disease.

Histological Verification: Large tubular adenoma.

Teaching Point

PET/CT does not overcome the limitation of FDG-PET that benign tumors can exhibit markedly increased rates of glucose utilization. Normal bowel activity can sometimes not be distinguished from benign or malignant disease.

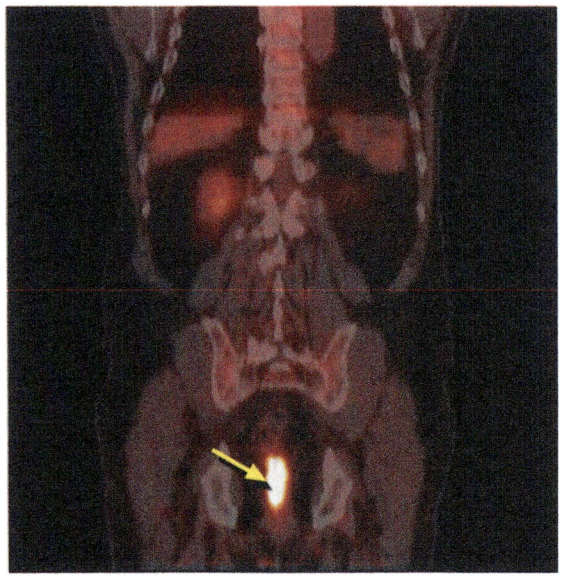

Image 1. Fused coronal image with large focus of increased FDG uptake in the recto-sigmoid region (arrow).

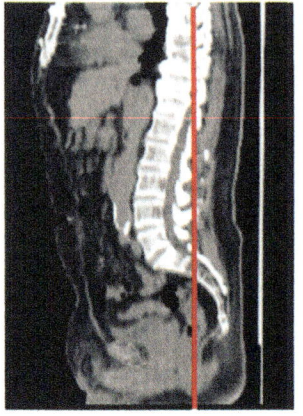

Image 1 (coronal)   **Localizer**

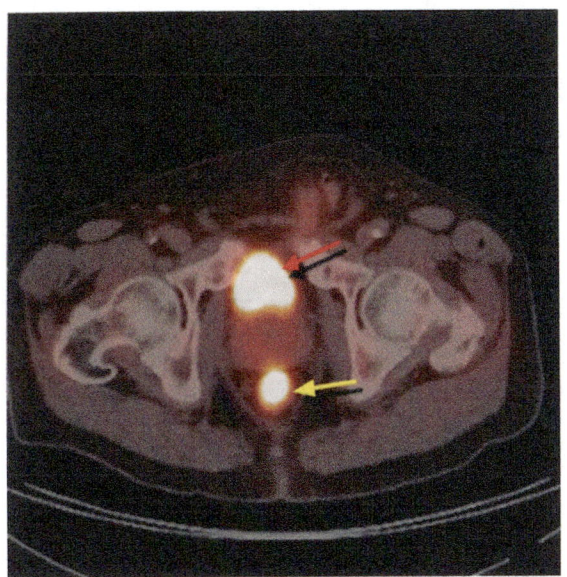

Image 2 (axial)

Image 2. Fused axial image demonstrating the urinary bladder activity (red arrow) and recto-sigmoid activity (yellow arrow).

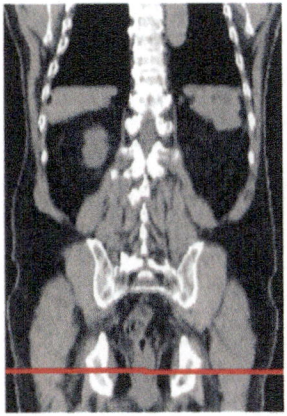

Localizer

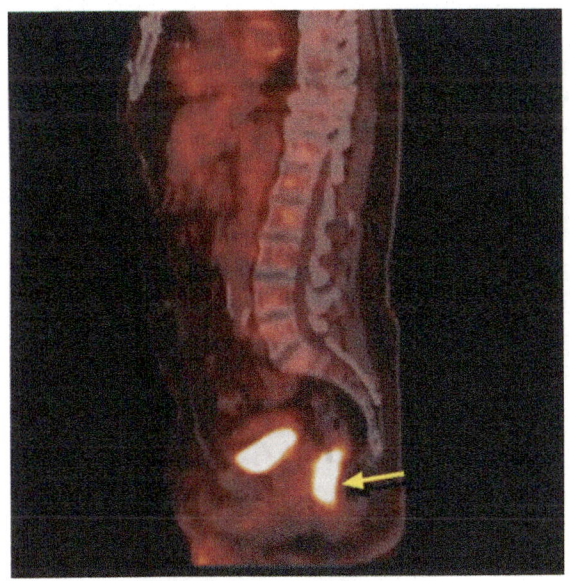

Image 3 (sagittal)

Image 3. Fused sagittal image with intensely increased FDG uptake in the recto-sigmoid region (arrow).

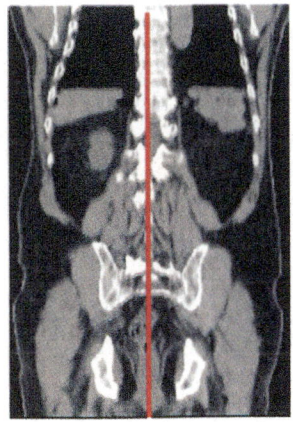

Localizer

Fibrous Dysplasia

Clinical History

63-year-old male with pancreatic and gallbladder cancer.

PET/CT indication: Restaging.

Findings

Focally increased uptake in the right acetabulum corresponding to a sclerotic bone lesion on CT. This is consistent with fibrous dysplasia.

Teaching Point

Benign diseases involving increased numbers of fibroblasts can sometimes exhibit intensely increased FDG uptake.

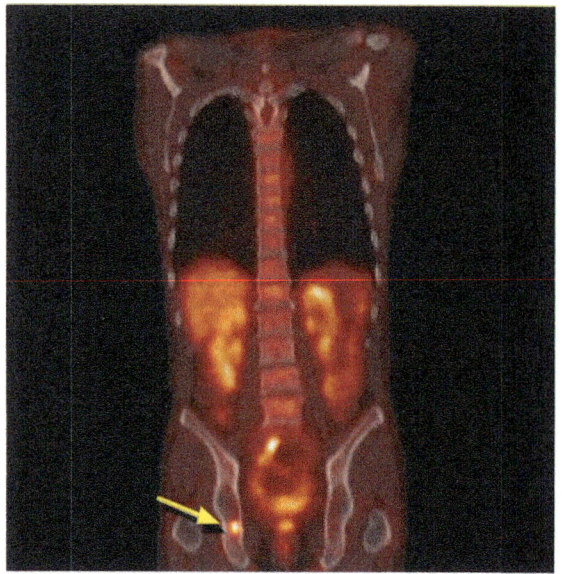

Image 1. Fused coronal image demonstrating increased uptake in the right iliac bone (arrow).

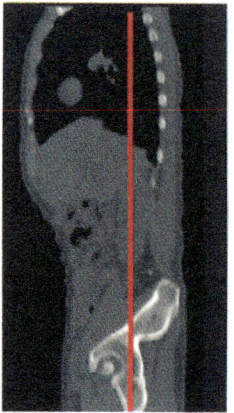

Image 1 (coronal)

Localizer

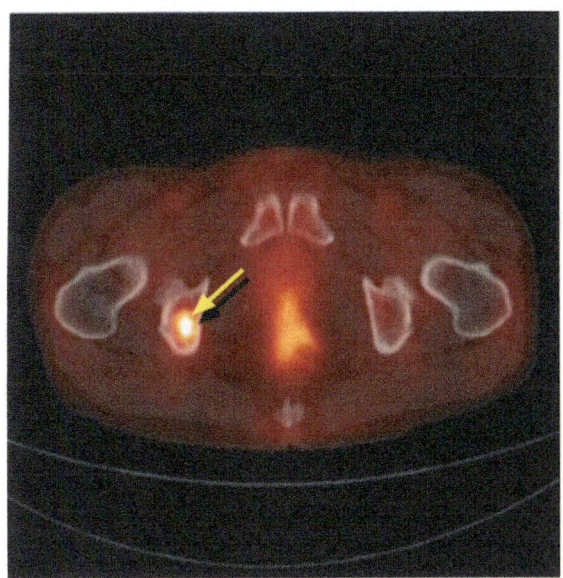

Image 2 (axial)

Image 2. Fused axial image demonstrating increased focal uptake which corresponds to a hypodense lesion in the right iliac bone (arrow).

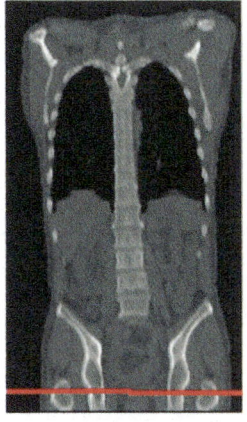

Localizer

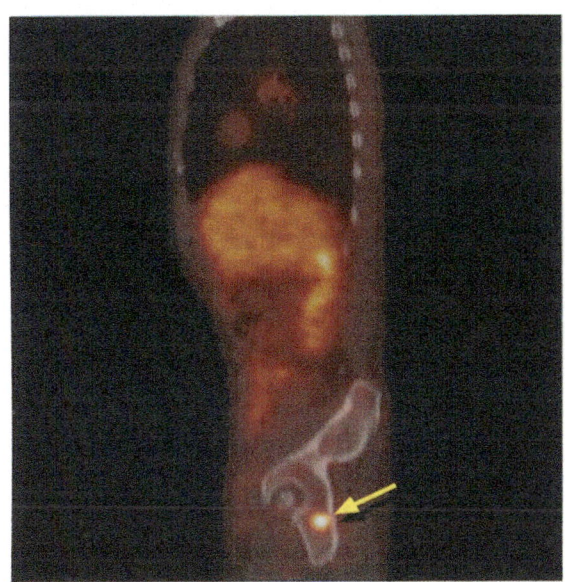

Image 3 (sagittal)

Image 3. Fused sagittal image demonstrating increased focal uptake matching a hypodense lesion on CT image.

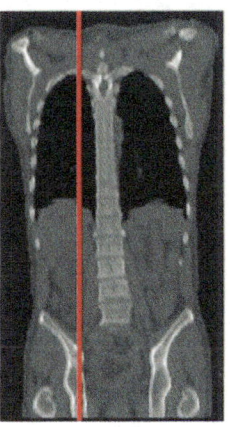

Localizer

Pneumonia

Clinical History

32-year-old female patient who was recently diagnosed with Non-Hodgkin's lymphoma. She underwent chemotherapy and treatment that ended 6 weeks prior to the PET/CT study. She developed systemic symptoms such as fever and night sweats suggesting residual disease.

PET/CT indication: Restaging.

Findings

Intense area of hypermetabolic activity in the left posterior lung base versus spleen. The CT appearance is more consistent with inflammatory process.

Teaching Point

PET alone failed to reliably assign the hypermetabolic area to the lung versus spleen. PET/CT ruled out the spleen as being tumor involved. Follow-up scan after antibiotic treatment revealed normal FDG uptake pattern. Thus, PET was false positive for malignancy, while CT correctly suggested benign, inflammatory process.

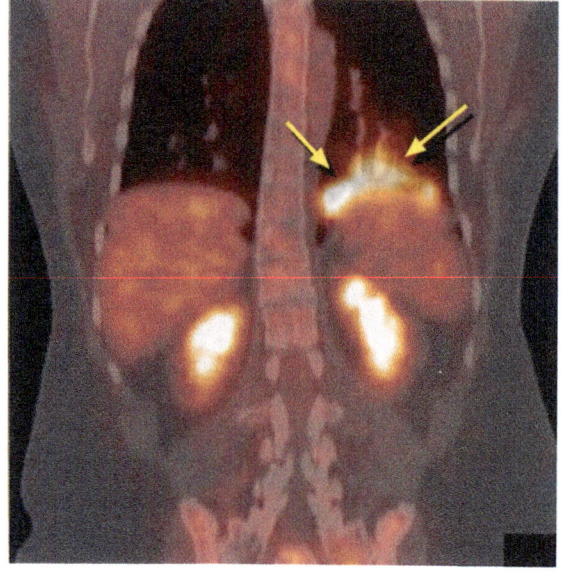

Image 1 (coronal)

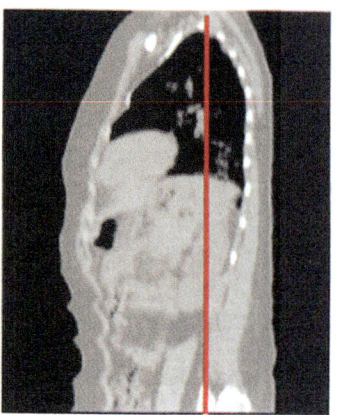

Image 1. Coronal fused PET/CT image demonstrating abnormal FDG uptake in the posterior base of the left lung (arrows).

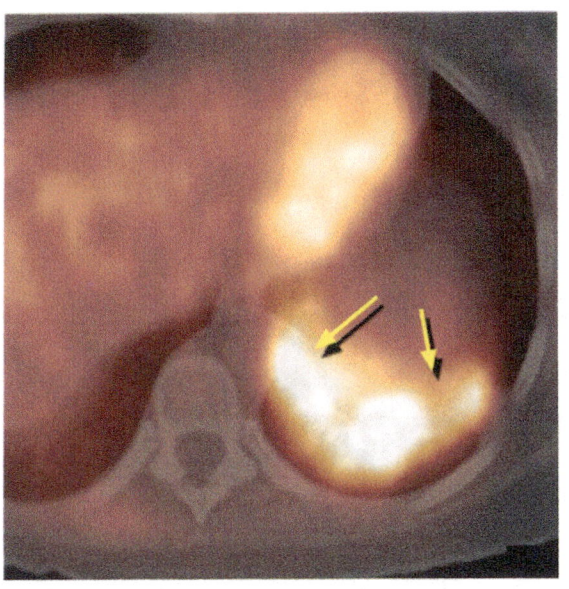

Image 2 (axial)

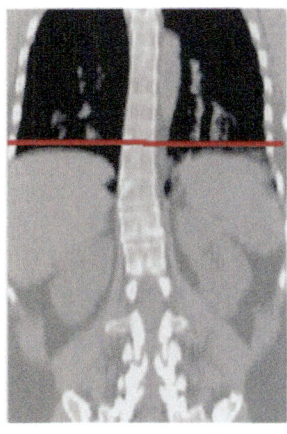

Localizer

Image 2. Axial PET/CT image demonstrating abnormal FDG uptake in the posterior base of the left lung (arrows).

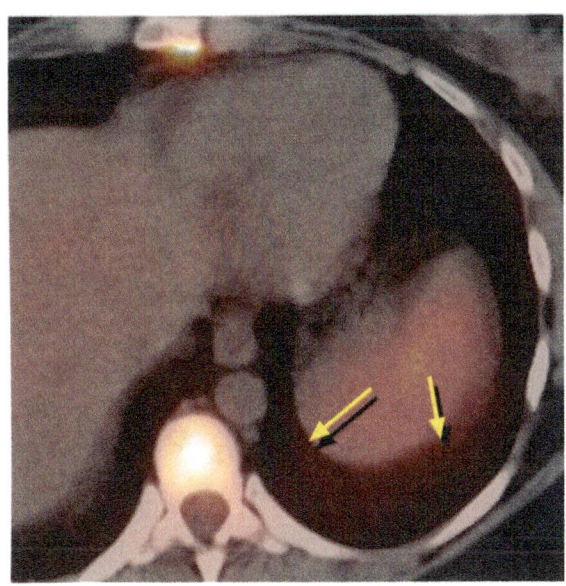

Image 3 (axial)

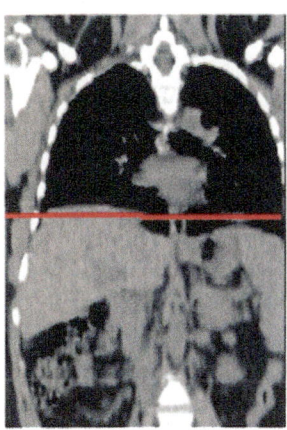

Localizer

Image 3. Axial PET/CT image obtained after antibiotic treatment. Note the normal anatomic and molecular appearance of the posterior left lung base consistent with resolved pneumonia (arrows).

Printed by Printforce, the Netherlands